FACULTY-CURRICULUM DEVELOPMENT

ABOUT THE AUTHORS

Helen Yura, PhD, RN, is eminent professor of nursing, graduate program director, Old Dominion University, Norfolk, Virginia.

Gertrude Torres, EdD, RN, is vice-president and dean, academic affairs, D'Youville College, Buffalo, New York.

Rose Marie Chioni, PhD, RN, is dean, University of Virginia, Charlottesville.

Edwina Frank, EdD, PhD, RN, is professor, Loyola University of New Orleans, Louisiana.

Eleanor A. Lynch, MSN, RN, is associate professor, Hampton University, Virginia.

Rose P. McKay, EdD, RN, the late chairperson, community health, University of Colorado School of Nursing, Denver.

Marjorie Stanton, EdD, RN, is professor and chairperson, division of nursing, D'Youville College, Buffalo, NY.

Sylvia Carlson, PhD, RN, is associate director of nursing education/staff development; corporate nursing services; New York City Health and Hospitals Corporation, New York.

Helen J. O'Leary, MSN, RN, has recently retired from her position as assistant director of nursing, Suffolk County Department of Health, Hauppauge, New York.

Jean A. Kelley, EdD, RN, FAAN, is assistant dean, graduate program, University of Alabama, Birmingham.

FACULTY-CURRICULUM DEVELOPMENT

Curriculum Design by Nursing Faculty

Pub. No. 15-2164

National League for Nursing • New York

The views expressed in this book reflect those of the
authors and do not necessarily reflect the official
views of the National League for Nursing.

ISBN 0-88737-337-2

Manufactured in the United States of America

CONTENTS

1 THE PROCESS OF CURRICULUM DEVELOPMENT

1 CURRICULUM DEVELOPMENT PROCESS

Helen Yura, PhD, RN

Curriculum development implies an ability to look into and predict the future for the practitioner who will be a graduate of a changing baccalaureate curriculum. Graduation will not occur for two to four years, to which must be added the time needed to develop the new curriculum. Nurse educators must have a grasp of the here and now, but they must also be solidly aware of the social and professional developments that will have implications for the future of nursing. Thus, there is a natural time gap which is necessary and which must be respected in determining what should be, what can be, and what needs to be in relation to nursing practice.

A focus on today only, or on the past is short-sighted and self-limiting and could have serious implications for the citizen. Cooperative determination of the future health care needs and nurse practice patterns by nurse educators, nursing service leaders, nurse practitioners and citizens is necessary so that changes needed in education can be made. Further, changes needed in health care agencies, which will be recipients of these future graduates, have to be made so that the graduates will be able to practice as predicted in an environment which is receptive to them and which fosters their continuing professional growth. The so-called gaps (or at times perhaps more accurately labeled "lags") between education and practice will be less likely to occur if the curriculum is designed to prepare the graduates as predicted and if the health care agencies make the needed changes to receive and utilize them. Since education precedes practice, it is strategic for

3

educators and practitioners to collaborate to determine the kinds and numbers of graduates required to meet the health care needs of citizens.

Curriculum development or revision is an ongoing process. Planned evaluation is an important component of curriculum development, not only in order to keep the curriculum viable, but in order to discharge our responsibility to the students enrolled in the program and to the citizens who will be the recipients of the service of the graduates. The curriculum that results from the utilization of the curriculum process to be outlined below *contains* the framework for evaluation.

Under the direction of the nurse leader who heads the nursing program, the faculty assume responsibility for the initial development and the continuing development of the curriculum. The focal point in this development is the student as an educated person and as a nurse practitioner.

Curriculum development is part of a nurse educator's role as a faculty member, which goes beyond his or her limited role as a teacher or an instructor. Curriculum development is a highly intellectual exercise in which the creative endeavors of the nurse faculty take form. Curriculum development involves a well-defined process which is logical and purposeful. A process is a blueprint for action; it is a continuous movement through a succession of developmental stages. This process is completed with the development of the curriculum design which, in turn, contains the framework for the evaluation of the total curriculum, specific course offerings, students, faculty and graduates of the program.

Simply, the process consists of six steps, namely: (1) philosophy development, (2) determination of objectives, (3) statement of terminal behaviors, (4) definition of a theoretic or conceptual framework, (5) statement of expected level behaviors, and (6) statement of expected course behaviors, with specification of particular learnings needed to meet the course objectives.

Philosophy

Philosophy can be defined as a study of the processes governing thought and conduct. The philosophy of the nursing program is the initial, and perhaps, the *most important* document to be developed by the nursing faculty. The philosophy contains the faculty's belief about man generally and, more specifically, about man the learner, the teacher, the nurse practitioner, the consumer. The faculty's belief about nursing, about baccalaureate nursing education, about the present and the emerging roles of the graduate of the baccalaureate nursing program, about the teaching-learning process and about other beliefs designated as significant to faculty can be included.

The stated philosophy of the nursing program should be compatible with the philosophy of the college or the university of which it is a part and should be developed within the framework of the philosophy and goals of the college or the university.

The philosophy of the nursing program should be reviewed periodically (1) for its relevance to social, cultural and professional needs in general and to the needs of students and consumers specifically and (2) to assure that the beliefs enclosed are inclusive and reflect the thinking of the faculty. Periodic review with needed revisions will enhance the viability of this important document. All other steps in the curriculum process have their roots in the philosophy and flow from philosophy.

Objectives

The objectives of the nursing program are broad statements of the goals of the nursing program. The objectives should be clearly stated and should be compatible with the stated philosophy of the nursing program. Since objectives are broadly stated, they are often few in number. Nurse faculty determine the content of the objectives. Objectives should be achievable.

Like the philosophy, the objectives need periodic review to assure that they are in keeping with the beliefs as stated in the philosophy. The key to the development or revision is broadness, clarity and relevancy.

Terminal Behavioral Statements

The statements of terminal behavior flow from the objective of the nursing program. These should be statements of observable terminal behaviors which, when taken as a whole, present a clear description of the graduate of the nursing program. These statements are strategic in that they serve as a point of focus and give direction to curriculum development. Terminal behaviors not only help to reveal to the faculty the range of specific behaviors with which they must cope, but enable each faculty member to relate activity in which he or she is engaged to a particular facet of the objectives of the school. Further, these behaviors provide the guide for the selection and organization of learning experiences. For the student, the terminal behavioral expectations give a focus for scholarly pursuits and a picture of the product resulting

5

from time, energy, and money invested. This is particularly significant for transfer students who come with varied academic and experiential backgrounds and whose credentials must be evaluated on an individual basis so that what they need in order to achieve the terminal behaviors in the baccalaureate nursing program can be determined. For the employer and the consumer, these statements lead to an awareness of what could be expected from the graduate of the baccalaureate nursing program.

The behavioral statements should be clearly, though broadly, stated. Additional behavioral substatements could be developed from the main behavioral statements.

Theoretic or Conceptual Framework

When the philosophy, objectives and terminal behavioral statements are developed, the nursing faculty is ready to select the theoretic or conceptual framework which will provide a system for classifying the knowledge of a theoretic field and the ordering of facts. This may be a single theory or a single idea or concept or more than one. The theoretic or conceptual framework selected is inherent in the philosophy, objectives, and terminal behavioral statements. The definition of nursing adopted by the faculty will be an important determinant in the selection of the theoretic framework. Numerous theories and concepts have been identified and developed by baccalaureate nursing faculties. Some of these center on the person, the family, the community, need theory, developmental theory, crises theory, systems theory, decision theory, adaptation theory, the nursing process, and levels of prevention, to mention a few. Faculty may designate any threads or strands flowing from this framework or reflected in the philosophy to permeate the curriculum. Strands or threads, as the leadership thread, research strand, health-illness strand, nurse-client-health team member relationships strand, and so forth may be included.

Level Behavioral Statements

In order to facilitate the realization of the terminal behavioral statements and to account for the theoretic or conceptual framework and any threads or strands that have been identified, behavioral statements should be developed for each level of the curriculum. Faculty need to designate what "level" means. Some faculty may designate four levels, some three and so forth. Such designation in no way lessens the opportunity for individual students to accomplish level behaviors in an earlier or later period of time than expected. The completed or fulfilled behaviors for one level become the expected entrance behaviors for the next level. Level behaviors flow from terminal behaviors and are stated in more specific terms. When all level behaviors are met, the terminal behaviors should be met. At this point the faculty should ask, "What must be learned by the student in order to fulfill each level behavior? What knowledge must be mastered? What kinds of learning experiences are needed to accomplish the level behaviors which, in turn, contribute to meeting the terminal behaviors? What learnings are directed toward the development of the student as a person, as a man or woman, as a citizen, and as a practitioner of professional nursing? What learnings are classed as general education? Which are scientific—representative of the physical, biologic, social, and behavioral sciences? What learnings are foundational to nursing? What learnings are nursing? Are there common groupings for these learnings? What learning should come first? What should follow?"

Course Behavioral Statements

Learnings are grouped into courses for which behavioral expectations are stated. These stated expectations are more specific than the stated level expectations. When all courses for a level have been completed, the level objectives should have been met.

The specification of learnings, deliberately selected, affect the planned behavioral change in the student that is needed to meet course behaviors. What are the specific learning experiences needed on a day-to-day, week-to-week, month-to-month basis? With whom are these learning experiences taken and where? Can one learning experience be planned to meet a number of behavioral expectations? Thus, all learning expeiences are specifically planned to meet specific objectives.

It is with the designation of course for each level of the entire learning experience that the curriculum design is completed. This is the operational outcome of the faculty's efforts relative to all components of the design. Learning experiences have been grouped into courses, and credit has been allocated. Some courses utilized may have been established by and are part of the total offerings of the college or the university. Some course offerings may be changed by the addition of learning experiences, the elimination of learning experience and/or changes in emphasis in content. Some new courses may be developed. Provision should be made for electives. The program of studies, approved by the faculty, needs to be interpreted to the nursing school's publics—prospective students, prospective faculty, parents, and employers.

Thus, the design incorporates general education courses foundational to the nursing major, nursing courses, courses to meet college or university objectives, and electives to meet the individual preferences and needs of the student.

The Development of the Design

The process used to develop a curriculum serves as a blueprint for action. A process—whether pertaining to curriculum, nursing or research—designates the steps by which to accomplish a task. The completed framework—the developed philosophy, objectives, terminal behaviors, conceptual framework, level behaviors, and courses—are a creative endeavor culminating in a unique design *appropriate to* the college or university of which the nursing program is a part, to the geographic area, to the vision the faculty has of the graduate of the baccalaureate nursing program. While there are standards for quality, there is no one curriculum design for everyone, and a curriculum design of one college or university cannot be transplanted to another.

As stated earlier, with the development of this framework the faculty have simultaneously developed the structure for evaluation of the total curriculum, each level of the curriculum, each course and each learning experience in a systematic way. It contains the basis for the evaluation of students, faculty, and graduates of the program. It provides the basis for the development of evaluation tools and the rationale for modifications and changes.

In order to accomplish the development of the curriculum design, a mechanism or structure must be set up. While curriculum development is the responsibility of the total faculty, a committee or a task force structure appropriate to the particular faculty group needs to be organized. Major responsibility may be delegated to a curriculum committee, with representation reflecting the total faculty as well as the student body. Subcommittees stemming from this committee should be designed as needed.

Or the faculty may designate a series of task forces to get the job done. A steering committee may be appointed to coordinate the work of task forces, to facilitate communication about plans, policies, procedures and progress, to locate assistance (e.g., resource people, clerical personnel, books) to maintain relationships with individuals and groups outside the committee, and to edit and prepare materials for consensus or majority vote by the total nursing faculty.

In some instances, one or more experts in curriculum development may be designated for initiating, facilitating, and directing the development of the curriculum. The selected person(s) may be called curriculum

8

project director(s). With input from nursing faculty and students, curriculum project directors serve as the working arm of faculty in curriculum development.

Advisory committees with members from the college community and the community-at-large can be a useful source of input for the curriculum as well as a public relations source for fostering understanding of the curriculum being designed. Nursing service leaders and consumers may serve as appointed members of task forces and curriculum committees or subcommittees in addition to serving in an advisory capacity. If a curriculum is to be revised, it is important to inventory what has been done and what is usable. The materials thus inventoried should be incorporated into the new design.

While small numbers of faculty may work on a specific aspect of the curriculum framework, the views of the larger faculty group should be continuously sought. These can be obtained through invitations to selected committee or task force meetings, through interviews with faculty members or through the use of survey tools for reactions to issues and ideas. Also, in addition to student representation on faculty committees, the views of the students should be sought through interviews, questionnaires, and meetings.

Membership of faculty on curriculum committees may be on the basis of areas of interest, knowledge and competence in a content area, broad understanding of the school of nursing and its characteristics as well as of the college or university of which the school is a part, and knowledge and understanding of a variety of teaching methods and materials which can facilitate the learning process.

It is helpful to be familiar with the literature available on learning, the learner, education, curriculum, and nursing education. Also, it is a good idea to develop an annotated bibliography of the survey of literature made by the faculty. The faculty should also develop a list of operational definitions of terms used in documents.

It is important that the minutes of committees be kept up-to-date and complete and include copies of any working papers and documents used by committee members, for it is here that the story of the design development unfolds and ideas evolve from the abstract to operational activities. Periodic reports of committee activity should be given to the total faculty group. Minutes, too, should be readily available for faculty review. All working papers, documents, and minutes should be dated.

An important activity in the development of a design for a baccalaureate nursing program is decision-making. Decisions must be made in order to complete the task. Among the many important decisions to be made are two that deserve mention. The first is whether to develop or revise the curriculum, and the second is when the new or revised curriculum will be implemented.

The designation of realistic deadlines for the accomplishments of tasks adds an important dimension to committee work by helping to maintain the interest of faculty members and by supporting the expectation of faculty that work will be accomplished and that a curriculum will be the result. It also implies good use of faculty time and resources by minimizing repetition of effort and discouragement caused by restudy of work previously accomplished. A realistic schedule will allow time for attitude change on the part of faculty and students, which is generally a concomitant outcome of curriculum development or revision. Too short a time allowance could be defeatist and may be viewed as a lack of consideration and appreciation of the amount of faculty time and energy that is needed to design a baccalaureate nursing program. Designing such a program is hard work.

To conclude, the design of the baccalaureate nursing program is developed upon determination of objectives, identification of the kinds and the range of learning opportunities pertinent to these objectives, selection of patterns through which these opportunities may be most effectively provided and the development of procedures for evaluation of the curriculum. It should reflect the intertwining of the separate strands of the curriculum into a consistent, comprehensive baccalaureate nursing program. The design may be compared to a mosaic in which the interrelation of the parts gives concrete form to the artist's conception. In this case the mosaic would portray an educated person as well as a nurse practitioner—a graduate of the baccalaureate nursing program.

2 CURRICULUM PROCESS—PROBLEMS AND CONCERNS

Gertrude J. Torres, EdD, RN

The following text will be devoted to *some* of the concerns and issues involved in the various components of the total curriculum process.

Philosophy

Some programs identify their philosophy as statements of beliefs. The difficulties encountered are:

1. *The incompatibility of the philosophy of the nursing program with the philosophy of the parent institution.* Frequently and surprisingly, universities and colleges either do not have a truly stated philosophy or the philosophy as stated is nonoperational. Here the nursing faculty need to work with other university faculty in further developing the institution's philosophy before refining their own.

2. *The philosophy of the nursing program should include the nursing faculty's beliefs about humankind, society, health, nursing, and the learner.* The emerging role of the nurse as well as the uniqueness of her role is frequently not clearly delineated. Often

faculty define nursing as a helping profession oriented toward man on a health-illness continuum; this definition, however, could apply to medicine or social work as well.

3. *The philosophy is often stated in terms of a health orientation, yet the major emphasis of the program is on disease.*

4. *The philosophy at times is nonoperational and idealistic rather than a realistic statement of beliefs.*

5. *The philsophy is frequently not considered when decisions regarding curriculum and course revision are made.*

6. *New faculty are not sufficiently oriented to the philosophy.*

7. *The philosophy is often stated in terms of authorities' beliefs rather than those of the faculty.*

8. *The philosophy is often not viewed as an "evolving" commitment to beliefs needing frequent review and possibly revision in order to reflect the changing needs of society and new knowledge and theories.*

Program Objectives

1. *Objectives usually include the nursing process, collaboration, comprehensive health care, leadership, change process, preparation for further education and learning, utilization of research, critical thinking and functioning as a professional nurse in any setting and as a citizen within the society.*

2. *Frequently there is a lack of objectives in the affective domain although values and nursing are closely related.* Can we encourage values in the philosophy unless we have objectives pertaining to them?

3. *The terminology related to objectives often requires definition, yet a glossary of terms is seldom included.* Such a glossary would clarify objectives of the nursing faculty and increase effective communication among themselves and with others.

5. *Frequently the objectives are redundant and duplicate one another.* Is utilizing the nursing process the same as critical thinking? Are accountability and acceptable of the need for continuing education somewhat similar?

6. *The objectives, when reviewed, need to be carefully compared to the philosophy, since they support it.* Similar, defined terminology might be used throughout the curriculum to prevent confusion of terms.

7. *Program objectives and graduate objectives are sometimes separated.* Program objectives may be discussed in terms of the purposes of the program while graduate objectives reflect what the practitioner will be able to do. The faculty need to decide if they want to combine program and graduate objectives or separate them. When separate objectives are developed, it is necessary to ensure that they support each other.

8. *Program objectives should closely relate to the objectives of the parent institution.*

Conceptual Framework

Conceptual frameworks are being developed by most baccalaureate programs today. Let me give you some idea of this subject which is gaining much interest.

A *concept* is a general notion or a symbol. Thus a conceptual framework is a notion or a symbol that gives structure to the curriculum and reflects the faculty's philosophy and objectives. A *theory*, on the other hand, is a hypothesis involving an assumption or an opinion. Its meaning is akin to conjecture. It differs from principles, or laws, in that the latter are based on scientific or empirical data. Thus, we are dealing with terms of different meaning when we use the words *concept, theory,* and *principle* or *law.* Theoretic formulations are based on broad concepts and support those concepts. For example, the concept of man has theoretic formulations such as development and need. Since concepts are similar in all baccalaureate programs—the concept of man, for example, of society, of health and nursing—the uniqueness of the program is identified by its particular theoretic formulations.

Some of the concerns and issues are:

1. *The lack of clarity in terminology.* The faculty needs to define terms for itself.

2. *The use of diagrams—circles, spirals, boxes—to represent the faulty's ideas on the relationship between concepts and theories often leads to confusion and misconceptions.*

3. *The conceptual framework does not sufficiently reflect the philosophy of the program, especially in relation to nursing and humankind.* Sometimes it reflects the sciences while leaving out the whole idea of nursing as a process. Should the uniqueness of professional nursing be identifiable within the framework?

4. *The faculty does not state its rationale for the utilization of a framework.*

5. *The students are oriented to the conceptual framework early in the nursing curriculum, but soon after the framework is often forgotten.* New faculty members have difficulty incorporating the framework into everyday teaching activities. If the framework is not truly functional, is it useful?

Level Behavioral Objectives

These are directed toward the terminal behavioral objectives, which obviously support the philosophy and program objectives.

1. *The objectives must be functional and clear so that they can be used for the development of nursing courses and should strongly influence the choice of the general and supporting courses required of the student.* A lack of clarity here can have an adverse effect on the individual faculty member's approach to her teaching. Each phase of the nursing process needs detailed objectives; otherwise one faculty member might stress assessment, and possibly only physical assessment, while another might emphasize intervention, giving priority to psychological intervention. Clearly stated, detailed objectives rather than broad ones can avoid confusion.

2. *Faculty frequently do not utilize the level objectives for evaluation purposes in the clinical area and in testing.* How many of us have created tests which do not reflect all the objectives for a particular level? If a level objective requires evaluation as part of the nursing process, how do we test this? Are students or faculty evaluating nursing care?

3. *Level objectives frequently are not stated in such a way as to build on one another from year to year in order to support the terminal behavioral objectives.*

4. *Objectives as related to society's nursing needs are based almost totally on the professional faculty's expertise and biases rather than on data.*

5. *The content and the type of level objectives are frequently not understood by the clinical agency, thus permitting education and service to remain wide apart.*

14

6. *The level objectives should dictate learning experience—both theoretical and clinical—rather than be fitted into them.*

Course Statements

These reflect the philosophy, all objectives, and the conceptual framework. Problems and concerns are:

1. *Often the course statements are not related to the philosophy of the problem, especially to the emerging role of the professional nurse and the faculty's beliefs about learning.* If the faculty members believe that the student learns through independence and self-motivation, why are so many classes organized around the large-group lecture method of teaching? Course outlines should support beliefs.

2. *Course statements frequently lack sufficient depth to identify differences in the various nursing courses and reflect the level objectives.*

3. *Course labels, statements and outlines need to allow for flexibility;* they should not be so specific as to stifle faculty creativity or neglect individual differences in student groups.

3 COMPOSITE OF PROGRAM AND/OR TERMINAL BEHAVIOR OBJECTIVES OF BACCALAUREATE NURSING PROGRAMS

Gertrude J. Torres, EdD, RN

The following composite of program and terminal behavioral objectives was developed by examining the objectives of forty-two baccalaureate nursing programs that had been reviewed by the Board of Review of the Council of Baccalaureate and Higher Degree Programs in 1973. The objectives are divided into major areas, or groups of characteristics, to be demonstrated by baccalaureate graduates. These areas can be utilized by others to develop specific objectives in terms of their own beliefs and recognized priorities.

Major Area: Professional Nurse Within the Social System

- Is a responsible citizen.
- Recognizes the impact of the social system on the delivery of health care.

17

- Advocates within the society the improvement of health care.
- Is aware of the influences of physical, social, and cultural forces on health care.
- Identifies changing health needs within the community.
- Recognizes interaction between the social system and the health care delivery system.
- Is aware of social and scientific forces affecting people and their environments.
- Exhibits awareness, concern, and a sense of responsibility with regard to contemporary social issues.

Major Area: Professional Nursing And the Change Process

- Understands the traditional and the future role of the professional nurse and can assist in restructuring this role within the health care system.
- Can analyze, synthesize and evaluate current nursing practices and theories and identify the need for change.
- Is aware of social and scientific changes and their influence on health maintenance.

Major Area: Nursing Process

- Utilizes biological, physical, and psychosocial principles and theories.
- Utilizes nursing theories.
- Utilizes the nursing process in a variety of settings with all age groups.
- Practices nursing to promote and maintain optimum health of individuals, families, and the community.
- Recognizes the patient's/client's position on the health-illness continuum.
- Utilizes the communication process with patients/clients, peers, and the public to establish and maintain a therapeutic and social relationship.
- Utilizes the nursing process by:
  - making a comprehensive assessment; collecting and categorizing data; taking down health and nursing history; assessing physical, psychological, and sociocultural aspects.
  - formulating a nursing diagnosis; utilizing critical thinking,

and making discriminatory judgments.
* nursing intervention; utilizing all resources; developing a plan of action establishing priorities.
* evaluating nursing care; modifying goals.

Major Area: Leadership

* Can foster independent and interdependent function of the professional nurse through critical assessment.
* Can utilize management principles.
* Collaborates, coordinates, and offers consultation as a colleague within the interdisciplinary health team.
* Is responsible for the quality and quantity of professional nursing care given within the health care system.
* Provides leadership for the improvement of health and nursing care.
* Directs, guides, and evaluates others who give nursing care.

Major Area: Professional Responsibilities

* Participates in professional and community organizations to improve standards of nursing care.
* Identifies and interprets concepts relating to the professional practice of nursing to society and members of the health and nursing team.
* Assists in identifying community health needs through participation, planning, implementing, and evaluating community programs.

Major Area: Personal Development

* Identifies learning as a lifelong process.
* Recognizes the continued need for personal and professional growth.
* Utilizes informal and formal methods of study.
* Can function effectively through self-motivation, self-direction, and self-evaluation.

Major Area: Research

* Contributes to a body of nursing knowledge through participation in scientific investigations.
* Makes decisions based on predictable and unpredictable results using scientific methods.

19

4 IDENTIFYING CHANGES AND PRIORITIES IN SOCIAL AND HEALTH CARE NEEDS

Rose Marie Chioni, PhD, RN

The changing needs and priorities of society for health care is a fascinating topic and one I have been attempting to learn something about for the past five years. To be certain, I have learned one thing very well—you cannot predict the future. As Popper states, you can only prophesy about the future, since there are no universal historical laws but only trends, and these may unpredictably switch direction at any time.[1] Therefore, I shall limit my remarks to what I believe may happen in health care in the near future and to how these will and should affect curriculum design in nursing education.

I have written the first several pages of this paper more than once, for I seemed to be caught up in what I hoped would happen or things I would like to see happen. In all fairness, it seems I should rather deal with things which are likely to happen. Being an optimist, I found this a very difficult assignment because in some respects the future looks very depressing indeed. I have attempted to strike a balance by examining some optimistic and some pessimistic trends.

I will divide the trends into societal trends and health care trends and discuss them separately and conclude with the implications of these trends for curriculum development.

---

[1] Karl R. Popper. *The Poverty of Historicism.* New York: Harper and Row, 1964.

General Societal Changes and Trends

It seems almost needless to say that one cannot speak of most, let alone all, the general societal changes and trends which will have a significant effect on nursing and nursing education. I have chosen eight such changes for brief mention in order to have a context within which to view curriculum change.

1. *Population growth.* The rate of population increase is so high that it surpasses even the norms of the exponential rate pattern. By the year 2000, the population of the United States will have risen to between 287 and 320 million; this will represent an increase of over 50 percent in only 35 years,[2] brought about to a great extent by public health services and improved nutrition.

2. *Move toward urbanization.* By the year 2000, 80 percent of the United States population will live in urban areas; 50 percent of the urban dwellers will live in three urban areas—the Atlantic seaboard, the lower Great Lakes, and California.[3] This will lead to increased density in residential and social interaction patterns. There will be more and more people in less and less space.

3. *Population patterns.* There has been an increasing migration of home dwellers from cities to suburban areas and a progressively rapid exodus of the middle class from the inner cities. At the same time there has been a steady migration of Blacks, Puerto Ricans, Mexicans, and Cubans to inner cities. This has led to changing needs for health care at a rate much more rapid than the rate at which health services have been modified or established.

4. *Consumption of natural resources.* At the current rate of use, our known petroleum resources will be exhausted in 31 years; the gold supply in 11 years or less; the copper supply in 36 years; the lead supply in 26 years; the natural gas supply in 38 years or less.[4] These resources are not merely lost but are dispersed in unusable form as pollution.

At the present productivity levels, agriculture will meet the total per person support needs only until 2003.[5]

Consumption of all resources is increasing while basic supplies are decreasing and polluting wastes are aggregating.

---

[2] John McHale. *World Facts and Trends.* New York: The Macmillan Company, 1972, p. 5.
[3] *Ibid.,* p. 81
[4] Meadows et al, *The Limits to Growth: A Report for the Club of Rome's Project on the Predicament of Mankind.* Washington, D.C.: Potomac Associates, 1972, pp. 63-78.
[5] *Ibid.,* pp. 58–63

5. *Supply-demand for services.* Affluence has led to an increased demand for personal services, including health services. Prepaid or voluntary health insurance has tremendously increased the demand for hospital and extended care services as well as for outpatient services. At the other extreme, poverty has also influenced supply and demand for health services. People in poverty are demanding health services, often in settings ill-equipped to provide minimal services.

6. *Production efficiency.* There is a clear trend steadily growing overall production efficiency, as we are becoming increasingly able to produce more goods in less time with less effort. This has been brought about by greater standardization and greater size of organization. However, these apparent requirements for efficiency tend to foster dehumanization and depersonalization.

7. *Technology.* Technologic innovation is causing rapid change as well as rapid obsolescence. For example, the space program alone has had spin-off effects in many areas, including food products, electronics, communication, education, and health care.

8. *Communication.* The methods of communication, as well as communication itself, are rapidly increasing in volume and intensity.

Results

Before I move on to health care trends I would like to draw some implications from these societal trends and the resultant issues.

It seems to me that trends in health care and nursing care are subordinate to the trends listed above. If these trends continue as projected, although there will be an increased demand for health care, it is probable that limited economic resources will be available to support such care. Therefore, the health care fields need to be committed to and active in the reversal of at least some of these and other large societal trends.

The scarcity of vital resources will require the setting of priorities for allocation of available resources. The priorities will necessarily involve value-based decisions. Conflict about and competition for scarce resources will increase. Accountability will become the key to minimizing waste and using scarce resources wisely and efficiently. Standardization and equality may have to be maximized; allocations may become arbitrary (e.g., When food becomes scarce and people cannot buy all the food they want or can afford, who will receive foodstuffs?

23

Will everyone receive an equal share? Will growing children have a higher priority for certain types of food? How can wastage of food be avoided? Or, will it be first come, first served? Or will the people with the most financial resources get priority?).

Living and working in deprived situations will involve and include levels of stress with which people may not be able to cope. The inability to cope will lead to unproductive responses, withdrawal, living in the good old days. This does not facilitate rational problem-solving and in turn increases stress which is a counterproductive response. Matek, a futurist, states that this spiral phenomenon will lead to a "further degeneration of the political processes upon which our society has depended for the resolution of such issues... And...there will be need and justification for giving power to a technological managerial elite..."[6]

Matek goes on to say that "given these conditions, the most pandemic health problems of the next three decades are very probably going to be physically, mentally or behaviorally related to stress. The management of stress and its consequences is therefore likely to become a major involvement for most health professionals."[7]

In order to solve these major problems, attitudes, roles, and perceptions will need to change. Changing current practice will be, at best, stressful, difficult, and looked upon with resentment. Such change will require improved and continuous communication, mediation, and revision. As roles change, for example, the groups involved will have to jointly plan and agree on the changes. This will mean give and take on the part of everyone involved and will require modification in our "ideal" plans.

Health Care Changes and Trends

Again, in the interest of time, I must limit the number of trends I can discuss. I have selected eight which, I believe, will have a major impact on nursing curriculums.

1. *Quality health care as a right.* Everyone, including the President, talks about quality health care as the right of all Americans. If this belief were to be operationalized, the implications could be either staggering or rather minor, depending on what is meant

---

[6] Stanley J. Matek. *Some Key Features in the Emerging Context for Future Health Policy Decisions in America.* Paper delivered at conference on Education on Nurses for Public Health. Washington, D.C., March 1973, p. 9.

[7] *Ibid.,* p. 10.

by the slogan "quality health care." What is quality? What is health? What is care? For some it means a response by a physician to an illness; for some it means elaborate systems for promoting health and providing for quality of life. The slogan is popular, however, and we will undoubtedly attempt to respond to the belief. It seems "American" to do so.

2. *Increasing involvement of the consumer in responsibility for their health care.* Hepner and Hepner list some of the reasons for this increased interest as awareness on the part of the consumers that they are paying for health care and health facilities through taxes, awareness of the qualitative differences in health services, impatience with the fragmentation of services, and the new image of the physician as an affluent businessman. For all these reasons the consumer is no longer willing to leave planning of health care to the professionals.[8] E.L. Brown indicates that the public is readier to accept innovation than are the health professionals.[9]

3. *International health care policies.* With the rapid changes in society and the speed of travel, it is no longer possible to think in terms of epidemics—pandemics are more likely to occur. The shortage of resources is not limited to the United States but is worldwide. Therefore, it seems that solutions to these kinds of health-related problems will require international policies. The difficulty in effecting such policies may long delay the process, but it seems futile for each country to have different, often fragmented and sometimes contradictory policies.

4. *Increasing government control in health care.* Although listed as a trend, this seems to be a way of life at the present. Governmental control leads to standardization, controls, and allocation of resources. Policies are often established by political, economic, and special-interest groups, which may lead to inequality and fragmentation within the system. HMOs and National Health Insurance are examples of such increasing control.

5. *Increasing need for health professionals to work with other professionals as well as the client system.* Role blurring is occurring at a very rapid rate with the profileration of new categories of health workers and the role realignment activities in medicine, nursing, pharmacy, and so forth. This interdisciplinary activity

[8] James O. Hepner and Donna M. Hepner. *The Health Strategy Game: A Challenge for Reorganization and Management.* St. Louis: The C.V. Mobsy Company, 1973, p. 31.
[9] Ester Lucille Brown. *Nursing Reconsidered—A Study of Change, Part 2: The Professional Role in Community Nursing.* Philadelphia: J.B. Lippincott Company, 1971, pp. 247-248.

may be a threat to professional autonomy and thus is more difficult to undertake.

6. *Increase in the professionalization of health workers.* The trend in nursing and allied health fields is toward professionalization. This implies a theory and body of knowledge based on scholarly activity and research. It implies the practitioner will engage in independent judgments and be accountable for his or her practice.

7. *Increasing specialization in the health fields.* This trend is based on a professional preparation for all practitioners, with the need for special training as knowledge and technology proliferate rapidly. As shifts occur and newly trained "specialists" perform functions once solely or primarily in the domain of another profession, grave confusion and insecurity result. The consumer is likely to view professionals and specialists as workers with a service to perform and will evaluate them by the level of services they perform or what they produce—this in place of evaluation by title or degrees held. Society may view specialization as less and less significant as man grapples with the scarcity of basic resources.

8. *Increase in the supply of health workers, perhaps resulting in oversupply.* Increasing numbers of students are entering health fields and new categories of health workers are finding their place in the health delivery system. As this occurs, consumers can be increasingly selective about who will deliver services and the degree of priority placed on funding health-related activities. Oversupply may also result in the availability of health services in locations not currently attractive to health professionals. If there are no jobs in suburbia, health workers may move to the rural or the inner-city setting.

9. *Rapid obsolescence of practice skills and knowledge level.* With the rapid expansion of knowledge and development of sophisticated skills for practice, the professional will find it increasingly difficult to maintain his or her competence and level of expertise. Continuing education will become the rule rather than the exception.

Curriculum Implications

How does one translate social and health care trends into curriculum development? We all seem to think such trends should be identified and used—or do we? Do some of us identify the trends and then file them away for "future" use? It seems one must raise several questions and answer them prior to deciding whether or not to engage in the process of curriculum designing based on changing trends. Some of the questions should include:

1. Do you really want to incorporate trends into the curriculum process? Trends change, trends are unpredictable, maybe we like the curriculum we have now.

2. Is the current curriculum flexible enough to incorporate trends as they evolve? Maybe we don't need to change anything but a little content. The content related to health statistics can be brought up to date fairly easily, for example.

3. Don't the professionals know what society needs? Can't we produce graduates who will help to modify the trends?

4. What do all the slogans really mean? We are already teaching "comprehensive patient care," "quality health care," and "total patient care." Or are we? What is total patient care? Who really wants it anyway?

5. Is interdisciplinary education worthwhile? Some will say we've been working together for years. It's so costly. The coordinated planning is very time-consuming. I'm not going to have any MD tell me what to do. We've struggled long and hard for our level of independence.

6. What is meant by nursing education? What is curriculum? Is it a prescribed set of courses and experiences designed to prepare a nurse who can really nurse—whatever that might mean? Is it presenting content necessary for "safe patient care"? Is it developing the individual learner? We really know very little in this area. Many nursing curricula aren't much different from those prescribed by the 1937 Curriculum Guide—how can trends be so important?—we still produce good practitioners.

7. What is the purpose of education? What is the purpose of professional education?

These are but a few of the questions one must raise and answer in designing any curriculum. You will find I am better at raising questions and providing answers. In order to proceed to the designing process I would like to assume you have answered the questions in the "right" way and are ready to commit yourself to curriculum change. I will try now to demonstrate how the trends I have identified might affect curriculum designing. I will not discuss these in any specific order of priority because it is impossible to rank the implications from my point of view.

1. If specific content and skills needed by the practitioner cannot be predicted, then it may follow that we focus too heavily on these today. It would seem much more feasible to focus on concepts and principles so that the practitioner has a base upon which to draw and recognizes that specific content and skills need to be added continuously throughout his or her career.

2. If content cannot be predicted, then the central focus of education and professional education should be to assist the student to recognize his own strengths and limitations, become inquisitive, a perpetual student, one who is accountable for his actions. From my point of view, this provides not only a safe practitioner but a quality practitioner.

3. If the most pandemic health problems are related to stress it would seem that stress, methods of coping and methods of managing stress would become a major focus in the nursing curriculum.

4. If nurses are to be involved in policy decisions regarding distribution of resources and other health-related concerns, the curriculum will have to provide for the expansion of thinking about such issues and for improvement in the judgment of nurses about priority setting. This could mean involvement in community affairs as a part of the instructional experiences during the educational program (e.g., legislation, health task forces).

5. If we believe the professional nurse practitioner will be prepared at the baccalaureate level, then it would seem essential that socialization into the profession, which happens haphazardly now, as well as professional concepts and skills, be incorporated (integrated) into the learning experiences (e.g., allowing the student to make judgments about his or her own program; to test ideas he or she may have—even though we might believe they won't work, no one thought Einstein's ideas would work either; and to be an independent learner—why must we foster dependence so, can't the learner go out into the community alone?). The faculty could also trust the student to use resources appropriately. At the present, we expect a professional product, but don't interact with the students as though they were budding professionals. This integration can be accomplished most easily by seeing professionalization as a continuing organizing element in the curriculum.

6. If the consumer is going to be a partner in health care delivery and decisions, then the nurse student must interact with the consumer as a peer throughout the program. It does *not* follow that the graduate will incorporate the consumer in the delivery of health care if the student has had no experience with the consumer.

7. If the nurse is to engage interdisciplinary activities as a graduate, then it follows that the nurse student must engage in interdisciplinary activities with other health professional students. Graduation in itself does not confer the ability to relate to or collaborate with other professionals—we seem to think it does. Likewise, in order to collaborate as partners, professionals need a common base of knowledge and skill which can be built into the curricular experiences. Schein states that "if the professions are to become more interdisciplinary...they will have to integrate both the applied and basic components of the behavioral and social sciences in the professional education and training."[10]

8. If increasing specialization is not necessarily going to best meet the needs of society for health care, then one must consider the degree of generalization or specialization that is appropriate at both the undergraduate and graduate levels. I contend that it takes more knowledge and skill to be a generalist than a specialist. Therefore, I would suggest that we look at the possibility of specialized areas of practice at the undergraduate level and generalized areas of practice at the graduate level (e.g., well-child care leading to family health care and community health or neurologic nursing care leading to long-term care).

9. If scholarly activity and research are essential for developing the body of nursing knowledge, then it follows that undergraduate students should be introduced to research concepts early—so that

[10] Carnegie Commission on Higher Education. *Professional Education: Some New Directions.* Edgar Schein, ed. New York: McGraw-Hill Book Co., 1972, p. 41.

they become a way of thinking, a way of solving problems, a way of generating new knowledge. For example, I am not implying that BS graduates can engage in independent research, but I do believe they can identify research problems, collect data, and cooperate or collaborate with a nurse researcher on a research project. Why not?

10. If the health care field changes as rapidly as predicted, then it seems necessary to avoid what I will call "cookbook" methods in the curriculum. Cookbook methods will fall far short of meeting the students' need for problem-solving, creative thinking. It is always refreshing to find out the spaghetti sauce I make without a recipe is better than that which I make with a recipe. Students may find the same thing if given the opportunity to do so (e.g., the nursing process can be viewed as a recipe—the product will be very standard; or a way of thinking about problems—the product can be very individualized). I believe it is of grave concern that many educators are viewing and using the nursing process as a "how-to-do-it" recipe.

Mayhew states that "professional schools can and have erred in the direction of overemphasis on practice, ending up with a 'how-to-do-it' procedure which limits members in adapting to changed conditions."[11]

11. If the population figures and the population trends are accurate, and if there will be an increased demand for health care by all groups, then it follows that students should have optional experiences to acquaint them with cultural and socioeconomic differences in the needs of groups for health care. To be able to take care of middle-class, white suburban dwellers is not the same as taking care of lower-class, white inner-city dwellers or Mexican rural migrant workers. It is not a question of the transfer of learning but rather of different concepts, values, and skills. Can a curriculum allow for students to indicate preferential experiences (e.g., on an Indian reservation in Arizona, with migrant workers in rural Wisconsin, or with inner-city dwellers in New York City)?

12. If the trends require mobility and flexibility for student learning, then it follows that regional or, at least, statewide curriculum planning should be done. This would permit me to send students to New York City and you to send students to rural Wisconsin. Can we ever hope for this development? Why not?

13. If we believe in "quality" or "comprehensive" or "total" pa-

[11] Lewis B. Mayhew. *Changing Practices in Education for the Professions.* Atlanta, Georgia: Southern Regional Education Board, 1971, p. 7.

tient care, then we need to develop measures of "quality," "total" or "comprehensive" care. We will have to be able to demonstrate that our care does make a difference. Somehow I don't believe the public will buy a statement such as: "It does make a difference because the graduates are professional." Or, "It makes a difference because they are graduates of the Unversity of ____ program." We'll have to do better than that.

These are but a few of the curricular implications that can be drawn from the trends. You may recognize that I was a bit biased in my selection of implications—the ones I believe in so strongly seem to always find their way into the list. However, one of the real advantages of using trends to assist in curriculum designing is that the designers, you and I, can be very creative in drawing implications. You will identify some I have not thought of and perhaps be able to use some I have identified. I hope we, in small groups and collectively, might find new ideas, new ways to place curriculum designing at the systematic level rather than at either the traditional or the prophetic level. I believe a brief quote from Galileo might give us the necessary support to be creative. "You cannot teach a man anything; you can only help him to find it within himself."

5 COMMENTS ON IDENTIFYING CHANGES AND PRIORITIES IN SOCIAL AND HEALTH CARE NEEDS

Edwina D. Frank, EdD, RN

Identification of the changing needs of, and the priorities for, health care is a multifaceted topic. It would indeed be overly ambitious to suppose that all aspects of the topic could be presented in this discussion. Assigning priorities to social and health care changes is often dependent on the position occupied by the viewer. For example, a consumer, a provider, an economist, an educator, a student, and a legislator might each begin from a distinctly different perspective. In all instances the priorities established would be speculative in that identifying them must of necessity include a certain amount of prediction as to what should be as a result of what is. The concern of this discussion is with exploring social and health care changes as they relate to the establishment of a context within which to view curriculum change. Although speculative, it is hoped that this discussion will proceed without the benefit of crystal-ball gazing.

Forecasts As An Essential Element In Identifying Priorities

There is currently on the social scene a newly developing science called forecasting.[1] Horvath proposes that the preparation of forecasts

---

[1] Joyce Travelbee. "Futures Research in Nursing Care." *LSU Graduate Newsletter,* 2:2, May-June 1973.

is an important and necessary part of program planning. The need for detailed estimates of future conditions arises from the desire to avoid obsolescence of new facilities and programs that are in the planning stage. As the pace of social change, knowledge, and technology accelerates, the need for timely and accurate forecasts increases correspondingly.[2] There are many ways of arriving at decisions in establishing priorities. Research relating to the future has as its goal the systematic examination of what can be as contrasted with what will be or should be. It is concerned with activities that improve understanding about the future consequence of present developments and choices and includes such processes as forecast planning and decision making. It is generally agreed, however, that the very futuristic nature of forecasting imposes limitations in that unanticipated events may occur, with the possibility of falsifying the forecast. Yet, in many instances validity for the approach has been established—witness the fulfillment of predictions made even ten years prior to the actual events. Forecasting scientists claim that the validity of such predictions can be measured in probability terms on the basis of what went into the predictions. There is consensus that the best forecast is one which manages to summarize current experiences and bends to choices which achieve present and future objectives.

For the purpose of this discussion I would like to utilize the simple guideline of summarizing current experiences as a basis for exploring the implications of current social and health trends. What, then, are the current social and health care needs? This discussion will be devoted to sources of change which seem immediately applicable to health care and educational planning.

Changes Evolving From Man's Needs, States, and Responses

One source of change evolves from the nature of man's needs, states, and responses. Although the comments presented here are limited, this area of change would be inclusive of population trends, developmental patterns, and life-styles.

Changing Family Roles

Change has been evolving slowly, but rather distinctively, in family role functions. Some attribute this change to the so-called sex revolution. We are approaching, whether we like it or not, more and more the

---

[2] William Horvath. "The Role of Operational Testing in Forecasting of Health Service Trends." *Health Services Research,* 8:3:179-183, Fall 1973.

idea of a unisex society, where male and female roles may not be as readily discernible as in previous times. The "spin-off" of shared roles and working mothers is reflected by a changing set of values surrounding such ideas as child rearing, motherhood, and so forth. We are experiencing an increasing trend towards the early introduction of children to peer groups and child care centers.

Other changing family roles include the development of the youth cult, with its rejection of the ideas and values of earlier generations; the advent of commune living and extended family groups; and a more viable and visible senior citizen population.

As we in the health fields plan our programs which focus on "developmental levels," we cannot ignore the changing family roles or the need for facilitating additional change.

Depletion of Natural Resources with Simultaneous Increase in Consumption

By 1990, the United States will probably have about doubled its present energy consumption. Domestic oil and natural gas, which today account for two-thirds of the nation's energy, will be able to supply only 40 percent of the demand. Nuclear, hydro, solar, goethermal, and other nonfossil fuel sources will take care of another 20 percent. To make up the 40 percent deficit, the nation will have to elect one of two choices—import much more oil and gas (and pay heavily in terms of both balance of payments and political dependence on foreign countries) or turn to coal, which now provides 20 percent of the energy of the United States (and pay heavily for developing the rich but problem-laden resources). Presently, it seems that there will be greater movement toward utilizing coal, with its related problems of occupational health hazards to miners and additional pollution.[3] As Dr. Rose Chioni has indicated, "Consumption of all resources is increasing while basic supplies are decreasing and pollution wastes are aggregating." The imbalance of available resources needed to meet human needs will indeed necessitate different decisions on the part of those in the health fields.

Health and Illness Trends as Determiners of Health Care Services

The health services of industrial societies, like other social services, are established on the premise that there is a level below which the well-being of citizens must not fall as a result of the routine workings of the economy.[4] Yet, in 1967, a National Advisory Commission on Health Manpower commented that the health statistics of certain

---

[3] "Fuel-Out of the Hole With Coal." *Time,* January 28, 1974, p. 32.
[4] J.H. Skalnick and Elliott Currie. *Crises in American Institutions.* Boston: Little, Brown and Company, 1970.

groups in the United States—the rural poor, the urban poor, migrant workers, and others occasionally resemble the health statistics of a developing country.[5] For us in the United States there seems to be more or less of a bimodal trend related to socioeconomic conditions. We must keep in mind that there are health problems resulting from deprivation as well as from affluence, excess stress, and substance abuse.

Recently there has been a proliferation of efforts to develop a health status index. Although the conceptual and methodological problems encountered are indeed complex, these efforts focus on developing indices that might be assistive in arriving at decisions about educational and service programming. A scan of the projected uses of such indices reveals several trends of thought on the part of the developers. It has been suggested that such computerized indices might serve as social indicators in comparing the health status of the populations of various geographic areas; provide criteria for evaluating efforts to improve the health status of a community or a target population; and assess the projected benefits of *new programs* competing for limited health resources.[6,7,8]

Weighted life expectancy indices as a health status index suggest interesting advantages both as indicators of current health status and as predictors of future status. Users of this tool indicate that such descriptive indices may provide a basis for estimating the social value of advances made in health status as a result of health team services and interventions.[6,7,8] Although development of such indices and their continuous utilization is rapidly growing (probably because they readily lend themselves to computer programming and the sorting of groups in the population), most investigators agree that the health status index also has the following limitations:[6,7,8]

1. In utilizing life expectancy and mortality as proxy measures of health a person either lives or dies—there are no measures which allow for gradations in the quality of life during the years lived.

---

[5] R.M. Titmus. "Ethics, an Economics of Medical Care." (Quoted from the Report on Health Manpower—United States.) In *Commitment To Welfare.* New York: Panther Books, 1968, p. 268.

[6] W.J. Horvath. "Need For Estimating the Influence of Techological and Social Changes on Future Health Facility Requirements." *Health Services Research,* 3:3, Spring 1968.

[7] D.F. Sullivan. *Conceptual Problems in Developing an Index of Health and Health Statistics.* Series 2, No. 17. Rockville, Md.: National Center for Health Statistics, 1966.

[8] I.M. Moriyanna. "Problems in the Measurement of Health Status." In E. Sheldon and W. Moore, eds., *Indications of Social Change.* New York: Russell Sage Foundation, 1968, p. 573.

2. There is no clear evidence that health status is a product of the health delivery system.

These newer approaches to identifying needs, states, and responses certainly offer us a number of alternatives in identifying priorities for planning. We must, however, keep in mind that there remains a need for methods and systems which permit the actualization of quality care at all levels of the health strata.

Changes Evolving From Knowledge, Power, and Technology

Another source of change seems to evolve from the availability and utilization of human resources, such as knowledge, power, and technology. Intricately woven throughout both sources of change is the influence of the humanity of the times (I am using humanity here in the philosophical context—inclusive of man's ideas about man) on final decisions about what will be.

Impact of Health Legislative and Governmental Control In Determining Priorities in Health Care and The Question of Who Determines Priority

We have recently felt the impact of several changes in governmental policy. First, there has been an increase in the involvement of state and local government in establishing health care priorities and effecting health care planning. A major and radical change has occurred in the functions of such organizations as HEW, NIH, NIMH. Federal budgeting and programming for health services and the education of health professionals have also undergone change. There has been a major reassessment with respect to the amount of federal expenditures for resolving specific health and human welfare problems. It would seem that a crucial question for nursing and other health professions might be, "How can we more directly influence or be involved in the determination of health and human welfare priorities at the national, state, and local levels?

The Role of Theoretical Formulations, Scientific Discoveries, and Technological Innovations in Expanding the Horizons of the Health Fields

We have in our times seen the impact of aerospace research, automation by computer, electronic instrumentation, and a knowledge explosion in the theoretical realm. As a result of such rapid expansion in knowlege and the consequent development of sophisticated skills in practice, there is an increasing trend toward rapid obsolescence. Futuristic researchers remind us that "although new technical and administrative methods may be available to solve health problems, there are some properties in our system of health care that might be expected to result in an inability to change."[9] The availability of innovations gives us no assurance that they will be used in practice. If change is to occur there must be built into the practice system methods for the ongoing assessment of relevancy of services, skills, and systems. We must also have ready access to methods for "junking" obsolete components, once identified. Of utmost importance is the incorporation of systems that offer opportunity for attitudinal change and continuing education.

Conflictual Coexistence of Humanistic and Behavioristic Ideologies With Reference to the Provision of Human Services

Science is steadily increasing our power to influence, change, and mold human behavior. It has identified variables which can be used to predict and control behavior in a new and increasingly different technology. At the same time, we in the human service fields adhere to a basic philosophy that focuses on individuality and the belief that the actions of men are free in some sense. The humanistic antithesis implies that scientific knowledge of man's behavior is impossible. Individual motivation and environmental influences are more related to the humanistic ideology which views man as having free will and the right to determine the course of his destiny, whatever the outcome may be.[10] I am not suggesting that it should be a matter of either or which value, but rather that we should provide health services in a pluralistic value setting. I shall not attempt an ethical analysis of the loopholes but rather illustrate a few of the related problems. There is a decrease in emphasis on one-to-one contacts between consumers and providers of service. The application of an automated and servo-mechanistic approach to health monitoring, diagnosis, and treatment has increased efficiency in terms of delivering needed services to greater numbers. Simultaneously, there is an acceleration of efforts to facilitate self-care (bio-feedback, autonomic nervous system control, programmed learning) and the provision of services for groups. The result of this is the loss of contact with a central health care worker. We are beginning to see what almost amounts to a counterattack approach by con-

---

[9] Horvath, *op. cit.*

[10] C. Rogers and B.T. Skinner. *The Self and the Drama of History.* New York: Charles Scribner's Sons, 1955

sumers to put "caring people" back into the system. Evidence of this lies in increased consumer criticism and involvement. There is also an increase in the incidence and variety of "self-therapy" groups. More than obvious is the need for the presence of health workers who deal with the person in the system. Who will it be?

Summary

If we can predict the future on the basis of current phenomena and trends we should be able to plan for attaining outcomes. An interesting question that we as curriculum planners might ask ourselves is, "Do we believe in the existence of miracles beyond our control that will affect the course of health events, or do we believe that our knowledges and understanding of the total scope of societal forces and health care can serve as a basis for developing the methods and systems needed to effect change in health care?

6 THE IMPLICATIONS FOR CURRICULUM OF CHANGES IN THE HEALTH CARE SYSTEM

Gertrude J. Torres, EdD, RN

Before discussing *The Implications for Curriculum of Changes in the Health Care System* specifically, there is a need to present certain background ideas.

Although the present health care system lacks much of what a system represents—"an interacting or interdependent group forming a unified whole and performing one or more vital functions"[1]—it does seem to be moving in that direction at a greater pace today than ever before. The fact that so many recognize the system or nonsystem of health care today as needing change in the direction of holistic functioning and in terms of the consumer of health care seems to indicate that we may well be on the road toward a viable health care system. For this reason, this presentation will use the term health care system with these facts in mind.

Change implies going from point one in time to point two, and that between the two points some noticeable alteration occurs. Thus, it might be said that if we are to prepare the nursing practitioner for tomorrow's health care system, we must change the way we prepare the practitioner today to something different for tomorrow.

Some would stress that our *major* responsibility is to prepare the practitioner to function in today's world, giving only some attention to

---

[1] *Webster's Seventh New Collegiate Dictionary.* Springfield, Massachusetts: G. & C. Merriam Company, 1963.

41

the future, since we cannot accurately predict what will occur. Others might conclude that at the present rate of change, we should forget today's health care system and focus on tomorrow's. This thinking leads me to wonder if their idea of tomorrow is three, five, ten or even 40 years from now. There are even those who feel history repeats itself, so why be concerned with any changes? They would probably agree with the old saying, *Plus ca change, plus c'est la meme chose* [the more things change, the more they remain the same]. For this discussion, let us take a central position, since that seems to make the greatest amount of sense: we, as nurse educators, need to prepare students for today, with emphasis on improving the present system of health care, and also, for tomorrow, utilizing present trends to predict the future. Some are fearful of making predictions, since the future is so uncertain; yet, it seems, fearful or not, we must do so, although with humility and caution.

Before continuing, let me clarify a point: the word *curriculum* in this particular discussion refers to the organized areas of learning and that which relates to them, such as the program's philosophy, its objectives, its course requirements and the learning experiences it provides.

One of the first questions that came to my mind in thinking about this topic was, "Should the curriculum change consistently as society's demands for health care change and the funcitons of the nursing practitioner evolve?" In other words, does changing the functions of the professional nursing practitioner to meet the changing health care demands require that educators today constantly change the total curriculum? Generally, it is wise to present a question and let the readers ponder the answer for a while in the hope that they would believe what Voltaire wrote, "Judge a man by his questions, rather than by his answers." In this case, however, it is best to answer the question, and the answer seems to be, "No, the total curriculum need not change."

Some new developments within the health care system may be here today and gone tomorrow. Idzerda encourages professional educators to realize that society has made decisions out of panic and rage and regretted them the next day.[2] Societal demands and priorities change at a rather constant rate.

We all know that total curriculum changes take time, money and much effort and require effective ongoing evaluation. There are those who feel that the curriculum should be changed every four years negating any chance for evaluation of the total curriculum. Understand, the word *change* here does not refer to revision. Revision means improving or updating the parts, rather than starting from the begin-

---

[2] Stanley Idzerda. "Evaluating Rhetoric of Curricula Change." In *Challenge of Curricula Change.* New York: College Entrance Examination Board, 1966, page 146.

ning because the old is totally inadequate. Few would disagree with the belief that the various components of the curriculum must be continually revised.

Educators who feel that the total curriculum needs changing as the health care system and the functions of the professional nurse evolve, should be encouraged to create a curriculum with flexibility. Flexibility here does not pertain to the open curriculum or to choosing courses to meet students' individual needs; flexibility in this context refers to curriculum revision performed in a scientific manner as society changes. Could we think of curriculum revision as a means towards an *evolving* curriculum which is nonstatic?

Let me point out that there are basic concepts relating to nursing that seem not to change, or at least not to change very noticeably. These concepts relate to our beliefs about man and his needs, and the function of nursing—that of caring or nurturing. That part of the curriculum that deals with these concepts—as expressed in the philosophy, the objectives, and the course requirements—might remain rather constant, while other aspects, such as the emerging role of the nurse and the specific contributions that nursing makes toward meeting the health care needs of society, require revisions. Thus, we might think of a curriculum as having *constant* and *inconstant* components.

The constant areas are those that relate to man and his needs—his physiological, emotional, social, and cultural needs among others. The way the professional nurse helps people meet these needs could be termed the *inconstant* component of the curriculum, the component needing revision. Let me remind you that this is not a discussion of the implications for curriculum of changes in health care needs, for we have a fairly developed idea of that; rather, it speaks to the health care system. Thus, as the health care system changes, the curriculum evolves, requiring revision but not total change.

Now let me talk about what the changing health care system implies for an evolving curriculum. One of the health care trends identified by Dr. Frank in her paper was increasing governmental control, which may have started with Medicare and may easily lead to a form of socialized health care—national health insurance. This trend might easily create a tremendous impact on health care and professional nursing. It has several possible directions. For example:

1. *Catastrophic national health insurance.* This would call for a continued emphasis on the care of the acutely ill and possibly those needing long-term care. The evolving curriculum with its emphasis on man and on nursing as care would remain *constant*, while specific learning experience and course content might emphasize man's needs during crisis and illness. This would be the

inconstant. It would also necessitate a greater need for nurses to function in environments requiring greater interdependence than would a more community-oriented program.

2. *Comprehensive national health insurance.* This would make necessary a greater emphasis on prevention, health maintenance, diagnostic, restorative, and protective services. The specific learning experience needed in working with this type of insurance would be helping people maintain their health and working with community groups. More numerous opportunities for independent action, with collaboration with other health professionals, would also have to be included among the major learning experiences.

The trend toward *blurring* of nursing functions will increase if nurses have to take on functions of other health care workers. This may affect the autonomy of the nursing profession. For example, professional nurses may become more involved in functions generally assumed by physicians, dietitians, and physiotherapists, which means that opportunities for students to provide for an assigned patient case load a scientific nursing care plan on a continuous basis in all settings need to be encouraged. The student should be permitted to evaluate her performance on her own with the help of guidelines, rather than be subjected to constant supervision.

With a comprehensive health care plan, nurses would probably function more autonomously in certain areas. Students might need simultaneous experience in different agencies or in different areas, possibly alone, or in small groups with other professional nurses. The often practiced fixed teacher-student ratio of 1:8 during a laboratory experience could become inappropriate and sometimes impossible. The teacher-student ratio must be flexible and should relate to the specific behavioral objectives to be achieved by the student in a given situation. The teacher need not necessarily be visible, but available, and also easily accessible. Insisting on a rigid ratio with a rotating system is as unreasonable in clinical experiences as is insisting that all course content be presented through the lecture teaching method.

Another health care trend is the recommendation on the part of some, and without significant study of the health manpower needs, that there be more types of health care workers—witness the introduction of the physician's assistant. Such a development would affect nursing curricula by influencing institutions of higher learning to create new programs for a variety of health care workers other than nurses, thus giving rise to many different administrative structures. Institutions are becoming increasingly interested in interdisciplinary courses.

Outside groups may pressure educators in nursing to revise their curricula in the light of this interest. Here, again, it would appear that the *constant* parts of the curriculum can stay as they are, while the *inconstant* parts can make way for interdisciplinary practices without the further clouding of the specific functions of the professional nurse. The question remains which knowledges are specific to professional nursing and which are common to other health care workers? The sharing of the science courses, which is an increasing practice, is probably as far as we can go until we have a much clearer understanding of the profession of nursing in tomorrow's health care system.

Still another trend is the consumers' ever-increasing knowledge and interest in having health care provided at a reasonable cost and with greater efficiency. We, the educators, must respond to this trend and prepare the student to be a community leader representing professional nursing, as well as an informed citizen. For this type of leadership, he or she needs a greater amount of sophistication in effecting political change. This may mean that the nursing curriculum should include specific behavioral objectives which reflect involvement in change and an understanding of how change occurs. Finding these experiences for students is not simple. Faculty need to identify themselves as active change agents and consumers of health care.

In summary, whatever organized health care system evolves in this country has significant implications for baccalaureate nursing education. As the health care system changes, various competencies within the occupation of nursing will need to be identified more clearly. It is essential that the professional nurse who is a graduate of a baccalaureate nursing program have distinct functions to perform— functions which can definitely be differentiated from those of other nursing and health care workers—otherwise his or her position in the job market will be questionable, and he or she may become extinct. My belief is she must become *distinct* or she will become *extinct!*

In *Ms. Magazine*, Luunda B. Fleeson, who had interviewed physicians concerning nurses, wrote:

> All the doctors I interviewed expressed, without hesitation, their dependence on nurses, their respect for them, the extreme value of nurses in the health team, and their personal liking for most nurses.
>
> Most revealing were the comments that followed these sentiments of admiration. Where nurses expressed problems, physicians did not see them to be critical. Where nurses had instigated new programs, the physicians saw no resulting differences. Where nurses felt that the thrust of nursing depended on increasing the number of educated nurses, physicians saw no differences between baccalaureate or diploma (or associate-degree) nurses. While the nurses sought "equality," the physicians viewed this as an impossible goal.[3]

---

[3] Luunda B. Fleeson. "Doctors Diagnose Nurses." *Ms. Magazine,* August, 1973.

45

Professional nursing involves a great number of separate and distinct abilities. Some of these are:

- Leadership within and outside the health care system, as a participant in change.
- An ability to use scientific theories that have been developed in the nursing process, together with an in-depth ability to perform assessment, nursing diagnoses, and interventions involving decision-making.
- An ability to lead others and participate in change in order to improve nursing care.
- An ability to function independently or interdependently, as the need arises.
- An ability to focus on health maintenance and health promotion in any setting.
- An ability to evaluate oneself, others within the health care system, and the plan of nursing care being carried out.

The acquisition of these abilities requires a strong foundation in general education and science, which is available only in a baccalaureate program. If this premise is accepted, then there is little validity to creating nurses who focus on technical skills prior to creating professional practitioners. Perhaps two *separate* careers is the answer—one in professional nursing and the other in technical nursing.

As the organized health care system changes, the nursing process remains a *constant*, but the environment or settings in which the nurse functions may change. In preparing for the future, we must not become overly involved with the *where* of nursing, but must concentrate on the *what*. Maybe we can truly socialize and prepare the professional practitioner better, and with fewer experiences, within the acute care setting. The professional experiences in this setting should serve the purpose of developing the leadership skills needed in relation to the nursing process, such as the ability to handle a 24-hour patient case load. I hope these ideas I have presented have given you some food for thought about the relationship between health care trends and baccalaureate education.

7 THE EVOLUTION OF CURRICULUM PLANNING

Edwina D. Frank, EdD, RN

All educators think about ways of getting their body of knowledge across to the learner. Nursing educators along with other educators in the practice disciplines have the added task of transmitting a body of knowledge that has as its ultimate aim the provision of a frame of reference within which those who practice can meet a particular need of society.

The health field and related disciplines today encounter a steady stream of changes. The sources of change might exist within the area of practice and reflect advances in educational and technological knowledge or new theories and different problems pertaining to the practice field. Or, on the other hand, outside forces might serve as change sources and evolve from events of a politico-socio-economic reactionary nature; also influential might be the emergence of new health-related occupations or changes in the practice of another discipline.

Where the ultimate goal of the educational process is to prepare a practitioner of nursing, the question of relevancy—who, what, and where—is an ever-present one and often makes the necessity of curriculum change a continuous, ongoing process. Evidence of the impact of curriculum change on nursing educators might be found in the not uncommon experience of hearing those involved express feelings of frustration at the complexities and the unpredicted events that occur once the transitional phase begins. There is the recurrent use of such terms as *resistance to change, faculty turnover, student dis-*

satisfaction, graduates not prepared for practice, lack of funds, and a host of other expressions with which we are all but too familiar. Such questions arise as, Are we really doing anything? Is change occurring? What went wrong—and where? With these questions in mind, we propose in the subsequent discussion that in our efforts to effect curriculum change we consider the curriculum process in broad perspective and ask the larger question, What approaches, methodologies, and systems are available to facilitate the required change?

The Curriculum Process As A Change Process

Although there are many definitions of curriculum process, some commonalities are found in all of them. There is general agreement that change in the curriculum is initiated by either dissatisfaction with existing education practices or the awareness of a more desirable or effective way of accomplishing the education program. The initiating agent may spring from within or without the organizational structure, or external and internal forces may interact to precipitate change. Another commonality is that whatever the approach, subsequent activities eventually involve development and implementation of the proposed changes and evaluation of the effects. Put so succinctly, the preceding descriptions may seem an oversimplification in view of the many forces involved in curriculum change and are possibly more definitive of methodology than of total process. They do not quite provide us with what we need for examining all of the components of curriculum change. The very obvious missing elements are the human elements in curriculum change or what behavioral scientists might refer to as *people technology, change agents, change strategies* or *cultural forces.*

People Change As An Essential Element

Whether we define curriculum as process or as content, the object of curriculum change always has as its focal point altering some characteristics of the educational program; and the student is the pivotal point around which the curriculum revolves. Whatever the priorities for change, there are usually the interactional influences of what Barnes[1] refers to as "Task, People, Technology, and Structure." We in nursing education have moved into an era where our Task, Technology, and Structure concepts include such terms as *conceptual*

---

[1]Louis Barnes. "Approaches to Organizational Change." In *The Planning of Change* (W. Bennis, K. Benne and R. Chin, eds.). New York: Holt, Rinehart and Winston, Inc., 1969.

48

framework, learning laboratories, simulated laboratories, teaching teams, dual appointments, multidisciplinary and a host of others we use depending on where we are and what influences we are responding to. The crucial factor, however, in the extent to which the "things" are accomplished is the extent to which the people component accepts and effects the proposed change.

Chin and Benne[2] view changes in educational practice in the same context as changes in any other system. Their emphasis is on planned changes—on "attempts to bring about change (that) are conscious, deliberate and intended, at least on the part of one or more agents related to the change attempt." In this frame of reference, the change problem which might arise from attempts to introduce new things and technologies is viewed as shifting to the human problem of dealing with the resistances, anxieties, threats to morale, conflicts and disrupted interpersonal communication which occur when people are confronted with prospective changes in patterns. If, then, we can accept the existence of the human problem as a necessary component of change in the curriculum process, we need to build strategies for dealing with "people change" in the same sense that we build them in dealing with change in content, methodology, and organizational structure. The solution proposed by Chin and Benne is that the introduction of change, whatever the focus, must be based on behavioral knowledge of change and must utilize people techonologies based on such knowledge. This concept is not new to us as nurses, and would certainly be incorporated in any plan of which the target was recipients of care. Chin and Benne propose a group of strategies, referred to as "Normative Re-education," which have as their aim changing the normative orientation to old patterns, attitudes, values, skills and significant relationships and the development of commitments to newer ones. Essential elements in this strategy include: improving the problem-solving capabilities of a system and releasing and fostering growth in the persons who make up the system to be changed.

An emerging trend in nursing education that seems to facilitate changing normative orientation has been for programs to pool their resources in developing strategies to effect curriculum change. Some rather interesting observations relative to change and curriculum process grew out of the discussion of a gathering of nurse educators held at Georgetown University in the summer of 1972 on the initiative of Rose Marie Chioni and Loretta Nowakoski.[3] The representatives of 14 pro-

[2] Robert Chin and Kenneth Benne. "General Strategies for Effecting Changes in Human Systems." In *The Planning of Change*. New York: Holt, Rinehart and Winston, Inc., 1969.
[3] Judith Bancroft. "Summary of the Proceedings of the Process Subgroup *Curriculum Workshop*." Washington, D.C.: Georgetown University School of Nursing, July 6-7, 1972.

grams from various regions of the country and all involved in USPHS-funded curriculum projects met to share experiences in developing models or strategies for effecting curriculum change. It was possible for the group to identify three recurring themes which related to the curriculum process—Change Process, Organization, and Instruction:

1. The theme of *Change Process* seemed to pervade the other two themes. The issues and problems related to the very process of change within the institution. The effects of change and resistance to it were noted throughout the institution and in various ways affected the organizational structure of the school, the administrative approaches, the teachers and the students.

2. The *Organization* theme identified a number of different approaches used during the preparation of a proposal; the structuring of hierarchical levels within the organization to accomplish the various tasks; the use of faculty and consultant manpower and the phasing of major work activities, usually referred to as planning and implementation.

3. The theme of *Instruction* related primarily to the question of decision-making regarding instructional approaches and continuity. The specific ideas expressed had to do with instructional decisions regarding multidisciplinary teaching, promotion of self-direction among students, curriculum patterns, course content and patterns, and faculty loads.

Although this discussion cannot do justice to all of its implications, the report of the meeting at Georgetown University has been cited here because commonalities identified by the group might possibly reflect trends in other programs undergoing curriculum change. The group has continued holding meetings over the past year; its recent activities focus on identification of factors that enhance the curriculum process.

The Cultural Context

Another approach to examining the curriculum process has been advanced by Gordon Mackenzie,[4] who, after analyzing descriptions of curriculum change in elementary and secondary educational settings, arrived at a conceptualization of the curriculum process in a cultural context. Mackenzie defines curriculum as "the planned engagements of learners" and the focal point of curriculum change as the modification of one or more of six components that he refers to as "determiners of the curriculum." (The six components are teachers,

---

[4] Gordon Mackenzie. "Curriculum Change—Participants, Power and Process." In *Innovation In Education* (Matthew Miles, ed.) New York: Teachers College, Columbia University, 1971.

students, subject matter, methods, materials and facilities, and time.) The cultural context of the curriculum change process described by Mackenzie includes four components: (1) participants in curriculum change; (2) their sources of power; (3) phases of the process of change; and (4) the determiners of the curriculum. This conceptualization depicts participants in change as both internal and external—those having a direct connection with the social system and those outside of the immediate social system under consideration. Similarly, the various phases of the process might be initiated by either internal or external participants. What, then, are the implications of the "cultural context" for the curricular process in nursing education? Irene Pagel[5] applied Mackenzie's conceptualizations in studying the curriculum process in three baccalaureate programs undergoing curriculum changes. Pagel's observations relative to the influences of the cultural context were similar to Mackenzie's. She found the "cultural context of the curriculum change limited in perspective." Mackenzie's observations were of programs undergoing curriculum change in elementary and secondary education; he found inequity in the influences of internal and external participants—much of the change was initiated from sources outside of the social system. Pagel's observations of the three baccalaureate programs indicated a tendency for nursing faculty "to accept responsibility for curriculum change. All other groups and agencies were seen as having limited influences." With regard to the determiners of curriculum, Pagel, like Mackenzie, found that "subject matter was the focal point most frequently cited as it was directly related to other determiners, teaching methods and facilities." Pagel further noted that "students were not a focal point of curriculum change." As a result of utilizing this approach to studying the curriculum process, both educators were able to identify side effects (positive and negative) and the consequences of the change efforts. With regard to nursing education, Pagel recommends that "nursing faculties need to articulate more clearly the educational goals and the cultural context of the society," and that "evaluation of the process and content of the curriculum change. . .be incorporated from the outset."

Summary

It is not within the scope of this paper to present all of the possible approaches to studying the curriculum process, but rather to illustrate the value of employing a deliberate, planned approach to examining its various aspects.

---

[5] Irene Pagel. *The Process of Curriculum Change in Three Baccalaureate Schools of Nursing.* Doctoral dissertation. New York: Teachers College, Columbia University, 1971. (Available on microfilm and xerography, Xerox Company, Ann Arbor, Michigan.)

At the outset of this discussion, reference was made to the implications of the multifaceted nature of education in a practice discipline. Educators must respond to the simultaneous existence of the concept of education as a process which promotes creativity, inquiry, and the development of potential and the concept of utilizing scientific knowledge with service to society as the end in view.

It is proposed here that, out of necessity, educational planners in baccalaureate nursing education be sensitive to influences arising from various sources (the idealized concerns of the academic world as well as the pragmatic concerns of the society). It would seem that a view of the curriculum process as a social process inclusive of people systems as well as method and content is essential if we are to facilitate educational change. Questions arising from this viewpoint might then be:

1. *Participants in the process.* Who are the "significant others"? To what extent do internal and external participants interact in initiating and implementing the desired change?

2. *Determiners in the process.* What about students as the targets of whatever modifications are sought? Do our efforts include their characteristics, expectations, and goals?

What of accountability? Are our people task, technology, and structure strategies appropriate to attaining the desired change? Combs,[6] for example, asks, Does a system of accountability dependent solely on prior definitions of behavioral outcomes promote holistic thinking and inquiry?

3. *Change Process.* If we really consider the act of education as a change process, how do we know who and what we are trying to change? What are the attitudes, resistances, and obstructions? Are our evaluative approaches holistic enough to determine the effects of curriculum change efforts?

---

[6] Arthur Combs. *Educational Accountability Beyond Behavioral Objectives.* Washington, D.C.: Association for Supervision and Curriculum Development, 1972.

8 HIGHER EDUCATION AND CURRICULUM ISSUES

Gertrude J. Torres, EdD, RN

There are many educational controversies today in higher education that have a strong impact on nursing education. There are, also, many educators who approach these controversies as though simple answers and solutions were readily available. This discussion attempts neither to relate to most controversies nor to give simple answers to complex issues. Thus, only some of those issues in higher education which seem to have a significant impact on nursing education will be discussed.

Issues are like polygons in that they have many sides. The side a particular individual takes depends on such things as his or her past experiences in relation to the subject, personal interest in or comfort with the ideas at issue, the political or social forces that, in his or her view, are involved, and especially understanding of the implications of the issue for himself or herself and others. In this discussion, an attempt will be made to bring out various sides of each issue. It might be interesting for you to identify which, if any, of the sides presented to you take on a particular issue and examine the reasons why. The issues to be discussed are educational funding, flexibility of curriculum design, and academic policies.

Funding

Higher education is becoming more accountable, especially in relation to cost. It is no longer capable of receiving financial support from governmental or nongovernmental agencies without giving attention to present societal needs, priorities, and demands. Society no longer is willing to support higher education simply on the premise that education is beneficial for the society and the individual. The question of *who* should pay for higher education for *what* purposes is being heard more often every day. Does the individual or society benefit from higher education? Should federal or local funding be encouraged? Should we continue to pay for educating certain types of professionals, such as physicians, dentists and nurses, when many of our citizens do not have access to health care?

Federal support for nursing education is said to be a major factor in increasing and improving health care because it results in an increase in the number of nurses at all levels of competency, and since the enactment of the traineeship program in 1956, it has been especially important to graduate education. A survey made by ANA showed that federal funds presently constitute 50 percent or more of the student-aid available in 81 percent of the masters programs, 77 percent of the associate degree programs, 63 percent of the baccalaureate programs, and 44 percent of the diploma programs.[1] The study also revealed that 16 percent of the responding nursing programs now receiving student assistance reported that they would become nonexistent if financial assistance cutbacks should be approved. These statistics demonstrate how dependent on federal funds nursing education has become within the last two decades. Reduced support would lead to the reduction of faculty, the elimination of special projects, and a shrinkage of several areas of the programs. Federal support has also been given for construction, with some 30 pecent of the studied schools applying for such grants.

Thus, if we look at the issue of who should support nursing education, it appears that until recently there has been little question that strong federal support is indicated. Nursing seems to be able to accept this idea easily, and this is reflected in many of the activities now being carried on by nursing organizations and leaders. It appears we should encourage the same type of support for another two decades.

The whole issue of support for nursing education relates to other issues. It seems issues beget other issues. Issues such as state or federal support for nursing education, identification of specific programs that should be supported by federal funds and for what purposes, whether the financial needs of nursing education should take a greater or lesser priority over the education of other health case workers, whether we as a society need to focus on issues other than those involving health care, such as ecological needs, welfare problems, and social ills—all

---

[1] "Impact on Administration's Health Budget Revealed." *The American Nurse,* 5(7):9, July 1973.

need to be discussed and priorities need to be established. Let me present some questions, for which I have no answers, that come to my mind on this issue of federal support.

- While federal support for nursing and nursing education has increased the number of special projects and research grants, has it benefited the consumer of health care? With millions of dollars being given to support maternal-child nursing and psychiatric and mental health nursing, for example, has the nursing care in these areas substantially improved?

- Has federal support dictated certain priorities that have been identified by others rather than by nurses? Have some of these priorities been established within a bureaucratic political system without specific regard to regional or local needs for nursing care?

- Has federal support tended to stifle other available support?

- Will continued federal support for nursing education create too many nurses at all levels of practice, resulting in a job market similar to those of teachers and scientists?

- Has federal support been given to graduate programs having only five to ten students, and should this continue? Are some 80 graduate programs needed for some 3,700 full-time and 1,200 part-time students?

There are many sides to the issues in federal funding and nursing education. Admittedly, some of the questions just asked have a negative connotation. So we should also recognize the positive side. Federal support has been instrumental in the following:

- In the last decade the number of student enrollments in masters programs has doubled, a fact that can be largely attributed to federal funds. With the present recognized need for additional nursing leaders, this is a welcome trend, for one is almost afraid to imagine what state nursing service and nursing education would be in without them.

- Nursing research has increased its level of sophistication in the last two decades.

- There no longer is a *national* shortage of registered nurses.

- Federal support to nursing education has encouraged institutions of higher education to develop nursing programs and take their rightful place within the educational setting.

• Federal guidelines have stimulated nursing educators to examine and evaluate their curricula in terms of such things as flexibility and meeting the needs of minorities, and have led to a greater commitment to the evolving role of the professional nurse.

There exists another approach to this issue of federal support for higher education and nursing. That is to look at it as basically neither positive nor negative but critically. We, as educators, often speak of encouraging critical thinking in our students, yet we frequently deal with issues on a subjective basis. Here, critical thinking can be thought of as synonymous with problem-solving and the use of logic.

Fundamentally, the problem is that nursing education has, for the past two decades, received a significant amount of federal support and may now have this support reduced substantially or totally withdrawn. The facts concerning the issue need further study. Questions regarding the purposes, methods, and evaluation of federal support need to be answered. In terms of the answers to these questions, we must find solutions which have as their emphasis the improvement of nursing education and thus improved nursing care for our citizens.

What I am proposing here, as a consumer of health and nursing care, as an educator and a taxpayer, is that we examine federal funding programs especially related to nursing with a view to their implications. We cannot go back in history and predict what nursing and nursing education would have been like today if we had not received so much federal support. But we can study the issue in the light of the past and come to grips with the future.

Flexibility

Another significant issue in higher education which has had a deepening impact on nursing education is whether there should be "flexibility" in curriculum matters. Colleges and universities are increasingly being charged with having *inflexible* curriculum designs and course requirements. Educational leaders and the public are encouraging them to loosen admission policies, to reduce the number of specific course requirements and to grant credit for life experiences. The idea of giving credit for fun is gaining greater attention. According to the July 16, 1973, issue of *Time* magazine, a Detroit news journalist compiled a 386-page directory of educational vacations for credit. Among such vacations were:

- An ecology study of the Amazon, sponsored by the University of California and focusing on the study of the flora and the human inhabitants of the region. The cost of such a vacation: $1,468.

- A course in golf at Temple University which includes an analysis of swing through instant video replay. The cost: $80.

- A European study tour offered by the University of Pennsylvania featuring visits to famed European restaurants and food markets. The cost: $1,153. This particular one interested me the most.

Do you want to follow this trend of thought with the title *Nursing Education for Fun?* We might have a course in International Nursing Care and take the students around the world to visit health agencies and compare the nursing care given.

The Carnegie Commission on Higher Education advocates flexibility in curriculum design and recommends that more opportunities be created for students to "stop out" at appropriate points in their educational career for the purpose of acquiring work experiences or for other reasons. They would like to see a reduction in the number of high school graduates who seek a college education immediately upon graduation and encourage some to obtain higher education later. Stimulating creativity through independent study and providing educational opportunities for all age groups while giving greater attention to creative approaches to teaching are ideas which are part of the whole educational push toward greater flexibility and change.

There is also interest in the idea of a "free university." The activities involved would be supplementary to those of the classroom and not too different from the university's other student-initiated extracurricular activities except that they would be offered for credit. Some colleges, in their 4-1-4 semester approach, are already granting credit for such activities.

Equality of educational opportunity, especially as it relates to minority groups, strongly tests the educators ability to be flexible. Open admission polices create a different kind of student population, which in turn requires the reevaluation of present approaches to counseling as well of remediation and course requirements and offerings. The emphasis here is, *Come as you are and leave as we would have you be.* The idea that a college education requires four years may need to be challenged if we admit the less prepared to our baccalaureate nursing programs. Some are asking, "If the graduate behavioral objectives are met, what difference does it make if it takes three, four, five or even six years for the student to meet them so long as she or he is willing to spend the money and the energy needed and the college has the available resources?'' Yet those who would encourage a more inflexible approach to admission policies might feel that it is better to admit students who, on the basis of statistics, have the greatest potential for success, since resources and qualified faculty are now scarce. There seems no simple answer here, but consideration and possibly action are needed to pave the way to greater educational opportunities for all groups with the present resources.

Inherent, also, in flexible admission policies is the need for educators to be more creative in identifying alternative ways of allowing students to meet the various level objectives in nursing. We frequently encourage students to treat clients and patients as unique individuals, yet we teach all our students within the course as though they were all identical in their ability and motivation to learn. If we had adequate evaluation tools to measure each of the objectives, we might allow students to learn at their own pace rather than assume they must all meet the objectives by the week of the final examinations. And if we do so, we will have to determine whether or not each student must have the same types and the same number of laboratory experiences and, also, whether they all require teacher supervision during all these experiences or can be permitted greater independence at certain times and in accordance with their individual needs and abilities.

of higher education and our beliefs regarding the way people learn. In looking at the issue of flexibiity, we must neither ignore the above-mentioned considerations in the hope that they are only a passing fancy nor incorporate all new ideas pertaining to the education of professional nurses today. Flexibility would reflect our ability to yield to influence and our capability to respond. Yet, to be so flexible as to bend into distorted shapes would serve neither the student nor the society. In 1865, Abraham Lincoln said, "Important principles may and must be inflexible." Yet, total inflexibility would deny the need for some changes and would reflect our uncompromising inability to deviate from our present rules, standards, and requirements.

If we believe our mission as nurse educators is to prepare the professional nurse practitioner, then our curriculum design by necessity becomes rather inflexible. For example, if we feel that courses in the sciences of anatomy and physiology are an essential base for the practice of professional nursing, then there seems little possibility that we can allow the student to enter the first nursing courses without this base. Yet, if we believe it makes little difference where and how she has acquired a knowledge of these sciences, we can become flexible by allowing transfer credit or credit by examination for *all* students, not just RNs. Thus, as nurse educators we need to decide when and where flexibility is appropriate in relation to our beliefs about higher education and how students learn.

58

Let me now turn to the issues pertaining to academic policies in higher education and try to demonstrate how they relate to nursing education. As educators, we, in our personal and professional lives, can be strongly influenced by academic policies. Areas such as governance, tenure, and contracts are having an ever-increasing effect on our lives. As a large group of women educators, we need to make a greater impact on policies in general, but especially on those policies relating to pregnancy, academic leaves, and different salaries for males and females. Both faculty and administrators must become more involved in personnel policies. At a recent meeting I attended of the American Association of Higher Education at which mostly administrators were present, there was an obvious lack of female representation. They say, by the way, the only want to become a college president as a female is to join a convent. Don't you think some of our "outstanding" nurse administrators should seek positions in institutions of higher education as academic deans, vice-presidents or president? Policies such as tenure, which was instituted in this country in 1915, have recently received much attention. Such questions are being raised as: Does tenure assure society that the faculties of its educational institutions will be made up of free minds, independent in thought and courageous in advocacy?[2] If tenure insures academic freedom, is this academic freedom for blacks and women, too? Does tenure ignore the interest of students?

As nurse educators, we have tended to move from institution to institution and have not truly identified tenure as a significant issue to us. Tenure policies have generally been closely associated with the concept of academic freedom. Our ability to teach students controversial subjects such as abortion and euthanasia has not, seemingly, been stifled, and we apparently have not felt the great need for increasing our academic freedom. Yet, as we become more active politically, as society focuses more on health care and the issues involved, we may by necessity need to take a closer look at tenure.

Unionism is also gaining impetus. About 10 percent of the nation's 900,000 college teachers are affiliated with faculty unions. Unions have the ability to assist faculty in winning greater participation in governance, better salaries and job security, yet they can cause a greater rigidity and standardization of policies relating to teaching load, hours, sabbaticals, and research. This can have a significant influence in nursing education in relation to curriculum design, teaching methods, and laboratory experiences.

If, for example, union contracts, which focus on the needs and demands of the majority, state that the faculty-student contact load is

---

[2] Florence Moog. "Tenure is Obsolete." In *Expanded Campus Issues in Higher Education,* Vernilye W. Dyckkma, ed. San Francisco: Jossey-Bass, Inc., 1972, p. 136.

15 hours per week, and the nursing courses are planned so that faculty have 14 or 16 contact hours, what problems does that create? The curriculum design has a rationale to it and may not be that easily or properly revised to meet faculty requirements regarding teaching loads. Might there be a need for a more flexible approach, such as a range of hours for each semester and possibly a yearly requirement for contact hours? Many nursing curricula offer differing amounts of nursing credit during the fall and the spring semester. With unionization there is always the possibility of a strike. What implications does this have to the nursing curriculum which is highly dependent on laboratory experiences planned months ahead of time? Nursing educators should weight carefully the pros and cons of unionization and take an active part in decision-making.

In conclusion, it should be recognized that there are many other issues in higher education that affect the nursing curriculum. Issues such as the decreasing value placed on the university by society and the reassessment of the value system seem significant at this time in our history, especially in relation to present governmental activities. Higher education needs to come to grips with technology.

9 SUMMARY OF DISCUSSIONS

Participants in the Faculty-Curriculum Development Workshop Series, New York, New York

Topic: Identifying Changes and Priorities in Social and Health Care Needs

Major Responses

To bring about change there must be:

- Identification of the need for change and the process involved in creating change.

- Identification of the external forces for change, such as funding, consultation, legislation, revisions in criteria, changing consumer demands, and research findings.

- Recognition of the internal forces for change, such as peer evaluation and students.

- Increased collaboration among nursing service, other health professionals and consumers of health care.

- Changes in the image of nursing owing to changing faculty, students and consumer attitudes.

The major health care trends relative to nursing that will affect the curriculum are:

• Increased sophistication of consumers concerning health care, resulting in their greater participation in planning and identifying their own needs. Students need to be offered a greater number of experiences relating to the consumer as an individual and within groups.

• Increased political forces affecting the health care delivery system and the availability of funds for nursing education. This should encourage experimental nursing curricula, innovative teaching methods, increased flexibility within the curriculum, and accountability on the part of the student for his or her own actions.

• Less expansion of clinical practice facilities with an increased student enrollment, requiring creative ideas and the need for master planning.

• Greater emphasis on prevention and health promotion as opposed to illness.

• Increased "blurring" of the roles of the various health care workers, requiring that nursing examine its specific role within a given situation.

Topic: Curriculum Trends and Process

Major Responses

Aspects of the curriculum process which are most difficult to accomplish are:

• Faculty commitment to be change initiators of the curriculum and utilize the process.

• Faculty concensus on the various aspects of the process.

• Development of the philosophy, conceptual framework and behavioral level objectives, and the implementation of the design.

• Development of evaluation tools.

• Communicating curriculum process to related groups, such as general college faculty, students, and agency personnel.

• Faculty assuming responsibility for their actions once consensus is reached.

• Obtaining sufficient time to develop the curriculum.

Support systems which facilitate the curriculum process are:

- Effective administrator and curriculum leader.
- Built-in system of evaluation.
- Legislative and financial support.
- Approving accreditation bodies.
- Academic support from other disciplines.
- Understanding the end product of the program by the consumer and other health professionals.
- Informative feedback system.
- Faculty resources and knowledge.
- Clinical facilities and community resources.

Topic: Faculty Roles and Functions

Major Responses

One group developed a conceptual model (Figure 1) for faculty responsibility in changing the curriculum.

Leaders and/or change agents in nursing are:

- Nurse educators, administrators, theorists, researchers, consultants, and practitioners.
- Nurses functioning in governmental or voluntary organizations who have access to national communication channels.
- Those who have the ability to obtain power, have influence and are willing and have the ability to articulate and take risks.
- Those who know the strategies for change and can use their knowledge and expertise to affect the political scene.
- Those who are outside the field of nursing.
- All professional nurses who are baccalaureate graduates.

Specific functions of the faculty in the process of curriculum changes are to:

- Systematically assess, plan, implement, and evaluate the curriculum.

- Identify the need for change.

- Identify the change forces and resistors of change.

- Determine their specific needs in terms of their professional preparation and use of a consultant.

- Interpret changes to others where and when necessary.

- Identify the impact of the changes.

- Identify participants needed for change.

- Develop skill in group dynamics and the utilization of principles of change.

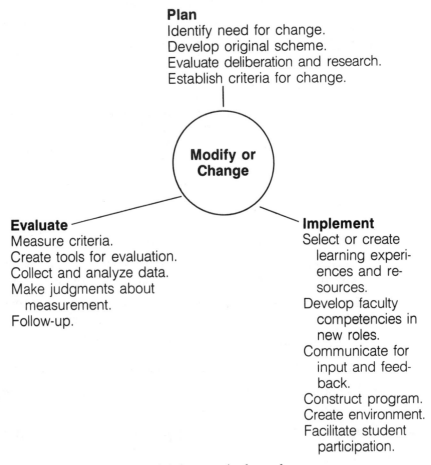

Plan
Identify need for change.
Develop original scheme.
Evaluate deliberation and research.
Establish criteria for change.

Modify or Change

Evaluate
Measure criteria.
Create tools for evaluation.
Collect and analyze data.
Make judgments about
    measurement.
Follow-up.

Implement
Select or create
    learning experi-
    ences and re-
    sources.
Develop faculty
    competencies in
    new roles.
Communicate for
    input and feed-
    back.
Construct program.
Create environment.
Facilitate student
    participation.

Figure 1. Conceptual model for curriculum change.

Topic: Curriculum Issues and Teaching Methods

Major Responses

Major issues in higher education which affect the nursing program are:

- Governmental funding and control.
- Decreased value placed on the university by society and reassessment of the value system.
- Increased interest in interdisciplinary education.
- Flexible approaches to admissions and curriculum designs.
- Greater opportunities for minorities at all levels.
- Shared decision-making by administrators, faculty, and students.
- Personnel policies within the institution, such as evaluation procedures and tenure.
- Utilization of advanced technology.

To determine teaching methods which will support curriculum change:

- Identify resources available, such as funds, space, equipment, faculty preparation and expertise, and clinical facilities.
- Consider methods utilized previously with the students in reaching objectives.
- Involve students more actively in determining, implementing, and evaluating teaching methods.
- Utilize scientific method when experimenting with new or innovative teaching techniques.
- Utilize the method which reflects the school's, faculty's, and the students' philosophy of learning.
- Develop a curriculum approach which will provide for a variety of learning styles as well as allow for the learner to progress at a different pace.

10 SUMMARY OF DISCUSSIONS

Participants in the Faculty-Curriculum Development Workshop Series, Chicago, Illinois

Topic: Identifying Major Health Care Trends Relative to Baccalaureate Nursing Education

Major Responses

The health care trends are:

- Society's changing ideas regarding life and death and a greater evolution of a social consciousness.
- Increased knowledge of the consumer regarding health care and his desire to participate in decisions relating to the health care system.
- Increasing mobility of society, which affects the health care system.
- Impact of health legislation and funding programs.
- Proliferation of health care personnel, which has caused a greater blurring of roles.
- Change in the expectations of society in relation to nursing roles which are less traditional.
- Rapid expansion of knowledge and technology, and the identified need of health care workers to continue to gain knowledge throughout life.

Topic: Major Curriculum Implications for Preparing the Professional Nurse to Function in the Year 2000

Major Responses

In preparing the professional nurse for the future, the curriculum implications are that:

- Environmental effects upon the holistic nature of man will require continual curriculum adjustment to meet changing health needs.
- Flexibility to change directions and areas of focus within nursing will be needed.
- Constants within the curriculum will need to be the nursing process and man and his holistic nature.
- The nurse will have to be prepared to function both independently and interdependently.
- Greater emphasis will be put on community health care.
- The focus will be on assessment skills rather than technical skills.
- Greater emphasis will be given to the nursing process as the *what* of nursing rather than the *where*.
- The graduate will have to function in different roles in nursing—for example, on state boards of nursing.
- Different kinds of practice for different competency levels within nursing will have to be identified.
- Different teaching methods will have to be utilized, such as permitting the student to assume a 24-hour responsibility for nursing care.
- The student will have to be assisted in understanding the concepts of change.
- The students' understanding of interdisciplinary methods of providing health care will need to be enlarged.
- The need to teach values within the curriculum will have to be identified.

Topic: Curriculum Process in the Evolution of a Curriculum

Major Responses

Advantages of utilizing the process are that it:

- Provides a logical feedback mechanism.

- Provides guidelines for curriculum development.
- Allows for greater faculty input.
- Can be divided into components that can be handled especially during curriculum change.
- Helps to prepare faculty at the master's level.
- Assists in creating movement and achieving the task of curriculum development more efficiently.
- Provides for accountability and evaluation within the curriculum.
- Clarifies to others what is operational within the program.
- Facilitates faculty selection and orientation.

Disadvantages in utilizing the process are:

- Changes in faculty may be difficult, especially in obtaining concensus about the philosophy, and so forth.
- There are limited resources to permit released time from administrative or teaching responsibilities.
- Can discourage creativity if not used effectively.
- Lack of decision-making power may be present on the part of the faculty in implementing the process and its results.

Problems and implications are:

- The need to free faculty for curriculum process and evaluation tools.
- Difficulty in getting faculty to utilize the process and accept change.
- The need for unseasoned faculty to be provided with means, both educational and emotional, to adapt to new roles and to ventilate frustrations or opinions generated by the process.
- The need for funds to be appropriated for implementing the curriculum process.

Topic: The Change Process and the Faculty

Major Responses

The forces influencing baccalaureate nursing education:

External
- Change in the public's attitude toward nursing as an occupation.
- Women's Liberation Movement.

- Influence of associate degree programs in nursing.
- Closing of diploma schools of nursing.
- Societal values—services as a life concept.
- Changes in elementary and secondary education.
- Economic changes—cost of health care and education.
- Changes in functions of other health care professionals.
- Proliferation of health care workers.
- National and state legislative trends and policies.
- Consumer attitudes.
- Technology and the greater use of knowledge.
- Available job opportunities.
- Accreditation and approval bodies.
- Community structure and agencies.
- Nurses within the community.
- Professional organizations.
- Changes in graduate nursing education.

Internal
- Faculty needs and preparation.
- Students' needs and reactions.
- Administrative personnel.
- Dissatisfaction with status quo.
- Emphasis on nursing research.
- Changing philosophy of the institutions.
- Economic factors.
- Core requirements.
- Consultants.
- Changing climate of institutions.

Change resistors and forces influencing faculty to act as change agents.
- Faculty overload.
- Economic factors.
- Clinical laboratories.
- Physical facilities.
- Faculty insecurity.
- Lack of communication.
- Inability to see the need for change.
- Unrealistic goals.
- Acceptance of status quo.
- Lack of motivation.
- Educational policies.
- Fear of the unknown.
- Self-image of faculty members.

- Societal attitudes toward nursing.
- Traditions within nursing and medicine.
- Faculty preparation for change.

Topic: Higher Education and Curriculum Issues

Major Responses

Higher education issues that have the greatest impact on nursing:

- Funding.
- Administrative support.
- Self-image and societal image of nurses as educators.
- Failure of nursing educators to enter into the full academic life of the university or the college.
- Decentralization of the university campus.
- Newer approaches to education, such as self-pacing, greater amount of independent study, proficiency examinations, open-door policies, and innovative teaching methods.
- Accountability of the educational system.
- Emphasis on continuing education.
- Research emphasis.

Nursing faculty can influence higher education through:

- Involvement in campus politics.
- Assisting women to obtain equal rights on the university campus.
- Involvement in legislative matters.
- Influencing professional organizations.
- Offering courses to students of other universities or colleges.
- Increasing the awareness of other educators as to the purposes of the nursing program.

11 MODEL FOR THE UTILIZATION OF THE CURRICULUM PROCESS

NOTE: The following model was used for discussion purposes by the workshop participants.

Philosophy of the College

Our commitment as a liberal arts college dedicated to the Christian education of women is expressed in the ideal of searching out and sharing truth, both natural and supernatural. This is inherent in our objective to educate the student to achieve the fullest development of her intellectual, physical, emotional, spiritual, and cultural potentialities.

In accord with the traditional ideas of liberal arts education—to free man by enabling him to understand himself, society, and God—the curriculum is planned to be sufficiently flexible to meet the changing needs of the student and of society.

The college aims to assist the student to develop into an intellectually responsive, self-directing, religiously oriented, responsible member of society; to prepare her to function efficiently in the field of her choice; and to provide an acceptable basic preparation for graduate study.

Philosophy of the Nursing Program

We, as a faculty, believe in the Christian philosophy of life and education. We subscribe to the philosophy of the college that liberal arts education frees man by enabling him to understand himself, society, and God.

Recognizing the tremendous increase of knowledge in all areas, we believe that nursing shares with other professional health disciplines the broad responsibility to provide for the health needs of society now and in the future.

We believe that professional nursing is charged with overall responsibility for giving care and for those who assist in giving care, wherever and whenever it becomes necessary to satisfy the nursing needs of people.

We believe that professional nursing practice demands a high degree of competency and responsibility and involves decision-making at a level which requires perceptual and cognitive ability. It includes creating and initiating new methods based on current research.

We believe that baccalaureate nursing education is based on a foundation in liberal education which gives the student an opportunity to increase her ability to think responsibly and to communicate sensitively and clearly; to better understand herself and others; to become more aware of the forces that mold society and how these forces can be modified for the improvement of society.

We believe that our conceptual approach to curriculum provides opportunities for relating scientific, abstract and professional knowledge in identifying and dealing with nursing problems, assessing health needs, making clinical judgments, and initiating or sustaining nursing intervention in the care of individuals and families. Courses are planned to develop independence, judgment, professional competence, and leadership.

Our program in essence is one in which the patient is seen as an integrated whole, not as a specific disease entity. The student thus becomes aware of the impact that illness has not only on the patient but also on the family and the community.

This type of orientation allows the student at every level greater mobility and increased facility to learn in many varied settings.

We believe that our curriculum is sufficiently flexible to provide for the changing needs of students and the consumers of nursing and will serve as an acceptable basic preparation for graduate study. We believe that the graduates of our program will be prepared to accept professional responsibility for the care of patients and to assume beginning leadership positions in hospitals and other health agencies.

Objectives of the Nursing Program

1. To provide a broad foundation of knowledge and understanding, derived from the major areas of learning upon which professional nursing education can be based.

2. To stimulate habits of critical thinking and to help students become increasingly self-disciplined and self-directed.

3. To help students develop the ability to plan, give, and evaluate nursing care for patients on the basis of their individual needs and to guide others in the giving of care.

4. To enable the student to cooperate with other members of the health team and other interested groups in identifying and solving the health problems of the individual, the family, and the community.

5. To aid the student in developing the ability to plan and work for the improvement of nursing care—as a citizen and as a professional nurse.

6. To help the student increase her understanding of the need for continuous personal and professional growth.

7. To help the student acquire a base for advanced study.

College Requirements for the Baccalaureate Degree

Degrees that may be earned at the completion of the four-year course of study in the liberal arts and sciences are Bachelor of Arts and Bachelor of Science.

The Bachelor of Arts degree may be earned by students who choose as an area of concentration biology, chemistry, English, French, history, mathematics, philosophy, political science, sociology, Spanish, or speech. Art and psychology will be offered as areas of concentration beginning in 1969-1970.

The Bachelor of Science degree may be earned by students who choose as an area of concentration biology, chemistry or nursing.

Upon completion of the nursing program, which has been registered with the New York State Department of Education, the student will be eligible to take the State Board Examination, for the license to practice nursing as a registered professional nurse in New York State.

The college offers a program approved by the New York State Education Department that leads to a five-year provisional certificate in the field of elementary or secondary education.

To fulfill our objectives as a Catholic liberal arts college, we offer the following program of basic studies:

	Credits
Theology	12*
Philosophy	12
English	12
History	6
Mathematics	6**
Modern Language	6 or 12***
Science (Laboratory)	6-8
Social Science	6
Art	2†
Music	2†
Speech	2†
Physical Education (two years)	0

*Non-Catholic students may substitute other courses to meet theology requirements.
**In the field of science, 6-9; in that of nursing 3.
***This depends on the language background of the student. May be taken as an elective by nursing students.
†May be taken as electives by nursing and science students.

In addition to the above program, a student must fulfill the departmental requirements in an area of concentration and elect courses for their cultural or professional value. The minimum number of required credits is 128. The departmental requirements for a concentration in Nursing is a minimum of 44 credits.

A course in Independent Study in Nursing is offered for 1-3 credits for junior and senior students who qualify and are interested. At the present time this is the only professional elective couse offered. A curriculum guide for nursing majors is provided by the department.

Rationale for Organization and Selection of Content

The rationale for organization and selection of content in the college of nursing program is the belief that nursing is a discipline, since it has a history and a tradition, a body of knowledge about a unique domain of things and events, and can be organized for teaching. The faculty, following Bruner's theories, also believes that the best way to organize content and teach for transfer is to teach the fundamental structure of the discipline. In nursing, this structure is a synthesis of the problem-solving mode of inquiry with the basic ideas or concepts which are essential to the solution of problems. One cannot act rationally without knowledge.

Although the total college environment contributes to the education of a professional nurse, a program here is limited to courses and learning experiences within the nursing department.

The nursing program consists of three consecutive broad courses of one year's length, each building on previous learning, including the liberal arts. There is a constant focus on showing relationships, similarities and differences, and on guiding the student in using problem-solving to synthesize basic ideas into more and more comprehensive and meaningful patterns of understanding.

The first course, *Family and Community Health*, is organized around the concepts of health needs (developed by the students and teachers jointly) and developmental tasks involving the principles, concepts, and skills basic to professional nursing care. The student is introduced to the framework of Nursing Diagnosis and Intervention in relation to the normal and more familiar health needs. It includes the promotion and maintenance of positive mental and physical health at all ages and in a variety of settings. Students are given an overview showing how these basic ideas and the nursing process will be built upon each year until they have acquired mastery of the discipline.

At this initial level the student spends most of her time in learning basic facts, terminology and analyses, as well as all the basic motor and cognitive skills used in communication, interpersonal relations, identifying needs, and giving hygienic care. Data are collected from observation of human behavior in the more normal setting of home and family. The student is introduced to the development of a written plan and the implementation of the plan by nursing intervention. All nursing action must be planned on the basis of knowledge of normal psycho-physiological responses of selected patients. Since integration takes place in the learner, opportunity is provided in learning experiences—for example, comparing and contrasting the providing of hygienic care and safety factors for a normal infant with that of a senior citizen. By guiding the student in identifying underlying facts and principles from the behavioral and natural sciences and from nursing content (related to health needs and the nursing process), the student can arrive at basic understandings and generalizations of care which can then be applied to new but similar nursing problems. The student then progresses to utilizing the nursing process and basic skills and knowledge in caring for the expanding family, starting with the familiar adolescent and proceeding through the normal reproductive experiences. An attempt is made to go from the known to the unknown and from the simple to the complex, as advocated by theorists. The faculty, however, believes that learning basic concepts and skills does not always proceed from easy to difficult, but often from general to specific.

The second nursing course, *Nursing Diagnosis and Intervention,* involves the learning of nursing care of patients and families in illness and deviations from the normal. The course is organized around four unifying concepts—Stress and Response, Metabolism and Alteration, Oxygenation and Alteration, and Awareness and Adaptation to Environment. Also, the basic concepts of health needs and developmental tasks are redeveloped within each of the above concepts in relation to their alteration in illness. By selecting concepts that cut across all of the "big five" subject areas and include all age groups and settings, the faculty hopes to provide a general framework into which new knowledge can be filed and organized by the student for use. It aims, as Bruner says "...to provide a general picture in terms of which the relations between things encountered earlier or later are made as clear as possible." Mednick describes concept-formation learning as a category-naming process.

The introductory concept of Stress and Response, for example, enables the student to organize her learning experiences in relation to the physical and emotional response of patients and their families to physical, chemical, biological, and environmental stressors in illness and hospitalization. Basic general ideas such as homeostasis-equilibrium, general response of illness (symptoms, diagnostic data), cellular responses (including inflammation, infection, and cancer) and emotional responses can be introduced in relation to the concept of stress and response to the individual. In class the student is taught the basic facts, principles, and generalizations about a class of particulars, such as infections and the general expectations of care, including the therapeutic and supportive nursing measures common to most infections. Concepts, however, have operational value only when the student sees relationships among elements in her own experience as she is given opportunity in clinical learning experiences to use previous and new knowledges in meeting the objectives of planning and giving individualized care to a patient with a specific infection. The patient selected may be a child or an adult and the setting may be in a home, a clinic, an area of the hospital, and so forth. If the patient chosen is to undergo surgery, the student would, in planning and giving care, follow the patient from surgical unit to operating room, to recovery room, and, if time allows, back to the surgical unit. Her learning is active, since, although she has a general expectation of the care involved, she must, with the guidance of the instructor, seek data relevant to the individual patient from the library, assessment of the patient, the record, the family, and so forth. She must then make a nursing diagnosis and develop and implement a plan of intervention which is then modified by continuous evaluation. Discussions in class and post-conference provide for a continuous sharing of experiences showing relationships among elements of care of patients of all age groups and in various settings. These discussions give opportunity for the student to analyze and interpret her plan of care and to understand that there is no one "routine" solution and that individual students will use different approaches in response to patient needs.

For the advanced senior couse in the care of ill patients, content is selected as it relates to the structure and methodology used in the previous course. Thus, content is selected within the framework of the same four basic concepts (stress, metabolism, oxygenation, and adaptation to environment) using the problem-solving approach (nursing diagnosis and intervention). New knowledge and skills are presented showing relationships to previous learnings and experiences developed in Nursing 21-22 and Nursing 31-32. In the advanced course students assume more initiative in learning, the problems become more complex, and the focus is on the leadership aspect of "working with groups." Further discussion is developed in giving examples of selection of learning experiences using the criteria.

Each of the concepts is developed by the team of teachers and student representatives of the class. Students are encouraged to question, to know the why, not only the how, of nursing action, and to feel free to disagree, but to express why they disagree. Their interests and suggestions are always recognized and considered and often utilized in planning. Faculty recognize that their own attitudes are important in engendering appropriate attitudes in the students and try to reach concensus in planning to transmit an enthusiasm and commitment to professional nursing to the students. Bruner believes that interest is created when the subject is rendered worth knowing, when it is meaningful.

Criteria for the Selection of Content and Learning Experiences for Nursing Courses

1. Are consistent with the theoretical framework of the total nursing program.

In order to teach for the future and to avoid fragmentation and artificial lines of demarcation, focus of the content should be on using relationships among the basic concepts and the problem-solving nursing process of nursing diagnosis and intervention (assess, plan, give and evaluate care) as a framework within which to organize new data and content. Thus, the same four major concepts of Stress and Response, Metabolism and Alteration, Oxygenation and Alteration, and Awareness and Adaptation to the Environment, plus the categories of content included under each, would be revisited. By continuing to reconstruct more advanced content within this pattern of concepts, there would be a review and reinforcement of basic ideas and skills which would be used as a basis for recognizing subsequent problems as special cases of the ideas previously learned. Use of the problem-centered approach enables the student to convert chaotic masses of facts into manageable problem situations. This is particularly vital in the nursing profession, since it is what Bruner calls an "unpredictable service," one in which action is contingent on a response made by somebody or something as a prior act.

   2.   Provides for continuity and sequence of curriulum development.

Balance of breadth and depth. In providing for sufficient range of breadth of content one could, for instance, present the commonalities of nursing problems of patients with chronic or advanced renal disorders under the concept of alteration in metabolism, but also provide depth and a model by having the students study a patient with a specific type of renal disorder, such as a patient with uremia; then one can provide opportunity in the clinical areas for students to use this model to generalize in individualizing care for specific patients with renal disorders.

Logical sequence. Vertical sequence would provide opportunity to build on past experiences. Thus, in the example above, the student would build upon an accumulation of previous learnings, such as cellular response to stressor agents and cellular defenses; behavioral responses to illness or hospitalization; fluid and electrolyte balance; knowledge of acute and simple infections (such as nephritis); knowledge of nursing ministrations in renal disorders, such as catheterizations, irrigations, dressings, diet therapy, and so forth. Analyses of similarities and differences in the care of specific paients would enable the student to see relationships and make inferences in new but similar situations.

Horizontal sequence would provide for progression in complexity. As the student is learning the nursing process and basic concepts and ideas, she is slow, unskilled, and needs more guidance and supervision (sophomore year). At this time, content and learning experiences are selected which are obvious, deal with judments about one patient, and focus on one specific nursing situation. As the student progresses in ability to observe, collect data, analyze elements in a problem situation, plan and implement nursing action, she is more able to cope with content and experiences which involve stress, require more speed, call for analysis of more elements in nursing problems and synthesis of a greater range of pertinent facts and generalizations. Advanced content would include what Holsclaw terms "Nursing in High Emotional Risk Areas."

Integration. Here the student is given models in class and opportunity to synthesize theory and principles from many courses, including courses in the liberal arts, and personal experience, both in class and in making clinical nursing diagnoses and interventions. Integration takes place within the learner, but only when she is given the opportunity to practice the classifying of situations and thus to see relationships between experience and knowledges which are separated in her experience.

3. Are consistent with learning principles.

Learning principles should be applied in selecting content and learning experiences. Such principles would include: (1) learning proceeds from familiar to unfamiliar, from simple to complex, from known to unknown; (2) anxiety interferes with learning; (3) learning takes place when the act that is performed is reinforced or rewarded; (4) learning is active—one learns the acts that are performed, the words that are repeated, the thoughts and feelings that are experienced.

4. Responds to social realities.

Max Lerner, in speaking of curriculum states that ". . .it is our function to respond to the great social urgencies, to direct the shaping of social goals and life purposes." Though a curriculum cannot respond to every passing social change, it should respond to the important realities of change in our culture as they affect nursing. Certainly there is a need to study international as well as local health and social problems and scientific advancements as they relate to health. Such problems include control of major world diseases, nuclear and natural disasters, automation, poverty, chronic and long-term illness, environmental pollution, population control, epidemiological studies, civil rights, and the delivery of health services, especially in our urban future.

5. Provide for professional competence.

Flexner, in setting up his criteria for a professional, said that it involves (1) intellectual operations with large individual responsibilities, (2) raw materials drawn from science and learning, (3) practical application, (4) an educationally communicable technique, (5) tendency toward self organization, and (6) increased altruistic motivation. Charles Russell, in commenting on these attributes, states in essence that the first, second, and fourth concern the intellect and can be developed by learning. Education designed to create a sense of social responsibility can also build the sixth—altruistic motivation, and study of a broad range of subjects including the liberal arts will form a student who is capable of intellectual operations, competent to perform individual responsibilities, able to grasp raw materials from science and learning, master a technique and develop an increasing altruistic motivation.

Thus, content and experiences should be selected which stress independent action, self-direction, freedom, mastery of the process of problem-solving, utilization of research findings, ethical behaviors, and value orientation.

In providing for professional competence in nursing, the senior course should include such functions as leadership, decision-making, working with groups, working with newer types of therapy (intensive care, hyperbaric oxygen, etc.) and advanced forms of patient assessment, including the use of monitoring and nursing history forms.

However, for the leadership potential of the student to be developed during her professional education, she must be encouraged and supported in her effort to be creative, innovative and critical in thought and action. All learning experiences must be planned to foster rather than stifle appropriate leadership behavior.

6. Are appropriate to the needs and interests of the students.

The student in a baccalaureate program has all of the needs of an older adolescent in addition to those of a nursing student. She still needs acceptance by peers, identification with a group, security, and independence. Mereness believes that educational freedom is necessary for learning. Therefore, an atmosphere should be provided where the student can feel free to disagree, to explore, to help choose her own goals, to experiment with alternate methods, and know the faculty as vital caring human beings. Students' needs and interests should be considered in individualizing assignments, in providing feedback to show the students that they are progressing toward their goals, and in giving support and encouragement.

12 SUMMARY OF DISCUSSIONS

Participants in the Faculty-Curriculum Development Workshop Series, Dallas, Texas

Topic: Identifying Major Health Care Trends Relative to Baccalaureate Nursing Education

Major Responses

The health care trends are:

- Increasing need for and interest in state/regional planning for the use of resources such as money, people, facilities, and hardware.
- Rapid development and changes in knowledge and technology.
- Increasing need to cope with stress situations.
- Increasing involvement and changes in the attitude of the consumer toward health care.
- Increasing governmental control of health care.
- Increasing need for interdisciplinary cooperation.
- Decrease in economic and national resources.
- Greater demand for specialization and the expanding of roles.
- Changes in health care from episodic to more distributive.
- Increased blurring of roles of health care workers.
- A search for an alternative health care delivery system which focuses more on primary health care.
- Increasing demand for "accountability" in terms of health care.

- A proliferation of health care professionals.
- A rapid obsolescence of skills and content.

Topic: Major Curriculum Implications for Preparing the Professional Nurse to Function in the Year 2000

Major Responses

The curriculum implications are:

- Need to take into account a greater amount of deceleration and/or acceleration by the students, allowing for greater self-pacing within the curriculum.
- Greater emphasis on health maintenance.
- Greater amount of articulation between nursing service and nursing education.
- Increased utilization of nursing research.
- Increasing efforts to socialize the student into professional nursing and to the concepts of change.
- Increasing opportunities for the student to utilize the nursing process as an independent practitioner.
- Greater involvement of the student with the community and the consumer of health care.
- Need to encourage learning experiences for students in which they will be managers of care rather than managers of units.
- Increasing opportunities for students in mobile clinics with teams of nurses and other health care workers.
- Greater use of demonstration units for teaching and delivery of health care, such as "nursing centers."
- Increasing emphasis on "discovery learning" and creativity.
- Greater emphasis on helping the student to adapt to change.
- Need for greater understanding by the student of the health care system and her contribution.
- Greater emphasis on the behavioral sciences to reduce the trend toward the depersonalization of health care.
- Greater emphasis on dmeeting the health care needs of people whenever and wherever the need arises.
- Increasing number of interdisciplinary courses.
- Greater emphasis on meeting the health care needs of people whenever and wherever the need arises.
- Faculty and students independently caring (preventive and curative) for a group of selected clients.

84

Topic: Curriculum Process—The Evolution of Curriculum Planning

Major Responses (See Model for the Utilization of the Curriculum Program, pp.73-82)

Major components of the philosophy and objectives:

- Man as an integrated whole.
- Nursing as based on a foundation of liberal arts.
- The student as a learner involved in self-individualization and self-direction.
- Nurses' responsibility to man and society, both in the present and future.
- The Christian ethic.
- The nursing process.
- Initiating or sustaining nursing intervention in the care of individuals and families.
- Decision-making, self-direction, and creativity on the part of the nurse.
- Interdisciplinary cooperation.
- Philosophy of learning as progression from simple to complex and from general to specific and the utilization of a conceptual approach.
- Flexibility to allow for changing needs of the student and society.

The following represent weaknesses noted in the philosophy and objectives:

- Lack of clarity in the definition of nursing.
- Inadequacy of the statements relating to the beliefs about the product of the program.
- Failure to note operational definitions.
- Lack of clarity as to area of emphasis—on health or illness.
- Lack of specificity as to the relationship between man and nursing.
- Objectives oriented toward teacher rather than student.
- Inconsistencies between philosophy and objectives—for example, with respect to beliefs about an independent thinker, leadership skills, and the care components of nursing.

Components reflected in the conceptual framework were:

- Lack of clear definition.

- The use of problem-solving approach as a mode of inquiry.
- An emphasis on health initially in the program without health maintenance appearing again later in the program.
- The nursing diagnosis and process and the four unifying concepts.

Components in the philosophy and objectives which were not reflected in the conceptual framework were:

- The spiritual aspect.
- Meeting the needs of society.
- Interdisciplinary cooperation.
- Change theory.

Components in the conceptual framework which were not in the philosophy and objectives:

- The philosophy of learning—from simple to complex.
- The promotion of health.
- Growth and development.

The conceptual framework as noted in the nursing course:

- Nursing process and the unifying concepts were noted at all levels.
- Family and community health were noted at the sophomore level.
- Diagnosis, intervention and the nursing process were noted at the upper division level.
- A greater emphasis on decision-making in dealing with the health status of individuals and families was noted at the upper levels.
- Emphasis on pathophysiology and relevant nursing intervention were noted in the upper division nursing course.

The groups developed the following behavioral level objectives in relation to the program objectives, "To enable the student to cooperate with other members of the health team and other interested groups in identifying and solving health problems of the individual, the family, and the community." The following generally relates to the areas covered within the objectives *only* and are not complete statements of the objectives:

Sophomore level
- Involve families and individuals in planning nursing care based on concepts and principles.
- Identify community resources.
- Understand health and health maintenance.

- Identify roles and functions of the various members of the health and nursing team.

Junior level
- Collaborate with health team member.
- Provide nursing care utilizing the nursing process in a variety of settings.
- Know principles of group dynamics.
- Evaluate nursing care.
- Identify health needs with individuals and families with deviations from normal.
- Recognize alterations of responses to basic human needs and developmental tasks in illness.

Senior level
- Utilize nursing process with groups of patients.
- Function as leaders on the health and nursing team.
- Utilize nursing process with patients who experience more complex problems of illness.
- Make patient/client referrals when necessary.
- Involve in community health activities.

Topic: The Change Process and the Faculty

Major Responses

Change forces influencing baccalaurate nursing education:

External
- Private foundations.
- Governmental assessment of health care needs.
- Regional and state accrediting agencies and planning commissions.
- Nursing organizations.
- Consumer attitudes.
- Mass media.
- Technological advances.
- Distribution of population—social mobility.
- Changing values and morals.
- Limitation of national resources.
- Economic restraints.
- Changes in higher education.
- Medical and nursing research.
- Health insurance plans.
- Allied health group.

Internal
- Faculty characteristics—prepration, attrition, teacher evaluation.
- Nature of administration.
- Budget.
- Available clinical resources.
- Available facilities.
- Student as consumers.
- Research reports.

Change resistors and forces influencing faculty to act as change agents:

- Job market—practice setting.
- Lack of evaluation tools.
- Resistance to becoming accountable.
- Faculty as clinical specialists.
- Student attitudes toward learning and nursing.
- Administrative commitments and philosophy.
- Lack of faculty power and authority.
- Physical setting within the educational institutions.
- Legislative factors.
- Textbooks.
- Accreditation bodies.
- Predominantly female professionals—lack of aggressiveness.
- Personnel policies, such as tenure.
- Community needs.
- Attitude of faculty to change.
- Consumer "power" groups.
- Lack of flexibility of persons involved.
- Lack of funds to support change.
- Bandwagon psychology.
- Changes in communication.
- Increasing interest in the concept of change.
- Faculty work load.

Topic: Higher Education and Curriculum Issues

Major Responses

Higher education issues that have the greatest impact on nursing education:

- Funding.

- Consumer involvement in planning and evaluating the curriculum.
- Use of technology.
- Increasing enrollment without adequate planning.
- Student responsibility for learning and power.
- Changes in tenure and academic policies.
- Credit for life experiences.
- Flexibility of curriculum design.
- Emphasis on continuing education.
- Junior college movement.
- Open-door remedial programs, especially for minority students.
- Change in core requirements.
- Increasing interest on the part of institutions of higher education to start new baccalaureate nursing programs.

Nursing faculty can influence higher education through:

- Involvement in academic policy committee.
- Increasing faculty credentials so that they will be more in keeping with those of other university faculty.
- Faculty involvement in research, studies, and community activities.
- Greater faculty sophistication in the use of multimedia.
- A demand by nursing faculty for salaries equal to those of other members of the academic community.
- Becoming more accountable.
- Developing a more flexible curriculum.
- Assisting in the further development of core curriculum requirements, especially in relation to other health care disciplines.
- Adhering to beliefs about nursing and nursing education.
- Greater involvement in legislative issues, especially those relating to funds.
- Working with different interest and power groups.
- Helping to unify nursing.

13 SUMMARY OF DISCUSSIONS

Participants in the Faculty-Curriculum Development Workshop Series, Atlanta, Georgia

Topic: Curriculum Process—The Evolution of Curriculum Planning

Major Responses

The "common threads" within the philosophy, objectives, theoretical framework, and course descriptions that were identified in the Model for the Utilization of the Curriculum Process (pp.73-82) were:

- Christian education.
- Problem-solving.
- Broad base of knowledge through liberal education.
- Self-directive individual who is responsible.
- Critical thinking.
- Development of self and one's potential.
- Understanding of self and the changing society.
- Concepts of illness.
- Leadership.
- Nursing process.

The following "threads" not reflected throughout the program were:

- Christian education for women.
- Man as an integrated whole.
- Lack of clarity in emphasis—whether on health or on illness.

- Concepts of society and nursing.
- Concepts of communication, stress, and metabolism.
- Student orientation.
- Flexibility within the program.

Topic: Identifying Major Health Care Trends Relative to Baccalaureate Nursing Education

Major Responses

The health care trends are:

- Energy crisis.
- Greater emphasis on distributive nursing care and primary prevention.
- Concept of the expanding role of the nurse.
- Changes in the health care delivery system, with greater decentralization.
- Changes in the financing of health care.
- Increasing sophistication of the consumer.
- Identifying health care as a human right.
- Increasing independent nursing functions within the community.
- Increasing the use of paraprofessionals with greater fragmentation of patient care.
- Increased government involvement in health care.
- Mandatory continuing education.
- Increased urbanization.
- Increase in knowledge.
- Increasing interest in the nursing generalist.
- Increasing interdisciplinary actions.
- Greater computerization affecting health care.
- Shift in age distribution of the population.
- Greater emphasis on problems relating to entry or access into the health care system.

Topic: Curriculum Implications for Changes in the Health Care System

Major Responses

As reported from each group incorporating a trend into a philosophy and terminal graduate objectives:

92

1. **Trend.** Health care moving out of the acute setting.

Philosophy

One of the human rights of man is optimal health. He is free and therefore has the right to choose. It is the responsibility of nursing to provide a means of meeting his nursing needs so that he can reach and/or maintain optimal health.

We believe the graduate of this program will be able to use nursing process based on a broad body of knowledge in providing nursing care to the individual. Special emphasis will be on prevention of illness and maintenance of health. Interdisciplinary collaboration is basic to meeting health needs.

The student has a right to an environment that stimulates learning and utilization of resources. It is our belief that the subject learns best by assuming responsibility for participation in the direction of his own learning. The faculty will act as facilitators of learning by assuming appropriate roles dictated by the situation.

Objectives

The graduate of this program will:

1. Effectively use nursing process based on a broad body of knowledge.
2. Initiate nursing at the point at which the individual needs nursing.
3. Collaborate in an interdisciplinary effort to provide optimal health.
4. Involve the individual in planning and providing nursing care.
5. Function independently and interdependently.

Philosophy

We believe that the graduate of the baccalaureate program will make an "impact."

Objectives

1. The student will make decisions based on facts.
2. The student will work in a variety of settings.
3. The student will work as a colleague.
4. The student will select and use the most appropriate communication behavior to accomplish a goal.

2. **Trend.** Nursing in primary care situations.

Philosophy

We believe that the attainment of the highest standard of health is a fundamental right of every individual.

We believe that the individual has the right to make autonomous decisions regarding his own health when these decisions do not interfere with the health and welfare of others.

We believe that the individual's decisions regarding his own health should be respected and that he has the right to expect that he will participate in those decisions which influence the health and welfare of others and receive help accepting them.

We believe that nursing is an involvement in the constant change of the health continuum of consumers.

We believe one responsibility of the nursing profession is to educate individuals as to possible alternatives to consequences of the decisions they make.

Objectives

To plan, implement, and evaluate health care in collaboration with the individual, the family, the community, and the multidisciplinary team.

3. **Trend.** Increasing ratio of aged in society.

Philosophy

We, the faculty, believe nursing is...We believe we have a commitment to the individual to respect his worth and dignity *throughout* his life span.

We believe that in view of the societal changes relevant to longevity, special emphasis should be placed on the independent function of the professional nurse practitioner in the areas of health promotion and illness prevention.

Objectives

The graduate will:
1. Utilize the nursing process in the guidance and teaching of individuals and/or community groups concerning the promotion and maintenance of health in its biological, psychological, and social aspects.
2. Utilize nursing process in providing, in various care settings, for individuals and their families during illness.

Learning Experiences

1. Include senior citizen centers, convalescent homes, nursing homes, and retirement centers.
2. Keep diaries of experiences.

3. Do process recording.
4. Engage in teaching projects.
5. Collaborate with health team in provision of health care.

Topic: Change Process and the Faculty

Major Responses

Identified a major health care trend and developed strategies for or approaches to change as follows:

Trend. The emerging role of the nurse and the physical assessment skills needed.

Strategies

1. Development of workshops for faculty to learn skills (internal).
2. Exploration of the idea by faculty first to see if there is recognition and acceptance (internal).
3. Exploration of the feelings of professional nurse practitioners as to the advisability of including this function in B.S. programs (external).
4. Collaboration with physicians in acquisition of skills (external).
5. Exploration with employer of the necessity for beginning graduate nurses to have these skills (external).
6. Deciding where and how this content should be placed in the curriculum (internal).
7. Collaboration with related disciplines within the institution (internal).

Philosophy

We believe that man is an open system constantly changing and being changed by his environment.[1]

The concept of nursing is a holistic approach which serves to facilitate this open system. Because of this, the holistic approach to nursing makes us a unique and distinct entity.

We believe, therefore, that the nurse should assist individuals wherever they are on the health-illness continuum to attain and maintain their optimal level of health physically, psychosocially, and spiritually.

We believe, that man's view of his needs must be utilized in plan-

[1] Martha Rogers, *An Introduction to the Theoretical Basis of Nursing.* Philadelphia: F.A. Davis Co., 1970

ning his care. This involves the nursing process, where the nurse and the health care recipient carefully assess the recipient's needs.

We believe, therefore, that the educational process for the learner should evolve from general concepts to more specific and refined concepts and skills.

Objectives

To be able to:

1. Utilize the nursing process.
2. Participate with the client in meeting *his* or *her* needs in any setting.
3. Assist the client in reaching *his* or *her* optimal level of health.

Topic: Higher Education and Curriculum Issues

Major Responses

Higher education issues that have the greatest impact on nursing:

- Financial support of university.
- Academic flexibility and admission policies.
- Faculty-student ratio.
- Student-faculty involvement in administration process of institution.
- Place of nursing within the university setting.
- Identifying differences in nursing within the university.
- Funding issues.

Strategies That Nursing Faculty Should Follow In Relation To The Issues Or Trends

Issue: Student-Faculty Involvement in Administration

Strategies

1. Participation of nursing faculty on committees in parent institution.
2. Workshops for nursing faculty on committees in parent institution.
3. Encouragement of students by advisors to belong to committees in parent institution.
4. Student involvement in faculty evaluation.

Issue: Flexibility Within the Curriculum

Strategy

Increased use of modules, self-study approaches, and challenge examinations.

Issue: Community Cost of Nursing Programs

Strategies

1. Locating variety of sources of funding.
2. Collaborating with other programs in region.
3. Exploring power structure (e.g., relationship between nursing and rest of university).
4. Communicating with clarity and force with nursing discipline and other departments.
5. Use of affirmative action program.
6. Utilizing "student power" in helping to establish nursing's place within the university.

Issue: Lack of Understanding of Nursing Within the University

Strategies

1. Getting nurse faculty to become more involved in university committees.
2. Utilizing informal contact with community groups.
3. Using people and self appropriately.
4. Becoming politically knowledgeable and involved.

Issue: How to Get Adequate Funding

Strategies

1. Proving and demonstrating our worth (on the local and federal levels).
2. Helping to create the atmosphere in which students or graduates will work.
3. Offering career orientation in the program.
4. Creating unity.

14 SUMMARY OF DISCUSSIONS

Participants in the Faculty-Curriculum Development Workshop Series, Wakefield, Massachusetts

Topic: Curriculum Process—The Evolution of Curriculum Planning

Major Responses (See Model for the Utilization of the Curriculum Process, pp.73-82.)

The "common threads" that were identified within the philosophy, objectives, theoretical framework, and course descriptions were:

- The need to assist the student to develop into an intellectually responsive, self-directing, religiously oriented, responsible member of society.
- The conceptual approach to the curriculum.
- The need to stimulate habits of critical thinking and to help students become increasingly self-disciplined and self-directed.
- The concept of decision-making.

Common threads that were *not* identified throughout the curriculum:

- The need to free man by enabling him to understand God, self, and society.
- The need to assume beginning leadership positions.
- The need to search for external truth.
- The need to understand self and society.

Topic: Identify a Major Health Care Trend Relative to Baccalaureate Nursing Education and Utilize the Trend to Develop a Philosophy and a Terminal Graduate Objective; Then Select Appropriate Learning Experiences

Major Responses

1. Trend. Well-informed health consumers

Philosophy

Individuals have the right to quality health care and along with it the corresponding responsibility of collaborating in the planning and evaluating of health care services.

Objectives

- To develop interactional skills with consumers in planning and evaluating health care services.
- Working with groups of health care recipients.
- Exposure to areas outside of nursing, such as nonprofessional materials and other media utilized by the consumers.

Philosophy

We believe that quality health care is the right of everyone in our society and should be made available to persons of all ages, races, and socioeconomic classes on an equal basis. Quality care is preventive, curative, restrictive, supportive, and continuous.

Objectives

The graduate of this program:

- Recognizes the impact of legal forces on the health care system.
- Mobilizes the consumer to become aware of the impact of legislation on the health care system.
- Participates in comprehensive health care planning.
- Takes an active role in legislative matters that affect health care.
- Participates in evaluation of health care services and agencies.

Learning Experiences

- Students participate in regional health care meetings.
- Students involve themselves with legislative matters.

Philosophy

We believe baccalaureate preparation in nursing should be geared toward helping man attain or maintain his highest level of functioning.

Objectives

The graduate of this program will be able to:

- Apply the nursing process in the promotion and maintenance of the health of all individuals.
- Function independently and interdependently with others.
- Collaborate on an interdisciplinary level.
- Include the client and his family in the planning of care.

Learning Experiences

Clinical Experiences

- In homes (family-orientation visits).
- In well people agencies
- In nursing homes, apartment complexes (for the elderly).
- With senior citizens.
- In schools.
- In industry.
- In hospitals (including home follow-through promotion).
- In data collecting (airports, laundromats).
- In day care nurseries.
- In screening programs.
- In family planning and with crippled children.

Other Learning Experiences

- Participation in seminars dealing with changing roles.
- The use of nursing process in doing all the above.
- Assessment and how to teach (these should be emphasized).
- Adapting procedures to home.
- Independent studies and self-directed activities.
- Participation in seminars devoted to group discussions on group dynamics.

2. Trend. Health care as a right.

Philosophy

All persons have an equal right to health care systems that give them an opportunity to maintain their own optimum level of health.

Objectives

Upon completion of this program the graduate will:

- Be able to identify the health care systems available nationally and locally.
- Be able to use the nursing process within a health care system perspective.
- Be able to identify and implement strategies of intervention within emerging health care systems.
- Be able to teach clients within her sphere of influence about existing health systems.

3. Trend. Increasing professionalization.

Philosophy

We believe that the needs of society change and that professional nurses have increasing responsibility for meeting these needs and should be held accountable.

Learning Experiences

- With a unit in a hospital agency.
- With a unit in a community agency ("neighborhood clinics").
- With a unit in mother-baby classes (M/S clinic utilizing).
- With a unit in day care centers.

Topic: The Change Process and the Faculty

Major Responses

The change forces that influence baccalaureate nursing education and the development of strategies or approaches pertaining to change.

Change Forces

Introducing wellness into curriculum rather than illness.

Strategies or Approaches

Internal Participants

- Introduce what is meant by level of wellness.
- Show how physical assessment may be part of maintaining wellness.

- Provide inservice or continuing education programs for faculty to expose them to physical assessment.
- Bring to faculty people who are role models concentrating on wellness.
- Involve values. Faculty might have to take a look at their own values and realize that everyone else doesn't have the same ones.
- Identify concepts of health and then identify health as a value.
- Have consumers come to faculty to point out their needs. There are norms of wellness from which individuals deviate. Consumers could help in identifying these norms.
- Teach the practitioner skills that would help in determining the level of wellness.
- Have someone as a change agent talk to faculty about the factors in change—how uncomfortable they may feel. Share with one another (with those with different clinical specialities).
- Involve students as internal participants.
- Identify needs (positive) rather than problems (negative).
- Give students a good course in human development so that they can then concentrate on wellness, rather than on illness. Other supportive areas would be involved (psychology, physical science). This may be where we can get our input into college or university philosophy. Identify courses that nursing could provide on wellness-health which might be offered to the entire college population.
- Use university or college facilities (day care center, infirmary).
- Set up learning activities (screening) which benefit the university community.
- Emphasize maintaining wellness in health assessment in geriatrics (housing for the aged).

External Participants

- Involve physicians and other community agencies (coffee hour) in what we are going to do.
- Communicate with legislators, since they are involved with appropriation of funds for things like well child conferences and national health insurance.

Change Force

Orientation to medical model versus unitary concept of health and disease.

Strategies and Approaches

Internal Participants

- Search out new "clinical" areas to use for teaching the concept of wellness.
- Use of the college population for experience.
- Offer core classes with students of other disciplines (e.g., social welfare students).
- Offer core courses with other disciplines (e.g., in growth and development, the family).
- Educate faculty to the concept of wellness (e.g., teach physical assessment skills).

Change Force

Primary care—greater emphasis on wellness, health, and illness prevention.

Strategies

- Orientation to faculty.
- Use of a consultant.
- On-site visits.
- Sharing opinion, expressing fears, anxieties.
- Finding out what change means to the individual.
- Group sessions on feelings with other internal participants.
- After selling concept to faculty, getting consumers of service (individual and agency) involved so that they know what our practitioners will be like.
- Small-scale experiments to find out possible problems.

Change Force

Expanding role of the nurse to meet the health needs of society and to fill the void in health care that exists in many areas of the country.

Strategies and Approaches

Internal

- Introduction of the expanding role by those nurses participating in it.
- Workshops for faculty in the development of skills.
- Opportunities to validate new learning.
- Resource materials for faculty.
- Conference with others within the university and college settings; use of other disciplines to increase learning.

External

- Involve advisory boards—practicing nurses, physicians, agency representatives.

Change Force

Change from episodic to distributive settings.

Strategies

Internal

- Encourage members of the group to feel comfortable with one another.
- See to it that graduate education prepares more generalists.
- Organize workshops to air feelings.
- Get people to see their role in the change process.
- Provide programs for faculty development—new teaching skills, methods.

External

- Employ consultants for ways to approach integration; for objective opinions.
- Provide inservice programs and workshops with agencies used—to assist them in understanding the new objectives.
- Make short-term contracts with agencies where faculty could work to increase their input into the agencies utilized.

Topic: Higher Education and Curriculum Issues

Major Responses

Identify a major issue or trend in higher education and develop strategies that nursing faculty should follow in relation to the issue or trend.

1. Issue. Flexibility—the "in" and "out" within programs for RNs and undergraduates.

Strategies

- Put some pressure on institutions for accountability.
- Identify ways to determine whether or not program objectives have been met.
- Provide for critical clinical testing periods.
- Provide simulated experience—client problem via videotape; utilize the nursing process.
- Give challenge examinations—test recall of knowledge.
- Give oral examinations to faculty group.

2. Issue. Cost of higher education.

Strategies

- Trim the fat.
- Know the university's budget and the school of nursing's share, as well as the indirect costs involved.
- Get quality for money—competitive salaries, alternative ways of education.
- Present nursing needs to governmental agencies.
- Get faculty to offer input into identifying the priorities for spending.
- Reevaluate faculty-student ratio and the use of the clinical laboratory (use of time).

3. Trend. Flexible curriculum design.

Strategies

- Increasing nursing electives.
- Mini-term nursing electives open to all students within the university.
- Multidisciplinary seminars—team approach to teaching.

2 CURRICULUM EVALUATION

15 THE "WHAT," "WHY" AND "WHEN" OF EVALUATION

Eleanor A. Lynch, MS, RN

Introduction

Every time I am faced with the preparation of a paper on an aspect of evaluation, I am more than ever aware of the enormous complexity of the topic—the growth of my awareness being more like geometrical progression than arithmetical. It is because of this awareness that I feel it necessary to comment briefly at the outset of this paper on the complexity of the evaluation of outcomes in nursing education.

The purpose of these introductory remarks is not to create an atmosphere of gloom and pessimism, but to establish a realistic frame of reference. I believe that by being realistic, nurse educators are more likely to arrive at approaches which are relevant to the multiplicity of problems associated with planning, directing, and assessing educational programs in nursing.

The evaluation of educational outcomes remains one of the stubbornest problems facing education today. However, when we are attempting to assess the complex skills involved in the effective practice of nursing, we have an even more difficult and exacting task. The processes involved in learning how to provide health guidance and care for clients and patients are all-inclusive and far-reaching. This is so because nursing practitioners must function in and assume responsibility for the health needs of persons, sick or well, in a variety of health-care settings. The multitude of variables involved in this dynamic, interactive process further complicate the evaluation of nursing education.

In the following remarks, I would like to consider three aspects of evaluation—the "What," the "Why," and the "When."

The "What" of Evaluation

Evaluation, in a general sense, is the process of describing some quality or characteristic of an individual, a program or an institution as the basis for making a judgment about that individual, program or institution. The emphasis in evaluation is on gathering data designed to delineate the salient, identifying features of the attribute under study. Close attention must be given to the evidence provided by the data before a judgment can be made.

There are many definitions of evaluation. I will mention a few which represent some current concepts of the term. Gronlund defines evaluation as a systematic process of determining the extent to which educational objectives are achieved by learners.[1] This definition has the particular advantages of being clear and concise and containing the essential ingredients from an educational standpoint. There are three aspects to this definition. First, it states that evaluation is systematic. This would negate casual or uncontrolled data gathering, and would also contradict the idea that every observation or judgment would warrant being termed evaluation. Secondly, it defines evaluation as a process—a *series* of actions, not a single, isolated operation. Thirdly, in this definition evaluation is concerned with goals, objectives or expected competencies which have been previously determined, and progress toward which is being judged. It acknowledges that our objectives may not always be attained.

Some popular concepts of evaluation, although concerned with educational goals and objectives, go beyond gathering data specific to these aspects. Some are broader in definition and some have special pertinence to the administrator's role in an educational program. Stufflebeam, et al. define evaluation as "the process of delineating, obtaining and providing useful information for judging decision alternatives."[2] Other related definitions focus on professional judgment as a requirement for making decisions about the merit or worth of a measure.

Sometimes "testing," "measurement," and "evaluation" are used interchangeably. If one's concept of evaluation is limited to testing, the evidence gathered would be primarily numerical and would represent

---

[1] Norman E. Gronlund. *Measurement and Evaluation in Teaching.* 2nd ed. New York: The Macmillan Company, 1971, pp. 7-8.

[2] Daniel Stufflebeam, et al. *Educational Evaluation and Decision Making.* Bloomington, Indiana: Phi Delta Kappa, 1971, p. xxv.

a concept of evaluation in the narrowest sense—representing just one aspect of a characteristic, quality or attribute.

Evaluation includes measurement, but goes beyond it. Evaluation is a systematic collection of evidence to determine whether or not specified changes are taking place in learners and in educational programs, involving the determination of the extent or degree of change.

Gronlund demonstrates his concept of the relationship between measurement and evaluation by two equations:

Evaluation = Quantitative description of pupils (measurement) + value judgments

Evaluation = Qualitative description of pupils (nonmeasurement) + value judments[3]

Gronlund further states that evaluation may or may not be based on measurement and that when it is, it goes beyond a simple quantitative description.

Evaluation and measurement are therefore not synonymous. Whereas measurement is concerned primarily with quantitative aspects, evaluation is a broad term including measurement *and* nonmeasurement aspects. Both are essential to sound educational decision making.

The effectiveness of evaluation can be promoted by keeping the following eight points in focus, the last six of which are delineated by Bloom, et al.[4] as being pertinent to the improvement of teaching and learning:

1. Evaluation is a process of analysis.

2. Evaluation is a means and not an end in itself.

3. Evaluation is a method of acquiring and processing evidence needed for improvement in learning and teaching.

4. Evaluation is an aid in clarifying goals and objectives.

5. Evaluation is a process of determining the extent to which goals and objectives are met.

6. Evaluation is a system of quality control in which it may be determined at each step in the teaching and learning process whether the process is effective or not, and what changes must be made to ensure the effectiveness of the process before it is too late.

7. Evaluation is a tool for ascertaining whether alternative procedures are equally effective in achieving a set of educational goals.

---

[3] Gronlund, *op. cit.,* p. 8.

[4] Benjamin Bloom, et al. *Handbook of Formative and Summative Evaluation of Student Learning.* New York: McGraw-Hill Book Co., 1971, pp. 7-8.

8. Evaluation is not merely gathering evidence and information from tests and other pencil-and-paper devices.

There are other aspects of the "what" of evaluation. I would like to expand on two:

1. Curriculum and student evaluation. The basic difference between curriculum evaluation and the evaluation of students is related to the decisions that are the outcome of the evaluation. If a decision is made about the degree to which a student has met course requirements or progressed toward stated objectives or expected competencies, we are concerned with student evaluation. A decision as to whether an experimental program is to be continued is curriculum evaluation. Although student evaluation is a part of curriculum evaluation, the latter is considerably broader in scope and involves other than students' progress toward goals. Such aspects as the evaluation of program goals, the assessment of the impact of curriculum on persons or groups other than students and cost effectiveness are only a few of the focuses of curriculum evaluation.

2. Norm-referenced and criterion-referenced evaluation. If the interpretation of a score made by an individual student on a test is based on the test results of a comparable group of students, or norms group, this would be *norm-referenced* measurement. If, however, the student's performance is interpreted by comparing it with some specific behavioral criteria, or proficiency, this would be *criterion-referenced* evaluation. Norm-referenced measurement focuses on how well a student performs in comparison with other students on a comparable level, while the focus of criterion-referenced evaluation is on what a student is able to do in terms of specific predetermined standards.

The "Why" of Evaluation

Education is a process of change. In educational programs, we are concerned with three components of behavior: *cognitive,* the knowing or thinking component; *psychomotor,* the physical or acting component; and *affective,* the emotional or feeling component. When program objectives are developed and stated in terms of this interpretation of behavior, the overall plan for curriculum development and evaluation should reflect all components insofar as is possible.

The purposes of evaluation in education are diverse. They can be categorized according to the groups for whom decisions are made or according to the kinds of decisions which need to be made:

1. Groups for whom decisions are made.
- Individuals (students, faculty)
- Institutions

2. Kinds of decisions.
- *Instructional.* Determining the effectiveness of instruction; obtaining information about entry skills of students; setting, refining, and clarifying realistic goals for the teacher and student; determining and refining evaluation techniques; determining grades.
- *Guidance.* Helping the learner; communicating goals; increasing motivation; providing feedback for the identification of strengths and weaknesses.
- *Administrative.* Setting selection, classification, and placement standards; hiring and firing of teaching personnel; continuing current plans; terminating old or new plans; modifying old or new plans; adopting new approaches.
- *Research.* Cuts across instructional, guidance, and administrative decisions.

Formative and summative evaluation are sometimes erroneously classified as types or methods of evaluation and considered as aspects of the "what" or "how" of evaluation. Scriven,[5] however, introduced these concepts as being descriptive of the purposes—the "why"—of evaluation.

Formative evaluation is intended to help in the development of curriculum, programs of study, teaching materials and methods of teaching. The basic meaning is exactly what the word implies—to get feedback so that the persons responsible for devising new curriculum materials and new programs and methods of teaching can determine how well their plans are working. If plans are not working, of course, the materials or approaches can then be revised and new methods tried.

In formative evaluation, the emphasis is on improvement. This would include the gathering of data for the purpose of guiding developmental educational processes. In the formative evaluation of nursing students, the main purpose would be to determine the level of mastery of given learning tasks and to pinpoint the parts of the tasks which have not been mastered. The purpose is not to grade or certify, but to help the learner and teacher focus upon the learning necessary for movement toward mastery.

---

[5] M. Scriven. "The Methodology of Evaluation." In *Perspectives of Curriculum Evaluation,* AERA Mongraph Series on Curriculum Evaluation, No. 1 Chicago: Rand McNally and Co., 1967, pp. 39-83.

On the other hand, summative evaluation is directed toward a much more general assessment of the degree to which larger outcomes have been realized over an entire course or some substantial part of a course. A further purpose would be to grade and report the summative results to appropriate authorities. Summative evaluation is the process by which an overall assessment or decision can be made with regard to a student or program on a terminal basis.

In summative evaluation, one is requred to have a curriculum (or program of study or method of teaching) already established. The evaluation is made after a refinement of methods and approaches, and after these have been put to use. The essential purpose of summative evaluation is to provide evidence of the effectiveness of processes and materials utilized. The methods and procedures used to gather the data would be the same as for formative evaluation, but the end result would not be revision. A final judgment would be made about effectiveness in terms of how much learning has taken place or how effective a particular curriculum model has been.

Both formative and summative evaluation are needed. As a curriculum is being revised, formative evaluation procedures should be used before the design or model becomes set. After all of the materials are developed and put into use and after students go through the curriculum, then judgments must be made as to whether learning has taken place and whether it represents the type of learning desired—this would be summative evaluation.

The "When" of Evaluation

The "when" and "why" of evaluation are intimately related. A problem that can develop from this relationship involves inappropriate timing in terms of the purpose of the evaluation.

If, for instance, the need is to determine the level of competence of a nursing student in a particular content area as a basis for planning learning experiences for a subsequent course, the timing of the evaluation is obvious, and it is likely that the purpose would be achieved with little difficulty. If, however, the need is to assess the progress of a nursing student for formative evaluation, the timing of evaluation can interfere significantly with the achievement of the purpose.

The frequency of data-gathering procedures needs to be correlated with evidence obtained from estimations of the student's level of mastery in specific areas of learning. If a student's deficiencies are not assessed on an ongoing basis, and measures to correct the deficiencies are not instituted, it is unlikely that the purpose of formative evaluation will be met.

As already mentioned, the timing of evaluation can be: (1) prior to an educational experience; or (2) at scheduled intervals during periods of learning (to assess progress toward the achievement of objectives). Other important times for evaluation include: at the end of a course, to assess competency for grading; at the end of a program, to assess competency for certification; and after graduation, to assess professional progress and the success of the instructional system.

The last aspects of measurement and evaluation to be considered in this presentation are validity, reliability, and practicality. If these aspects are not given strict attention, the information on which decisions are to be made will be either inaccurate or incomplete. For validity in evaluation, the question to raise is, "Does the tool or device measure what it is intended to measure?" In questioning reliability, one should ask, "Would comparable results be obtained each time the measure or device is used under similar circumstances?" Lastly, in terms of practicality, the question might be asked, "Is the tool or method so complicated that more time is likely to be spent in the administrative process than in the gathering of data?"

In conclusion, may I say that evaluation in its broadest sense involves appraisal of a school's entire program. An evaluation plan should be related to the broad aims of the total program and should begin with the selection of students. In order to keep evaluation procedures focused on the broad objectives of a program, the plan for evaluation of the curriculum should be made concurrently with the development and revision of that curriculum.

16 THE NEED FOR AND CONCERNS RELATING TO CURRICULUM EVALUATION

Gertrude Torres, EdD, RN

Evaluation of the curriculum of a nursing education program is more than mere evaluation of courses, students or faculty—this is too narrow a concept. Instead, it involves a compex set of principles related to the whole of the curriculum process and can be defined as the delineating, obtaining and providing of useful information and data for the making or judging of decision alternatives in relation to the totally organized and planned curriculum.

Curriculum evaluation is presently given little or no attention in either the nursing literature or the schools of nursing. The word "curriculum," in this presentation, refers to the organized areas of learning and their related aspects, such as program philosophy, objectives, course requirements, and learning experiences. There is no real issue regarding the presence or absence of evaluation in education; it is always present in some form or other. What we need is a systematically planned, ongoing evaluation of curriculum so that our decisions will be based on real data rather than on tradition, bias or rationalization.

First of all, we as educators often have strong beliefs resting on grand assumptions which are totally uninhibited by scientific data. This applies not only to nursing educators but to educators in general. For example, some of our beliefs are:

- Higher education is effective and essential in and of itself.
- Higher budgets improve the quality of education.
- The faculty understands and has expertise on the needs of society and students.
- Higher education should be one of the highest priorities in our society.
- Higher education is the key to improvement of nursing care.
- Faculty's beliefs about man, health, nursing, and society reflect appropriate concepts essential to society's need for professional nursing.

Some of these beliefs, and other similar ones held as truths by most professionals and experts, might be found to be basically correct. Even though there are no hard scientific data to support them, some have been held to be valid throughout history. At least, there are no data to refute them.

The need for curriculum evaluation may seem to be self-evident. Yet, if this is so, why do we not spend time, effort, and money in creating an organized and dynamic evaluation plan instead of putting our efforts into constantly changing and revising our curriculum? On what do we base our decisions to change curriculum?

Curriculum evaluation is essential to give us the data we need to make sound decisions. Nursing education seems to be in a constant state of curriculum change, frequently recycling approaches by repeating, as "new and innovative," what was done twenty years ago. Some changes seem due, not to some appropriate evaluation mechanism which demonstrated a need for the change, but to a feeling that it "seemed like the right thing to do." We will never truly move ahead in baccalaureate nursing education until we learn to evaluate before we change what we are doing. Changing our programs every four years takes time and effort away from performing a systematic, longitudinal evaluation. It may even be that changing curriculum is a way of avoiding proper evaluation.

With a scientific approach to curriculum evaluation, nursing education can become more accountable and possibly make greater demands for support. We could demonstrate how our educational process is effective and/or ineffective in meeting the nursing needs of society and assisting students to realize their potential. We could utilize the evaluation data to improve our thinking and increase our knowledge, to affect state and federal legislators, to speak to each other about future curriculum needs, to affect other curricula within the university and to understand what curriculum evaluation can or cannot achieve.

In considering some of the issues that affect curriculum evaluation, one of the first is the question of whether and how to evaluate. Some take the position that evaluation can help identify past successes and failures in education and aid in the decision-making process. Others feel that evaluation is a goal and relates to the mastery of facts. Some see systemic evaluation as essential.

The position one takes may be strongly influenced by one's educational philosophy. Compromise and interaction among differing philosophies are often present and desirable. Dressel discusses three interesting patterns of thinking about education: traditionalism, eclecticism, and relativism.[1]

In his discussion, Dressel identifies *traditionalists* as being oriented toward the past, offering an elite education to a few and giving the student knowledge through required subjects with the assumption that integration of content is the responsibility of the student. Evaluation for the traditionalist tends to be highly subjective and emphasizes oral and written procedures, with little data collection or empirical procedures.

The *eclectic* is oriented to the present, offers education that exposes the student to a brief contact with many courses for breadth and an extended contact with a particular body of subject matter for depth. Emphasis is often on the facts, concepts, and principles which differentiate disciplines.

Evaluation to the eclectic tends to focus on the mastery of factual knowledge and the intellectual skills needed to deal with it. Cumulative, comprehensive evaluation is deemed of little worth. Values are hypothesized but, since they seem intangible, provide a basis for rejecting systematic attempts to evaluate. Evaluation may be carried out to justify decisions made by particular interest groups. This seems to be our orientation in nursing education.

The *relativist*, in Dressel's analysis, is oriented to the future, sees education as an instrument for progress and improvement, and is devoted to the total person. Integration is a conscious concern, and professors are viewed as motivators and counselors. Here evaluation must show evidence of change in individuals, and all parts of the institution are under continuing study. Only the relativist sees evaluation as a vital part of every aspect of the educational program.

Although it is recognized that there are few, if any, pure traditionalists, eclectics or relativists, individuals do tend to fall, for the most part, within one pattern or another. Thus, the concern as to whether we should or should not try to develop a systematic, total curriculum evaluation will be better resolved when we come to grips with our own philosophy as nurse educators. If we accept Dressel's concepts about education philosophies, we can see that the traditionalists and possibly the eclectics will need to revise their thinking.

---

[1] Paul L. Dressel, et al. *Evaluation in Higher Education.* Boston: Houghton Mifflin Co., 1961, pp. 19-20.

Whether we feel we should or should not evaluate systematically also relates to such things as our previous experiences with the evaluative process. Evaluation of the wrong kind, at the wrong time or for the wrong reasons is frequent and leaves educators with a feeling of futility. Since clinical evaluation lacks the strong theoretical background which would allow it to be thought of as truly reliable and valid, total curriculum evaluation—with even less theory, or none at all, to support it—seems to some totally inappropriate.

Educators must establish priorities in terms of time and funds; while some might feel curriculum evaluation is important, they would prefer to spend time and money in acquiring better-prepared faculty, improving the environment in which the students and faculty function or giving greater support to the library. Our lives are full of decisions, especially about establishing priorities. Some believe that the present cutbacks in educational funds and the social ills that are increasing daily cause us to struggle just to survive, let alone allow us to engage in the luxury of systematic, total curriculum evaluation. Yet, it seems to me, we have failed to solve many social ills because we keep moving ahead without really evaluating what we have already done. We make decisions based on feelings, not on data. This might be the very reason why accountability and curriculum evaluation are so badly needed.

Another issue related to evaluation of the curriculum is whether or not we should have objectives and, if so, what kind we need. Objectives are basic to evaluation; if one does not spell them out clearly, evaluation will be difficult, to say the least. Huebner feels that objectives tend to stifle the creativity and motivation of the learner, while writers like Bloom and Mager strongly favor the development of objectives. Mager holds that objectives must be precise and detailed descriptions of students' behavior, but others argue that this is trivial and constrictive. Probably a few would feel that evaluating detailed, specific objectives has previously proved conspicuously successful or useful in improving the total curriculum. Eisner[2], Walberg[3], and Bloom[4] all feel that precise, predetermined behavioral objectives impede student learning.

We in nursing have gone from few objectives to objectives for every learning experience. This concept of program evaluation avoids the necessity of having to go back to orient ourselves toward broad objectives before attempting curriculum evaluation. Related to this issue are decisions concerning types and priorities of objectives. Should we

---

[2] Elliot W. Eisner. "Educational Objectives: Help or Hinder?" *School Review,* 75:250-262, Winter 1967.

[3] Herbert J. Walberg. "Curriculum Evaluation—Problems and Guidelines." *The Record-Teachers College,* Vol. 71, No. 4, May 1970.

[4] Benjamin S. Bloom. "Some Theoretical Issues Relating to Educational Evaluation: New Role, New Means." *Sixty-Eight Yearbook, Part II, National Society for the Study of Education.* Chicago: University of Chicago Press, 1969.

evaluate value-laden broad educational objectives? Or should we be more concerned with objectives related to the intellectual, social, personal or productive dimensions of education? Do objectives sometimes become so broad that we feel immobile in terms of evaluating their achievement?

Our approach to curriculum evaluation presents another choice: whether we should be norm-referenced or criterion-referenced. A norm-referenced measure is used to identify an individual's performance as related to the performances of others, while a criterion-referenced test is used to identify an individual's status with respect to an established standard. We might say that accreditation, with all its criteria or standards, is a form of a criterion-referenced approach and that NLN achievement tests, used for the evaluation of students' performance, are norm-referenced. In developing a systematic curriculum evaluation, we must identify which approach we need to use. In evaluating the student's ability to think critically, should we use a given standard developed by faculty and representing a minimum of success, or should we compare the student to his or her classmates and to a given norm?

Most of us are familiar with norm-referenced measurements, since we grew up with them. Yet we need to ask ourselves if this approach is adequate and whether identifying a student's performance in relation to others' does truly guarantee the minimum standard of success essential in nursing.

The last issue I wish to discuss concerns whether we give priority to formative or to summative evaluation. Formative evaluation is valuable in supporting on-going revisions of the curriculum, while summative evaluation gives a feel for the whole. Some educators feel that formative evaluation is all that is essential, since they are constantly making judgments about what they are doing and then making improvements.

In nursing we use formative evaluation in developing new curricula and in testing ideas and planned approaches on a day-to-day basis. Without such an approach, we might postpone making appropriate revisions. Yet, we need to ask ourselves if it is sufficient to assess the isolated parts of the curriculum in an unorganized manner? We are frequently asked to look at the whole of a nursing program for accreditation purposes. Does this end as truly a report of what is, or is it a form of summative evaluation of the whole, in which changes may later take place? Maybe now we need to give a greater priority to a systematic total curriculum evaluation which is summative in nature but allows for formative changes.

Let me review the issues in the form of questions:

- Do we need curriculum evaluation, and should we engage in it?
- What are our priorities in terms of the different types of objectives to be measured?

121

- Is formative or summative evaluation more appropriate for curriculum evaluation? Or do we need both?

We need seriously to engage in systematic curriculum evaluation to demonstrate our effectiveness or ineffectiveness in meeting the professional nursing needs of our society. Our responsibility is to evaluate our curriculum prior to making changes, so that the decisions we make will be based on scientific data. We need to share, through both written and verbal communication, any ideas we have concerning approaches to curriculum evaluation. We need to stop giving evaluation a lower priority than the development of program and stop thinking of evaluation as merely the end product of a curriculum process. We need to identify ways which will allow us to spend a greater amount of time in total curriculum evaluation. And, finally, we need to be more future-oriented in our thinking.

17 CURRICULUM EVALUATION FOR TODAY AND TOMORROW

Gertrude Torres, EdD, RN

Although we are constantly struggling to make evaluation in nursing education as effective as possible, we generally limit ourselves to the evaluation of faculty and students. In the literature, little is written on the total curriculum evaluation process in either nursing or general education, and what is written is often confusing and contradictory. Thus, I would like to try to fill that gap by presenting some of my evolving ideas, which will perhaps provide a base or beginning for the concept of total curriculum evaluation in nursing.

My approach in this paper will be twofold. First, I wish to present the basic components of curriculum evaluation and, second, to take several specific objectives which seem common to most baccalaureate programs and identify ways in which we can measure our success or failure in meeting them.

Since evaluation at this point in time relates to achievement of objectives, curriculum evaluation speaks to the attainment of program and/or terminal behavioral objectives which are the essence and purpose of the total curriculum. Both Dyer[1] and Foley[2] have identified the basic components of an evaluation system in education.

---

[1] Henry S. Dyer. "Can We Measure the Performance of Educational Systems?" *N.A.S.S.P. Bulletin,* May 1970, p. 99.

[2] Walter J. Foley. "The Future of Administration and Education Evaluation." *Educational Technology,* July 1970, pp. 20-25.

Dyer identifies four groups of variables (input, educational process, surrounding conditions, and output)[3] while Foley identifies three (input, process, and output).[4] We can apply these components to the nursing educational process. In Figure 1, Total Curriculum Evaluation Model for Change, we can identify three major components—input, educational process, and output. These components reflect the concept that students enter the educational process with certain knowledge, skills, and beliefs and are expected to have changed when the process is completed. Within the process are forces influencing the potential for this change. We as educators are involved in both the external forces and internal forces, with our major impact on the latter.

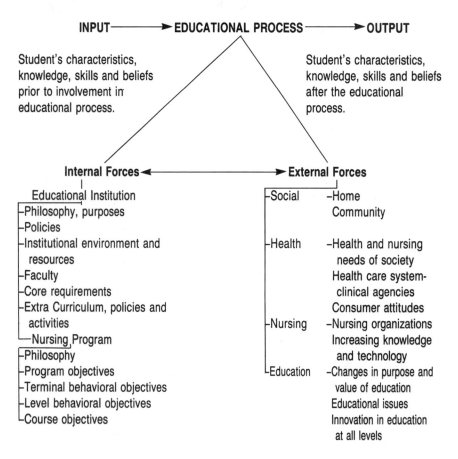

Figure 1. Total curriculum evaluation model for change.

---

[3] Dyer, *loc. cit.*

[4] Foley, *op. cit.*, p. 24.

124

Many external forces affect the student and her educational institution: the economic and social conditions of the home and community, value systems, resources and the state of society in general, with its varied economic, political and energy crises. Society's increasing demand for more and better health and nursing care, changes in priorities of care and in the health care system and consumer attitudes—especially as related to cost and accountability—have a tremendous effect on our clinical agencies and on the type of learning experiences we give our students. Increasing amounts of scientific data and technology affect the practice of nursing and constantly add to the body of knowledge that is incorporated into our curricula. Nursing organizations also frequently affect the student's beliefs and understanding about his or her profession and its place in society. In addition, general education, with its changes, issues and innovations, affects the nursing curriculum.

Internal forces which affect the achievement of the objectives in the nursing education process include the college or university philosophy, policies, resources, faculty and requirements.

As members of a community, as consumers of health and nursing care and as members of our professional and educational organizations, we are among the forces which have impact on the educational process.

As nursing educators, we are also strongly influenced by the total educational institution in which our nursing programs are found. Whether we are successful in meeting our program and terminal behavioral objectives can be influenced by a host of related variables— such as the institution's philosophy, objectives, and resources.

In Figure 2, which attempts to apply these same ideas to curriculum evaluation in nursing, the philosophy is seen as the foundation of the nursing program; from it flow the objectives of the program. These objectives are identified as program and terminal behavioral objectives rather than course, teacher or specific student objectives. The latter are useful for teacher and student evaluation, but this is too narrow an approach and is not total curriculum evaluation.

The process of evaluation can be said to include the following:

The assessment of variables. These influence the achievement of any objectives and are related to the external and internal forces.

The identification of constants and inconstants within the program. This is done through an historical survey of the program's previous objectives. The "constant" areas usually relate to man and his needs, the nursing process and society. These aspects of the philosophy and objectives remain constant with time, even though the exact terminology may change. Other aspects, such as the emerging role of the nurse and the specific contributions that nursing will make toward

125

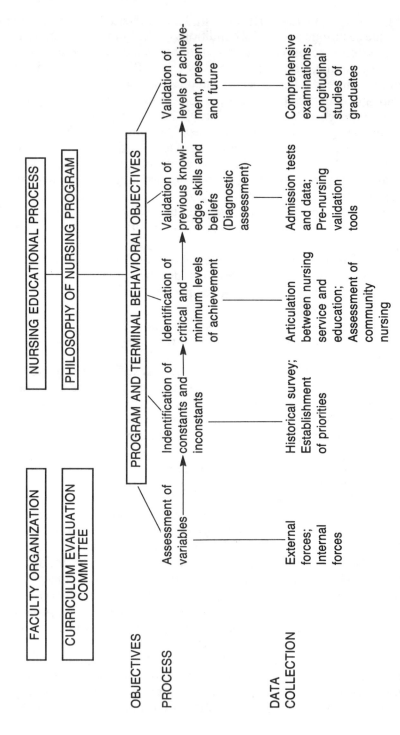

Figure 2. Curriculum evaluation in nursing.

meeting the health care needs of society, require revision and are the "inconstants." Inconstants also relate to how we achieve our objectives and include teaching methods and learning experiences. In identifying the constants and determining those which need to be measured at a given time, we create a base of information on which we can perform curriculum evaluation.

We also need to establish priorities within the terminal behavioral objectives. Faculty may decide to evaluate the achievement of all objectives or focus on a few which seem most essential or significant at a given time.

Identification of critical and minimum levels of achievement. Our educational process not only must provide opportunities to the students for the meeting of program and terminal behavioral objectives, but also must validate the achievement of a minimum level of accomplishment. This is what is involved in that overused word "accountability"— what we as professionals owe society and the student. In order to gather data as to the acceptable minimum levels of achievement, we need to articulate with nursing service personnel in all types of health care facilities for the assessment of community nursing needs.

Validation of previous knowledge, skills, and beliefs. This can be thought of as a diagnostic assessment of the student at the point of entry into both the total educational institution and the nursing program. If we define education as involving a change in the student, we must ascertain what she knows prior to her learning experiences so that we can later measure any increase in knowledge and skills and any changes in beliefs which have occurred as a result of her educational experiences. Admission tests and prenursing validation tools are essential to this task.

Validation of levels of achievement, both present and future. For present validation of the achievement of objectives, comprehensive examinations—in both theory and practice—can be used just before graduation; for the validation of future achievement, longitudinal studies of graduates are necessary.

The process of curriculum evaluation is an ongoing activity. This may be considered as more summative than formative evaluation in principle, but it actually includes both types of evaluation. This process does not negate the significance of teacher and student evaluation nor the evaluation of course objectives; these relate mostly to the "inconstant" parts of the curriculum—those that require frequent revisions and therefore a formative evaluation approach.

Although the whole faculty is involved in the process of total curriculum evaluation, it may be easier, depending on the size of the faculty, to have a committee on curriculum evaluation; this can be either a standing committee itself or a part of the regular curriculum committee. Activities of such a committee need to be planned with a careful eye to identifying priorities within the program, in which faculty can offer the greatest expertise.

Evaluating Objectives

Let us now turn to the second part of this presentation, which is focused on the utilization of the evaluation process in relation to specific terminal behavioral objectives. In 1972, some forty nursing educational programs, and/or their terminal behavioral objectives, were studied by the Board of Review of the Council of Baccalaureate and Higher Degree Programs. It was evident that most of these programs related to the student's ability to think critically. Henderson points out three general levels of critical thinking—becoming critical (finding fault) is a layman's concept; problem-solving and thinking logically are educators' concepts.[5]

The programs studied utilized a variety of terms which relate to critical thinking, such as "solve problems," "analyze," "evaluate," "synthesize," "scientific method," and "judgment." Two objectives which relate to critical thinking and the nursing process, were frequently found:

> 1.Ability to think critically and make discriminatory judgments in the assessment and diagnosis of nursing needs and in the implementation and evaluation of the care of persons in a variety of health care settings.
>
> 2.To develop critical attitudes and skills in evaluation and problem solving as a basis for effective nursing practice and as a basis for contributing to the development of professional nursing.

Let us take these two objectives and see how they can be evaluated in terms of the curriculum evaluation process as we have identified it.

The assessment of variables. Variables which can affect the student's ability to achieve these objectives relate to such forces as:

---

[5] Kenneth B. Henderson. "The Teaching of Critical Thinking." *The Educational Forum,* 371:45-46, November 1972.

- The attitude of faculty (both nursing and others) toward students' increasing their ability to think critically and how these attitudes affect student learning experiences and involvement in making decisions (e.g., in the area of program and curriculum revisions).
- The faculty's own definition of critical thinking, which frequently needs to be established.
- Policies within the institution which sometimes cause faculty to treat students as children rather than adults who can logically and critically make decisions about their own lives.

Identification of constants and inconstants.

- The faculty may identify this objective as pertaining to the "constants" within the curriculum and requiring little or no change in the near future.
- Historically, faculty may consider previously stated objectives which used such terminology as "problem-solving approach," "decision-making," and "judgment" as tied to critical thinking. Or they may decide that the objective is of recent emphasis and that it cannot be evaluated in the summative method until several groups of students have graduated from the program after the development of the objective.
- Faculty may identify critical thinking as part of the nursing process and give it increasing priority.

Identification of critical and minimum levels of achievements.

- Faculty will need to identify the narrower objectives that relate to critical thinking, such as identifying the critical issues in nursing, recognizing assumptions, identifying relevancy, determining if facts support generalizations, and drawing appropriate conclusions.
- Faculty will need to identify and establish minimum levels of achievement in relation to critical thinking and the narrower objectives. This would mean that *all* the students who graduate would be able to handle problem solving or decision making at a certain level. These levels may relate to leadership ability, analyzing certain issues, and so forth.

Validation of previous knowledge, skills, and beliefs.

- Admission tests related to making decisions and judgments may be helpful in validating previous skills in critical thinking.

- Identifying the student's ability to analyze current social and health care issues may give clues as to the student's ability to think critically. Prenursing examinations may be used.

Validation of levels of achievement, present and future.

- Comprehensive examinations may be used to test the student's ability to solve problems or think critically about a complex client or family situation. Longitudinal studies of graduates specific to identifying relevant health and social issues might be carried out.

Let me take one more objective and briefly apply the curriculum evaluation process to it. This objective is: To demonstrate an understanding of the research process through the critical analysis of research studies.

Assessment of variables.

- The amount of research being carried out within the educational institution by the faculty.
- The amount of funds provided for nursing research.
- The availability of the results of nursing research, as published in the literature, to students and faculty.
- The faculty's expertise and attitudes in this area.

Identification of constants and inconstants.

- Has a research component been identified historically or is this a new concept in the program? The faculty need to review previously stated objectives to answer this question. If it is recognized as a relatively new addition to the objective list, the faculty may decide to wait until there are sufficient graduates to measure the program's success in this area.
- Does this objective have enough priority to warrant effort to measure the program's success in meeting it?

Identification of critical and minimum levels of achievement.

- Faculty need to identify the desirable differences in understanding and knowledge of research between undergraduate and graduate education in order to identify minimum levels for their students.
- Minimum levels related to research may include the ability to utilize statistics.

Validation of previous skills and beliefs.

- Admission tests related to mathematical ability, comprehension and word associations may be helpful in validating previous skills related to research.

Validation of levels of achievement.

- Use of comprehensive examinations related to a critical analysis of research as related to a client/patient care situation.
- Longitudinal studies of graduates in relation to their future studies of and engagement in research.

These are some samples of how the curriculum evaluation process might be used in terms of broad terminal behavioral objectives. The process has not been refined and may require adjustments and revisions. There is no doubt that the process is time-consuming and frustrating. It is not important whether a faculty utilizes this approach or creates its own in order to perform more effective curriculum evaluation; what is important is that curriculum evaluation should take place.

We must recognize that there are reasons, both valid and invalid, for resisting the process of curriculum evaluation. Faculty may fear the possible results and their implications. They may perceive curriculum evaluation as not having top priority among their responsibilities at all. They may not see curriculum evaluation as anything more than student evaluation, or they may not be able to identify a valid methodology for curriculum evaluation.

Whatever may be said for or against it, I believe that effective curriculum evaluation, by increasing the "accountability" of nursing education, can benefit both society at large and nursing itself, through the improvement of nursing education and therefore of nursing service.

18 CURRICULUM EVALUATION—METHODS AND TOOLS

Eleanor A. Lynch, MS, RN

In order to assess nursing education programs, which focus on the utilization of the process of nursing along the general health-illness continuum with consideration given to individuals who need help in attaining, maintaining and regaining health, we need a broad variety of tools. This variety of devices is also mandatory in order to evaluate the synthesis of content and processes necessary to achieve the objectives of such programs. The basic question is how to evaluate effectively an attribute or group of attributes of students or of the educational program.

The method of evaluation used depends upon what it is you are evaluating; method and object of evaluation are intimately interrelated. If an educational system were to follow a narrow orientation toward subject matter, then the focus of its evaluative procedures would be greatly simplified. On the other hand, if the objectives or goals of an educational program are broad and go beyond subject matter, and if the learning structure is performance-oriented, the "how" of evaluation becomes more complex.

Any method used to assess student progress or the effectiveness of the curriculum has a greater likelihood of success if a systematic approach is followed. In this paper, we will consider the methods and tools for student and curriculum evaluation in the order of the following five steps:

1. Examine the objectives or goals to be assessed in terms of the content and implied behaviors or outcomes.

2. Identify situations which are likely to provide opportunities for the demonstration of the behaviors or outcomes to be assessed.

3. Examine available evaluation instruments or experiences to determine the extent to which they may satisfy the purpose of evaluation desired.

4. Determine the aspects of behavior to be evaluated and the terms in which each aspect will be summarized.

5. Establish means for collecting, interpreting and using data and results.

In discussing the first three of these steps, pertinent material about the fourth and fifth will automatically be included because of the close interrelationship of the last two steps with each of the first three.

Examine the Objectives or Goals
To Be Assessed In Terms of the Content and
Implied Behaviors or Outcomes

Educational objectives or goals need to be studied so that constituent elements and essential features can be identified. Behaviors or attributes must be reduced to their least common denominators. Synthesis does not serve the purpose of the evaluation of objectives; analysis does.

In nursing education, we are concerned with judgments pertaining to student attainment in terms of the three components of behavior: cognitive, psychomotor and affective. All three components can be identified by studying objectives or goals commonly found in nursing education programs. It is because we can identify these components that we can look for specific changes in relation to students' behavior in each of these three domains.

Let us consider Figure 1, Some Outcomes and Representative Behaviors Requiring Evaluation Procedures Other Than the Typical Paper-and-Pencil Test, in terms of the three behavioral domains.

Under the first column, entitled Outcomes, are listed some general attributes: Skills, Work Habits, Social Attitudes, Scientific Attitudes, Appreciations and Personal and Professional Adjustments. These attributes reflect some general outcomes that one could expect to find in objectives in nursing education programs. The second column lists some behaviors which would require evaluation procedures other than the typical paper-and-pencil test.

Outcomes	Representative Behaviors
Skills	Adapts teaching to the client's and patient's level of knowledge; relays pertinent information to appropriate personnel; maintains effective interpersonal relationships with clients and coworkers; provides problem-oriented care based on scientific principles; picks up cues from clients and patients indicative of possible subtle or unexpressed needs; works collaboratively with members of the health team; assumes an effective leadership role in guiding and directing health care.
Works Habits	Formulates, implements and evaluates nursing care plans based on individual needs; anticipates and provides comfort and safety measures specific to individual health care problems; utiizes appropriate resources in the solution of problems; demonstrates such traits as initiative, creativity, persistence and dependability.
Social Attitudes	Demonstrates sensitivity and concern for the welfare of clients and patients; demonstrates sensitivity to the influence of physical, social and cultural forces on health care; accepts responsibility for participation in community activities geared to promoting health care; demonstrates personal responsibility for community wellness.
Scientific Attitudes	Suspends judgments until all facts are available; uses facts and principles of the natural and social sciences in analyzing and solving new nursing problems; reassesses client and patient needs on the basis of objective data; distinguishes between objective data and opinions; draws conclusions from appropriate data; validates findings.
Appreciations	Uses the potential of individuals to promote their independence; respects and accepts persons as they are; is non-judgmental in the assessment of human behavior; reflects in own behavior belief that man is the focus of nursing; incorporates new and appropriate behaviors in nursing action; demonstrates commitment to nursing and to the service it renders.
Personal and Professional Adjustments	Examines possible effects of personal traits and qualities on nursing practice; uses pertinent data to modify or change beliefs about self; seeks guidance from appropriate sources; identifies own strengths and weaknesses; accepts responsibility for own behavior; seeks assistance when uncertain about effectiveness of nursing practice; encourages suggestions from peers and instructors in self-appraisal; sets realistic goals for own self-improvement; uses specific criteria to assess the performance of self and peers; seeks opportunities to increas skills and knowledge.

Figure 1. Some outcomes and representative behaviors requiring evaluation procedures other than the typical paper-and-pencil test.

135

Let us consider the first outcome, Skills. This is, of course, too global to assess. There are, however, cognitive, psychomotor and affective aspects of this attribute which do lend themselves to assessment:

Cognitive. Identifies the level of a client's understanding of care needed to promote his health.

Psychomotor. Adapts teaching to a client's level of understanding of health care.

Affective. Uses a client's potential for decision-making in regard to his health care.

Each of these aspects represents different abilities, and it is possible for a nursing student to demonstrate different levels of achievement in terms of each one. If behaviors are not considered in terms of constituent elements, judgments about the behaviors are likely to be invalid.

Identify Situations Which Are Likely to Provide Opportunities for the Demonstration Of Behaviors Or Outcomes to Be Assessed

Let us consider the Representative Behaviors listed in Figure 1. The question that needs to be raised here would be, "What situation or situations will elicit these representative behaviors in nursing students?" Situations could be selected that would allow the assessment of a single behavior or multiple behaviors. Notice the overlapping of the representative behaviors between outcomes; for example, "draws conclusions from appropriate data" under the outcome Scientific Attitudes and "uses pertinent data to modify or change beliefs about self" under Personal and Professional Adjustments.

Examine Available Evaluation Instruments or Experiences to Determine the Extent to Which They May Satisfy the Purpose of Evaluation Desired

Written Tests

Most behavior has identifiable components constituting abilities which are measurable by written tests. When desired cognitive abilities have been identified, they can be arranged in a hierarchy of knowledge ranging from knowledge of terms and simple facts to comprehension, application and on to evaluation. Test questions can be developed in accordance with the taxonomy developed by Bloom and others.[1]

Although written tests can measure scholastic achievement, they will never provide information about what a nursing student will do in a given situation. Test results can only tell what a student knows about the particular sample of items in a particular test.

Teacher-Made and National Standardized Tests

Teacher-made tests have a specific value because they reflect course emphases and can be tailor-made to reflect the specific objectives of courses. In addition, these tests can better serve to motivate students, because they pertain more directly to a particular course and can therefore provide more reliable information about the strengths and weaknesses of students. Teacher-made tests provide a basis for grades and feed back to the teacher information about the effectiveness of teaching.

National standardized tests, such as NLN's Achievement Tests, are especially useful to schools by enabling them to examine themselves in terms of comparable programs. This is possible because standardized achievement tests help to measure the extent to which students are meeting goals that are sufficiently accepted nationally to be reflected in the tests. However, standardized achievement tests are not developed in terms of the specific course offerings in any particular school and therefore cannot be used as course-end tests. Faculties can use standardized achievement tests in curriculum planning and evaluation: (1) to identify the level and range of ability among students; (2) to identify areas of instruction needing greater emphasis; (3) to evaluate experimental programs; and (4) to clarify objectives.

It is important to keep in mind the need for faculty members to review standardized achievement tests in terms of their content and objectives, to compare their own objectives with those reflected by test items, to determine when it is best to use the tests and to use test results appropriately.

Objective and Essay Tests

Objective tests allow for wide sampling of material and objectivity in scoring and can be used to test almost anything in the cognitive domain, the exceptions being the ability to select appropriate knowledge and ideas, without clues, and the organization and expression of ideas. Ingenuity and creativity are given rein in this kind of exercise. While objective tests are easy to score, they are not easy to construct. One well-known problem is the possibility of ambiguity in wording.

---

[1] Benjamin Bloom, et al. *Taxonomy of Educational Objectives, Handbook II: Cognitive Domain.* New York: Longmans, Green and Company, 1956.

137

Essay tests require students to recall information without clues and to present their response to the question in writing. The freedom of response generally permitted in essay questions varies considerably. Restricted-response questions are phrased in terms of words such as "list," "define" or "outline," whereas in the extended-response type, the action verbs take the form of "compare" and "explain." Major limitations of essay questions are limited sampling of content and subjectivity in scoring. An interesting point to note about the scoring of essay questions is that the problem is comparable with that of performance evaluation, that is, in the need to establish criteria for the assessment of the product. Criteria are needed to serve as the basis for assigning credit for essay questions.

Computerized Tests, Problem-Solving and Simulated Types

Another type of pencil-and-paper test is the computerized test for assessing decision-making skills, such as is reported by Sumida.[2] McIntyre, et al.[3] and de Tornyay[4] have developed simulated nursing tests to assess problem-solving abilities in nursing. These are paper-and-pencil tests, which present some or all of the content in a scrambled or branched fashion. Another simulated test, which involves much of the same characteristics as those developed by McIntyre, et al. and de Tornyay but adds to realism by the provision of films and slides, is the one developed by Curtis and Rothert.[5] These innovative evaluation devices have much merit; however, the development is complicated and costly, and much time, expertise and money are involved.

Although a large number of educational outcomes can be adequately measured by paper-and-pencil tests, there are significant areas and important behavioral changes which require the use of other methods and devices. Learning outcomes implied by the representative behaviors listed in Figure 1 can at best be only partially evaluated by paper-and-pencil tests.

Let us take a look at Figure 1 again to examine more carefully some of the outcomes which *cannot* be measured by typical paper-and-pencil tests. Other methods available for measuring or assessing such outcomes include: nursing care plans; patient-care studies; conferences; interviews; nursing diaries; nursing process recordings; self-evaluation

[2] Sylvia W. Sumida. "A Computerized Test for Clinical Decision Making." *American Journal of Nursing,* 20:458-461, July, 1972.

[3] Hattie McIntyre, et al. "A Simulated Clinical Nursing Test." *Nursing Research,* 21:429-435, September-October, 1972.

[4] Rheba de Tornyay. "Measuring Problem-Solving Skills by Means of the Simulated Clinical Nursing Problem Test." *Journal of Nursing Education,* 7:3-8, 34-35, August, 1968.

[5] Joy Curtis and Marilyn Rothert. "An Instructional Simulation System Offering Practice in Assessment of Patient Needs." *Journal of Nursing Education,* 11:23-28, January, 1972.

techniques; checklists; peer-evaluation techniques; patient reports; role-playing; rating scales; video tapes; nursing audits; seminars; and statistical studies.

Performance Evaluation

Another evaluation method is the direct observation of nursing performance, which, although the principal tool for the acting or doing component, is also considered to be one of the most expensive and difficult techniques. How a nursing student performs is ultimately the acid test of the educational program. The chief and all-encompassing purpose of performance evaluatin in the curriculum is to determine the degree to which program objectives have been achieved as demonstrated by the actions or behaviors of students in health care settings.

Direct observation is also the principal tool for assessment of aspects of the affective component. Because of the relative expense and difficulty involved, evaluation by direct observation should be reserved for those aspects which cannot be evaluated by any other means. The chief problems of performance evaluation are related to the techique of direct observation, which is inherently subjective. The technique amounts to what one individual thinks about the performance of another, and only to the extent that subjectivity in direct observation can be reduced, can the reliability and validity of the technique be increased.

The validity and reliability of performance evaluation can be promoted if the following four questions are raised and answered satisfactorily:

1. What objectives or functions of the individual or group are to be evaluated?

2. What observable and measurable qualities, abilities, traits, behaviors or skills are essential to the effective performance of the individual or group in terms of the objectives or functions to be evaluated?

3. What criteria or standards are to be used in defining levels of performance in relation to each of the qualities, abilities, traits, behaviors or skills to be evaluated?

4. What specific behaviors or activities appropriate to the functions of the individual or group will demonstrate each of the qualities, abilities, traits, behaviors, skills or objectives to be evaluated at the various levels of performance?

As a last consideration under the third step in the evaluation process, *Examine available instruments or experiences to determine the extent to which they may satisfy the purpose of evaluation desired,* I would like to talk about four methods used in curriculum evaluation: (1) statistical studies and surveys; (2) self-evaluation techniques; (3) peer evaluation; and (4) interviews.

Statistical Studies and Surveys

Statistical studies and surveys can contribute significantly to the maintenance or improvement of the quality of education within an institution. Such studies can provide reliable bases for decisions related to the effectiveness of educational programs. Some areas for study which are likely to provide significant data for curriculum development are the effectiveness of teaching strategies, the effects of curriculum change and the competence and professional progress of the program's graduates.

The methodology for such studies and surveys would depend upon their purpose and on the type of data desired. A number of the evaluation tools previously mentioned could be used as means to gather data. Important responsibilities of persons participating in such research studies would be: (1) to determine specifically what information is desired; (2) to utilize a research design that will provide pertinent, relevant and accurate data; (3) to establish criteria for assessing data; and (4) to impart the resulting information or data in readily understood terms to the appropriate person or persons. It would be particularly important to impart to all persons making decisions based on such data information which will enable them to weigh all possible alternatives, to be aware of possible outcomes of alternatives and to be knowledgeable about the probabilities and utility of outcomes.

Self-Evaluation

The development of the ability to evaluate one's own performance or achievement objectively is probably the highest aim of an educational program. It can also be stated that this ability is likely to be the most worthwhile, enduring accomplishment of an educational program.

In the Palmer study,[6] students were taught to judge their behavior (performance) and rate or grade themselves on the basis of faculty criteria defining levels of performance which were established for eight objectives in medical-surgical nursing.

---

[6] Mary Ellen Palmer. *Self-Evaluation of Nursing Performance Based on Clinical Practice Objectives.* Boston: Boston University Press, 1967.

Self-evaluation—the ability to look objectively at oneself and identify strengths and weaknesses—involves the ability to set realistic goals, to bear with imperfections, to know what one knows and to know what one doesn't know or knows inadequately. The ability to practice objective self-evaluation is difficult to teach and to learn, which may explain, in part, why so many people who have completed educational programs do not practice it. It can be very uncomfortable. It can also deflate the ego and disturb one's sense of security, if proper support is not provided. However, these problems are not insurmountable and should not discourage those who see its value. In order to develop this ability in students, the idea of self-evaluation must be introduced early, and faculty members must be committed to the importance of the concept.

Being able to encourage self-evaluation in students requires a sense of security on the part of the faculty. Because self-evaluation also sharpens the ability to evaluate other persons and things, the faculty will probably be subjected to more penetrating analysis by the students as a consequence. The problems associated with the development of this ability are likely to be more than compensated by the changes that can be seen in the behavior of the student who becomes increasingly able to evaluate strengths and weaknesses objectively and to utilize this ability further in evaluating the performance or achievement of others.

Peer Appraisal

Peer appraisal in general education has primarily involved sociometric techniques designed to evaluate social relationships within a group. This approach can be used in the assessment of various aspects of personal development, such as leadership ability, concern for others and social attitudes. The basic underlying premise is that peers (in this case, students) view each other on a different basis from instructors and that there are aspects of the behavior of students which would be better known only to other students. The question that would need to be raised is the purpose of using the method—as a means of formative evaluation or as a means of summative evaluation? If the purpose is to understand students better and to provide a more complete basis for guiding the learning activities and development of the student, this implies a use for formative evaluation. Burnside reports a study[7] in which each student both supervised and was supervised by another student. Handled properly, this can be an excellent

---

[7] Irene M. Burnside. "Peer Supervision: A Method of Teaching." *Journal of Nursing Education,* 10:15-22, November, 1971.

teaching and evaluation procedure. Each supervising student must evaluate the performance of the supervised student, identifying both positive and negative aspects of her performance. The use of this approach can be helpful in developing observation, communication and evaluation skills.

Interviewing Techniques

Interviewing is a particularly useful technique for the measurement of progress toward the meeting of objectives in the affective domain. In a face-to-face contact, using either a structured or unstructured format, data about the interests, attitudes and values of students can be obtained. The structured interview is built on a fixed schedule of questions and is therefore less flexible, the respondent being limited to specific response patterns. On the other hand, the unstructured interview is more likely to elicit ordinarily covert behaviors and attitudes, since the interviewer, by using a non-directive technique, can stimulate more spontaneous responses. When unstructured interviews are used, it is essential that the interviewer keep in mind the possiblity of bias in obtaining and interpreting data. The unstructured interview is more time-consuming than the structured interview, but it does provide data that would be difficult or almost impossible to obtain from some of the more common methods of evaluation.

A structured interview can also be used in the evaluation of knowledge of nursing practice and is particularly useful in assessing students' ability to relate theory and practice. Chuan[8] developed a guide for the use of structured interviews which have been taped. The focus of the evaluation is on the level of students' comprehension and their application of the components of the nursing process to patient care.

In conclusion, the selection of methods and tools for use in curriculum evaluation should be neither haphazard in approach nor limited in scope. Critical analysis of objectives and goals in terms of implied abilities should serve as the basis for the selection of evaluation methods. Decisions regarding the utilization of results obtained from evaluation devices should reflect agreement among all responsible parties.

---

[8] Helen Chuan. "Evaluation by Interview." *Nursing Outlook,* 20:726-727, November, 1972.

19 THE "WHO" IN CURRICULUM EVALUATION

Helen Yura, PhD, RN

Determining the "Who" in curriculum evaluation is the keystone to effective evaluation. Picture the faculty—those with graduate preparation in teaching nursing in the specific areas of their education and experience and those teaching the general education content; picture the students, committed and receptive to baccalaureate nursing education and hoping to become both educated people and skilled practitioners of nursing; picture the nurse leaders in health care agencies, who are partners in the education of practitioners and the major employers of these graduates; picture the consumers of health care, who will be receiving the services of these graduates and who increasingly want a say in health care delivery, in both the services available and who delivers them; picture the influential community leaders, who designate the allocation of funds for the support of education; and finally, picture the parents, who directly and indirectly pay the costs of education. This is a composite of the "Who" in curriculum evaluation.

If this picture seems crowded, it is, nevertheless, a picture of active participation. Each of these groups is concerned about the graduate of the baccalaureate nursing program and how this graduate is prepared. Each group is aware of the contribution and role of each of the others, in terms of their unique and common contributions to curriculum evaluation.

There is a great variation in participation in curriculum evaluation today, ranging from no evaluation by any of the "Whos" through a great number of variations of participants and levels of participation.

I hope to focus on the situation as it *should be,* with the goal of participation by *all* the persons mentioned. In looking at her own situation, the reader can determine where she is, as a first step in knowing where to go.

Basically, there are three "Who" groups in curriculum evaluation: the nursing faculty, the significant others and the influential others. The first and most important group is the nursing faculty. They have the ultimate responsibility for the product—the graduate of the baccalaureate degree program in nursing. The nursing faculty make a major impact upon curriculum evaluation, which is focused on the curriculum framework, with its stated philosophy, objectives, terminal behavioral expectations, its conceptual framework, its level and course behaviors—the "What" that is to be evaluated.

Curriculum evaluation is the responsibility of all faculty members. If you have input into the curriculum, you share responsibility for the output. Being passive or disinterested does not allow you to escape this responsibility. Of course, the amount of involvement differs among faculty members, and the type of involvement differs with the portion of the curriculum framework to be evaluated. For example, the broadest portions of the framework are the philosophy, objectives, terminal behavioral expectations and the conceptual framework. All faculty should be involved in the development of these areas. Once they are operational and have been approved by the faculty, a date can be set for evaluation of their purposefulness and viability. Some faculties choose to do this biannually and some annually, generally at the end of the academic year.

One plan is to appoint a task force to make a preliminary review and formulate recommendations. Then the total faculty can react to the results and recommend changes or affirm the work of the task force. Once this task force has completed its work, it can be disbanded, with a new task force being appointed when the broad framework is to be reevaluated.

Some faculty groups prefer to establish an evaluation committee as a standing committee with responsibility for the development of the plan for the evaluation of the broad, intermediate and specific aspects of the curriculum framework. This committee may collect data needed for evaluative judgments by the total faculty.

An evaluative plan is directed to validate the statements in the curriculum framework and to collect evidence that all behavioral expectancies are met. All faculty participate in the evaluation of the broad framework.

144

The intermediate aspects are the level behaviors, and the selected faculty teaching at a particular level will be responsible for the evaluation of the fulfillment of these level behavioral expectations, after which all faculty will review the totality of level behaviors as they relate to the broad framework of the curriculum.

Specific aspects of the curriculum framework refer to the course behaviors and the day-to-day learning experiences planned to achieve these behaviors. The faculty teaching a specific course will be involved in evaluating the course behavioral expectations. Formal evaluation of the specific daily or weekly learning experiences, the course behaviors and the level behaviors should come at the completion of these.

The evaluation of ongoing learning experiences may be done through planned post-conferences, through formal end-of-the-week meetings or evaluation of past learning experiences may take place at the same meeting at which future learning experiences are planned, thus providing data for such future planning.

In this manner, nursing faculty are intermittently involved in the formal evaluation of the broad framework of the curriculum but are consistently involved in the intermediate and specific aspects of the curriculum. All faculty contribute both formally and informally, though a select group may be designated to organize and collate faculty thoughts and ideas and make recommendations to the total group. This select faculty group, in fact, coordinate the evaluation of the broad, intermediate and specific behaviors. Curriculum evaluation is *always* made in terms of behavioral statements and beliefs inherent in the curriculum framework.

Second of the three groups we are considering as important to curriculum evaluation are the "significant others." These include: the faculty who teach the general education component of the curriculum, which has been designed to meet the objectives of the college or university as well as to provide the foundation for the nursing major and contribute to the meeting of the program's behavioral expectations; the students who will be the graduates of the program and who are directly involved as participants in and recipients of the educational program; the previous graduates of the program; the consumers who are the recipients of health and nursing care to be provided by graduates of the program; the employers of the graduates of the program; the nurse leaders; the influential political, legislative, educational, religious and social welfare leaders in the community; and the parents of the students.

Faculty teaching the general education component should be sought out for their participation in evaluation of the content of foundational courses designed to meet course, level and terminal behaviors designated by the nursing faculty. This participation presumes that a designation has been made concerning the content needed to serve as a foundation to the nursing major and the content upon which nursing intervention will be based and that communication is maintained with faculty teaching courses in which this needed content is contained. The frequency, intensity and focus of the involvement in evaluation by the general education faculty must be determined and incorporated in the evaluation plan. Participation may take place in conjunction with other parties in the significant other category.

Students should be involved in all aspects of evaluation—evaluation of the broad, intermediate and specific aspects of the curriculum framework. Representatives of the student body should hold committee membership with voting privileges. The views of the student group as a whole should be sought through surveys, questionnaires, rating scales, reaction sessions and other means. Evaluative views should be sought in relation to specific behavioral statements—whether for a specific learning experience, a course or a level—or in relation to the terminal behavioral expectations. Information unrelated to these behavioral expectations will have little or no value in the evaluative process and may, in fact, arouse feelings of unfairness or suspicion on the part of evaluators and evaluees. Thus, it is important that the focus of evaluation is clearly placed on a stated behavioral expectation, whether the expectation itself is being evaluated or whether it is the persons involved in the fulfillment of the expectation (students) or the evaluative tools that are being evaluated. No other criterion measure is valid.

Thus, although students should be involved at all levels, they are most pertinently involved at the course level. Their role at this level is ongoing and involves all components—themselves, the faculty involved, the specific learning experiences and any tools being utilized to evaluate the fulfillment of specific objectives.

The involvement of the consumer varies with quantity, quality, formality and timing in relation to the broad aspects of the curriculum framework. Other community leaders, as mentioned previously, may also be selected to serve on the evaluation committee or task force. The numbers and composition of the committee can be designated by the nursing faculty. Whether these persons will participate in all meetings, or only in selected meetings and whether they will have a definitive vote or serve in an advisory capacity should also be determined by the faculty. Whether views will be sought via questionnaires, through interviews or by other methods will be decided, also.

Seeking the views of these significant others gives faculty first-hand information on what is expected of the graduates of baccalaureate degree programs in nursing. Furthermore, it provides a medium for clearing up misconceptions about baccalaureate nursing education and clarifying for the consumer the educational and practice differences between technical and baccalaureate education. The involvement of the significant others, in accordance with the plan for evaluation designated by the nursing faculty, should include appropriate orientation to the purpose of participation and the role of the significant others.

In terms of the evaluation of level and course behaviors and day-to-day learning experiences, involvement of these significant others differs and becomes more specific. Suggestions and recommendations they have made in relation to the broad framework must be considered for their influence on level and course behaviors. However, the views and participation of general edcuation faculty, nurse leaders, health care agency representatives and specific community leaders who affect the provision of learning experiences or are partners in providing these experiences should be sought where their specific involvement would be relevant. Their involvement can be direct, indirect or a combination of the two. Direct participation might include meeting formally with the committee at specific intervals; indirect participation might involve seeking their views at random intervals throughout the experience of learning. Dialogue can be initiated by faculty, students or significant others. Review of contractual agreements would be part of the focus for evaluation as it stems from behavior to be achieved.

The significant others involved in evaluating the broad curriculum framework may be different from those involved in the evaluation of the level behaviors, course behaviors or specific behaviors for a specific learning experience. The significant others involved in the specifics may be those more closely tied to the rendering of health care services, while those involved with evaluation of the broad aspects of the curriculum framework may be those in community and health care service planning and funding. The recipient of nursing care can be directly involved in the evaluation of learning experiences and can provide direct feedback for judgments about the kind and level of learning necessary to the student, reflected in the behavioral expectations and placed within the curriculum framework. The recipients of nursing service can also rate the service they receive in terms of its person-centeredness, goal directedness, economy and utilization of human and clinical resources. Furthermore, it is the anticipated behavioral changes within the client that provide evidence of the correctness of nursing judgments, the appropriateness of planned strategies and the success of the implemented strategies. Thus the recipient of the health and nursing services of the student (whether an individual, a family or group of individuals or families) can function in the role of evaluator as well as providing the mechanism for evaluation.

Some of the tools used in evaluation include examinations, self-evaluations, rating scales, formal course evaluations and faculty evaluations. All evaluations are based on prestated behavioral expectations for a specific learning experience or for a specific course.

The third group to be considered in the "Who" of curriculum evaluation can be termed "influential others." These include members of such bodies as local, state and federal educational agencies that approve programs, provide grants and funding for programs and/or prescribe standards for programs. For example, the Board of Nursing in a particular state may withhold approval if specific components of a program do not meet prescribed expectations or if the needs of the state are not met by the particular program.

Other influencers are the agencies of the local, state and federal governments which, through their legislative and funding activities, influence the direction of the role of health care practitioners and new types of practitioners within the health care scene as well as influencing the quality of nursing education by providing or withholding funds, approving and awarding grants, initiating new health service coverage for citizens and specifying who shall provide services (as in the many Social Security amendments which have a direct impact upon nursing).

Also included among the influential others are the regional accrediting associations which determine the quality of the academic environment of the colleges and universities where nursing education takes place. This is an example of peer evaluation. Inherent in regional accreditation is self-evaluation based upon a stated philosophy and objectives. Peer evaluation for nursing education is accomplished through the accrediting services of the NLN and is based upon stated criteria; these criteria are determined by faculty from academic agencies throughout the United States which are members of the NLN Council of Baccalaureate and Higher Degree Programs.

In summary, the nursing faculty are ultimately accountable for the fulfillment of the terminal behavioral expectations set for the baccalaureate degree program in nursing. Nursing faculty and students are involved in the formal and informal evaluation of the broad, the intermediate and the specific aspects of the curriculum framework. A specific plan should be made for the evaluation of these three aspects of the curriculum framework. The broader aspects of the framework require formal evaluation less frequently than the specific aspects. In addition to nursing faculty and students, two other groups—"significant others" and "influential others"—are concerned in curriculum evaluation. "Significant others" participate in evaluation of all aspects of the curriculum framework in accordance with the evaluation plan. The significant others may differ according to the aspect of the curriculum under evaluation. The role of the significant others may be direct, advisory or both. "Influential others" include representatives of societal organizations on local, state, federal, and national levels. These groups are influential by reason of their powers in designating needs, granting or withholding funds, specifying standards to be met for permission to operate and protecting the citizens. Regional and specialized accreditation bodies are influential because of their function of reviewing colleges, universities and programs to determine quality through peer evaluation.

Those who are accountable for the effectiveness of the curriculum must be designated; they must be receptive and accepting of their responsibility. Otherwise, evaluation is likely to be ignored or, if attempted, fall short of its goals.

20 ACCREDITATION AND THE EVALUATION PROCESS

Helen Yura, PhD, RN

From the 1600s, when education began in a formal way for the citizens of the United States, to the present day, much effort has been exerted to preserve the quality of our education by allowing the private sector to manage the accreditation of colleges, universities and programs. This is a form of peer evaluation and is highly regarded by faculty in academic settings. Accreditation also influences the selection of an educational institution by prospective students.

Government interference is constantly guarded against in accreditation, and government agencies, whether local, state or federal, are more interested in the funding aspects of education and in assuring that institutions provide for the needs of the citizens. These governmental bodies acknowledge the value of and strive to foster the nongovernmental accreditation process. The Federal government does, however, sanction particular accrediting bodies and gives recognition to those which meet specified standards, including: being well-established, having specific criteria developed by membership, following a code of ethical practices, providing for appeal of decisions, giving evidence of integrity, currency and willingness to look at themselves as well as to subject themselves to review by an outside agency. These accrediting bodies receive approval by the Office of Education, U.S. Department of Health, Education, and Welfare, and are included in a published list of such agencies. Inclusion on the list indicates quality in the functioning of the accrediting agencies and designates that the programs accredited by these agencies will be eligible for federal funding and various other negotiations. NLN is among the agencies having this recognition.

There are two types of accreditation practiced by nongovernmental agencies in the United States at the present time, namely, institutional accreditation and specialized accreditation. Institutional accreditation is performed by the six regional accrediting bodies and is concerned with the quality of the total institution. The six regional associations are:

New England Association of Schools and Colleges
Middle States Association of Colleges and Secondary Schools
North Central Association of Colleges and Secondary Schools
Southern Association of Colleges and Schools
Western Association of Colleges and Schools
Northwestern Association of Secondary and Higher Schools

The regional accrediting associations have organized themselves into a Federation of Regional Accrediting Commissions in Higher Education (FRACHE). The purposes of this federation include (1) the formulation and promotion of a set of common principles, policies and general procedures to be used by members in their operations and (2) the review and coordination of the activities of the accrediting commissions to assure consistency with these principles, policies and general procedures.[1]

Specialized accreditation is concerned with the quality of a particular field of study, such as nursing, architecture, optometry, engineering, dentistry or medicine. A newly formed Council of Specialized Accrediting Agencies aims to strengthen the effectiveness and quality of postsecondary professional and specialized education through accreditation and related activities and to collaborate with other postsecondary accrediting agencies for this purpose.

Many institutions hold accreditation by both institutional and specialized accrediting agencies. Accreditation of the institution as a totality by an institutional agency is not generally interpreted as equivalent to the specialized accreditation of a part or program in a particular college or department. Institutional accreditation does not validate a specialized program in the same manner nor to the same extent that specialized accreditation does.

---

[1] Jay Miller. *Organizational Structure of Nongovernmental Post-Secondary Accreditation: Relationship to Uses of Accreditation.* Washington, D.C.: National Commission on Accreditation, p. 153.

The need for coordinating and, to some extent, regulating nongovernmental accrediting agencies gave rise to the National Commission on Accrediting (NCA), which was founded in 1949. This is an independent educational agency support by the colleges and universities of the United States to improve the operation and effectiveness of accreditation in higher education. The NCA was created to eliminate objectionable practices and policies of accrediting agencies, while preserving their contributions to higher education. It has enjoyed a cooperative working relationship with the regional associations but has never assumed authority over them. NCA also maintains a close relationship with FRACHE, although a proposed merger between the two organizations was withdrawn.

The National League for Nursing is the designated accrediting agency for standard-setting and evaluation of all educational programs in nursing and is recognized as such by the NCA and the U.S. Office of Education. Since the early part of the twentieth century, accreditation has been considered essential to the improvement of nursing education programs. When the American Society of Superintendents of Training Schools for Nurses changed its name to National League of Nursing Education (NLNE) in 1912, it was the purpose of the new NLNE to improve nursing education. This is also the overall purpose of all kinds of accrediting agencies. The National League of Nursing Education published its first list of accredited schools in 1941.

In 1920, the National Organization for Public Health Nursing published the first list of accredited programs in public health nursing. The association of Collegiate Schools of Nursing came into being in 1932. While it was not established as an accrediting agency, its requirements for membership were such that it actually performed an accrediting function. In 1938, the NLNE inaugurated an accrediting program for schools offering basic nursing programs. Also in 1938, the Conference of Catholic Schools of Nursing of the Catholic Hospital Association inaugurated its own accrediting program.

It gradually became evident to leaders in nursing that accreditation, when carried on by such a number of autonomous organizations, resulted in: (1) duplication of effort and cost; (2) confusion on the part of educational institutions, the profession, prospective students and the public; and (3) fractional rather than comprehensive evaluation. For these reasons, steps were initiated that finally led to the establishement of the National Nursing Accrediting Service in January 1949. Then, in 1952 the National Nursing Accrediting Service became part of the National League for Nursing.

The accreditation process for programs in nursing continues to the present day to develop and improve in order to maintain its viability and relevance. The accreditation process of NLN is frequently cited as a model by other accrediting agencies. NLN's willingness to cooperate with regional accrediting bodies, its clearly formulated criteria and sound policies and procedures for guiding the process of accreditation have contributed to its being recognized by both the NCA and the U.S. Office of Education.

The criteria and the policies and procedures used in accreditation have been revised throughout the past twenty years. Today, programs are evaluated in relation to their own statements of philosophy and purposes and in relation to their overall strengths and weaknesses; programs are accredited when their strengths outweigh their weaknesses. The criteria have been consolidated and have become more concise and precise, with less direction to faculty. Presently, criteria are stated under five headings, Organization and Administration, Students, Faculty, Curriculum, and Resources, Facilities and Services. The criteria in the past two decades have become more qualitative than quantitative. Emphasis is placed on the involvement in the evaluation process of all persons connected with the educational enterprise—students, faculty and administrators. The criteria permit greater flexiblity in the development of the program and in the preparation of the self-study report. Presently, there are 225 baccalaureate and 64 masters programs accredited by NLN.

The criteria of the Council of Baccalaureate and Higher Degree Programs are developed by an Accreditation Committee composed of faculty from the Council member agencies. The Committee does the initial work of criteria development based upon needs and trends. The draft of the revised criteria is sent to Council agency members for review and reaction. Feedback from the membership is sent to the committee, which reviews and studies the suggestions and recommendations, making appropriate additions, deletions or editorial changes. The second revision is then sent to the membership. The criteria are then presented at the next scheduled Council business meeting; opportunity for open discussion is afforded the membership, after which the criteria are subjected to voting by members from NLN-accredited baccalaureate and masters programs. The vote may be contingent upon certain changes to be included in the final draft, or members may vote to return the criteria to the Accreditation Committee for reconsideration and inclusion of desired changes. This process is followed until the criteria is approved by the Council membership. There is one set of criteria for baccalaureate and masters programs, all of which must be validated by both programs, with the exception of criteria that refer specifically to one or the other. An interim period is set for phasing in the new criteria. Generally, this is a two-year period, after which the new criteria are to be used.

If you look at the criteria as a whole, by the way, you will note

154

that they can serve as guidelines for curriculum development and revision, in addition to serving as the basis for program evaluation.

The most significant document in the accreditation process is the school's self-evaluation report. This report should be prepared by the faculty and should contain all the evidence available to validate each of the criteria. The development of the self-evaluation report is the end result of an intense self-study by the faculty of the existing baccalaureate and/or master's degree program in nursing.

In order to insure that the accreditation process is truly an evaluative experience, the following questions seem pertinent:

1. Were the faculty involved in all activities incorporated in the report? Have all criteria been considered, with specific evidence presented to designate fulfillment or lack of fulfillment of the criteria?

2. Was an intense *evaluation* of the entire framework for the curriculum done (i.e., review of the philsophy, objectives, terminal behavioral expectations, level behaviors, course behaviors and the conceptual framework) in contrast to merely reporting the state of things?

3. Did the faculty evaluate the relationship of the parts of the curriculum framework to the whole? If no relationship was found, were immediate steps outlined to rectify the situation?

4. Was the curriculum framework used in selecting course content and clinical laboratory experiences, or is there no relationship whatsoever between such learning and the curriculum framework?

5. Have the faculty clearly spelled out their beliefs about man, teaching-learning, health and nursing in the philosophy?

6. Did the faculty include their beliefs about the nurse practitioner of today and clearly indicate their beliefs about the emerging role and future functions of the graduate of the baccalaureate degree program in nursing?

7. Were the program's *publics* (students, health care agency representatives, consumers, prospective employers) involved in the evaluation of the curriculum and its products and in what way?

8. Have the faculty made specific plans for the ongoing evaluation of students, faculty and graduates and will this plan be implemented?

9. Have the faculty made specific plans for the ongoing evaluation of the theoretic and clinical experiences planned to meet course behavioral expectations?

10. Have the faculty made specific plans to evaluate whether the courses for a level contribute to meeting level behavioral expectations?

11. Do the level behavioral expectations for each designated level contribute to meeting terminal behavioral expectations?

12. Do these stated course, level and terminal behavioral expectations contribute to fulfilling the philosophy and objectives for the program and implement the conceptual framework?

13. Does the conceptual framework fit the philosophy, objectives and terminal behavioral expectations for the program as stated by the faculty?

14. Are the philosophy, objectives and conceptual framework truly utilized by the faculty and evident in the day-to-day, week-to-week learning experiences planned for students?

15. Is the foundation of physical, biological, social and behavioral sciences which has been specified by the faculty as the base for nursing intervention truly utilized in this way and evident in the theoretic and laboratory aspects of course offerings?

16. Are the physical, biological, social and behavioral sciences progressively developed throughout the program?

17. Is the nursing major concentrated in the upper division and is there evidence of the synthesis of all learning as the student progresses through the program?

18. Is there clear evidence in the curriculum framework, as well as in the day-to-day and week-to-week learning, that critical thinking, problem-solving, making nursing judgments and independent thinking permeate the learning opportunities and expectations and that they are not limited to an experience with an independent study project?

19. Is the awareness and interpretation of the research process evident in the utilization of the nursing process throughout the nursing major or is it nonexistent or limited to a minimal orientation at the termination of the senior year?

20. Is the leadership process truly developed throughout the learning experiences or is it limited to an observational experience of a hospital team leader?

21. Do students have the opportunity to take electives?

22. Are students who are admitted with previous academic and/or nursing experience evaluated on an individual basis for appropriate placement within the curriculum design to assure meeting course, level and terminal behavioral expectations for the product of the program?

23. Do the teaching methods utilized by the faculty contribute to the meeting of learning expectations for courses and levels?

24. Are the evaluative tools needed to test the meeting of specific behavioral expectations for stated courses and levels developed, utilized and periodically reviewed for their viability and validity?

25. Are the support services needed by the nurse administrator, the faculty and students to fulfill the program's objectives available in the kinds and numbers needed?

26. Are the clinical learning resources varied and selected to meet stated objectives and behavioral outcomes?

27. Have procedures been outlined and are they operational for input and output from the nurse administrator, the faculty and students for program and total college or university involvement?

28. Do the faculty truly function as faculty or do they have the more limited view of themselves as teachers?

29. Do the faculty fulfill their obligations by involving themselves in scholarly pursuits, in maintaining and increasing their clinical and functional expertise?

30. Do the faculty have the academic and experiential expertise to fulfill the roles for which they are responsible?

31. Do the faculty meet the stated college or university requirements related to appointments, promotion, tenure, and so forth?

After completion of this self-study period and the self-evaluation report, the program will register with NLN a petition for an accreditation visit. This means that the faculty wish to invite peer evaluation as a means of judging the quality of the program and that they are willing to abide by the decision and recommendations of the Board of Review of Baccalaureate and Higher Degree Programs. The onsite accreditation visit is made by two or more peers to verify, clarify and validate the evidence. The report of the visitors, prepared at the conclusion of the visit, is read to the head of the nursing program and anyone else she may designate.

The Board of Review then meets to consider all the materials concerning the program under evaluation; these materials include the self-evaluation report, the visitor's report, the school bulletin and any supplementary material sent in by the school. The Board meets twice a year, in April and December, and is made up of nine regular and nine alternate members. The Executive Committee of the Council of Baccalaureate and Higher Degree Programs selects the members of the Board of Review from names suggested by member agencies of the Council. Selection is made to insure a representation from the various geographic areas, clinical and functional specialties, colleges and universities of different control and size, baccalaureate and masters programs; all persons selected must be actively employed in NLN-accredited baccalaureate or masters programs. The Board of Review may be expanded to twelve members when the program review schedule is especially heavy.

The visitors are also selected from faculty of NLN-accredited programs in Council member agencies. They are selected to assure a representative group and receive preparation for the role of visitor at an annual intensive two-day visitor's conference generally held in January. New visitors accompany a senior visitor until they are completely oriented to the visitor's role. Visitors are expected to be keen observers, to be able to verify the evidence given to validate criteria and to be able to discriminate between evidence that supports specific criteria and information that does not. It is the function of the visitor to verify, clarify and amplify evidence. The visitor must be able to focus completely on another program. This means that the program from which the visitor came is completely out of the picture and is not used for comparison nor brought into any discussion. One of the visitors is present at the Board meeting when the program is reviewed and serves as a resource person or source of information about the school.

Following their review of the program, the Board of Review can make a number of decisions: that the program be given initial or continued accreditation with recommendations, without recommendations, with a request for a progress report, with a warning and a time limit or with other specified conditions; to defer initial accreditation; to deny initial accreditation; to withdraw accreditation. Every effort is made to mail the decision of the Board of Review to the nursing

158

program at the end of the review session, and all letters are mailed at the same time to assure an equal chance to hear. This initial letter states that a second letter including the Board's recommendations, if any, will follow in a few weeks. In my observations of the Board in action, I have been impressed with the thoroughness and honesty of its members and by the commitment of the Board to uphold quality nursing education at the baccalaureate and masters level. There is a collective wisdom inherent in the Board in much the same manner as in a jury. Beyond this, however, the Board members have the expertise in nursing education to make judgments and recommendations about programs, all of which are based on the criteria set by the Council.

The accreditation process is voluntary; it must be sought by nursing faculty. If faculty do not wish to submit the fruits of their efforts to peer evaluation, they need not. However, since nursing faculty members of the Board of Review are also informed members of the higher education community, evaluation is highly valued and sought after. The accreditation process rewards quality by withholding or awarding accreditation based on the meeting of specific criteria. On the other hand, accreditation is not a policing process. It cannot legally dictate which programs can develop where—this is the authority of state or regional planning commissions.

It is important for nursing educators to make input and impact in the state and the region where they live. Likewise, accreditation imposes on the faculty the responsibility of maintaining the quality of the nursing program during the interval between accreditation and follow-up visits, which may occur at any interval, the maximum being eight years. Accreditation also presupposes that the integrity of the baccalaureate and masters nursing programs will be maintained and that sound principles of learning and teaching will prevail. The end result of the accreditation process is verification of the program's accountability to the students enrolled and to the citizens who are the recipients of the care given by graduates. It verifies the collective belief of nursing education that the graduate of the baccalaureate nursing program is different from the graduate of a technical education program in nursing. It also verifies the beliefs that the graduate of the BSN program is a generalist and that preparation of the specialist in clinical and functional areas should be at the masters level. Specialized accreditation—such as is granted by NLN—is directed primarily at institutions granting the first professional degree and the masters degree, mainly in health areas, to ensure that the graduates meet society's expectations and that institutions hold the line on quality.

Doctoral programs in nursing, which at present number only eight, and certain other academic areas in nursing are not subjected to specialized accreditation.

In order to avoid repetition, every effort is made by NLN to cooperate in planning joint visits with the regional accrediting associations, when such joint visits are requested by the nursing program in question. Joint visits are also planned with representatives of the Board of Nursing, if requested.

In addition to the designation and affirmation of quality based on criteria set by peers, accreditation enhances: eligibility for federal and state funding, grants, and so forth; the public relations value of being included on a list of accredited programs in nursing that has national coverage; the ability to attract qualified faculty and interested students; the employment opportunities of graduates; and the ability of students to proceed into advanced study in nursing.

In order to be eligible for accreditation, the program must be in a college or university that is regionally accredited and the program must have the full approval of the State Board of Nursing (if this is a requirement in the state). Also, the program must be fully implemented so that students have graduated or are near graduation at the time of the visit. It is important to note that the visit for accreditation purposes is scheduled when the program is operational (i.e., when classes and clinical laboratory experiences are in progress). Thus, no visits are scheduled during registration week, final exam week or vacation periods.

All matters relating to accreditation of nursing programs are considered confidential. NLN refers all matters relating to the accreditation of a specific program directly to the dean of the school. The only information NLN will divulge is whether a program is on the list of NLN-accredited baccalaureate and masters programs.

To conclude, NLN, and particularly the Council of Baccalaureate and Higher Degree Programs, will continue to strengthen accreditation policies and to specify criteria with the intention of improving nursing education for nursing service. Every faculty member in a member agency has a responsibility to contribute to the goal of improving nursing education through participation in the Council and its activities, and to help maintain the integrity of the baccalaureate and masters degree in nursing through influence in the state and region where her nursing program is located. Faculty, students, administrators and citizens all have a large stake in the evaluative process generally and in the accreditation process specifically. Our right to peer evaluation must be safeguarded. It is through this process that we exercise our accountability for the education process and the kind of graduate who emerges from our programs.

160

3 CONCEPTUAL FRAMEWORK—ITS MEANING AND FUNCTION

21 THE MEANING AND FUNCTIONS OF CONCEPTS AND THEORIES WITHIN EDUCATION AND NURSING

Gertrude J. Torres, EdD, RN
Helen Yura, PhD, RN

The motives for the preparation of this paper were pure: the authors hoped to be able to clarify the terminology used in relation to the conceptual framework. However, the more we researched the literature, the more our comfortable state of simplistic clarity in relation to the terminology became an uncomfortable, albeit more informed, state of confusion. Yet, given the challenge, it seems appropriate to attempt to evolve some kind of clarity in the use of terms such as "concepts" and "theories" and to establish some common notions about these terms so that we can feel more secure about what we are communicating to each other when we use them.

Although the words "concepts" and "theories" are by no means new to nursing, it is recognized by most nurse educators that there are no standard uses of them. In the 1917 *Standard Curriculum for Schools of Nursing*[1] it was noted that the weaknesses in nursing programs at that time related to an overemphasis on the practical aspects of

---

[1] National League for Nursing Education, Committee on Education, *Standard Curriculum for Schools of Nursing*. Baltimore: Waverly Press, 1917, p.6.

training and a neglect of the theoretical foundation on which good practical work is built. What exactly was meant by the word "theoretical" at that time is not clear, but it seems to have indicated the knowledge and principles needed for the understanding of the practice of nursing.

Dock and Stewart in 1920 discussed the changing "concepts" of nursing as going from care of the well child, to care of the sick and infirm, and then to the promotion and conservation of health and prevention of disease.[2] These cyclic concepts of nursing seem all too familiar.

The New York League of Nursing Education in 1933 offered the concept of nursing as "using skillfully scientific methods in adapting prescribed therapy and preventive treatment of the specific physical and psychic needs of the individual."[3] One year later, Effie Taylor wrote that the prevailing concept of nursing was practical, having real depths through love, sympathy, knowledge, and culture.[4] These may not exactly represent our concept of what nursing is today, but they do represent a kind of conceptualization about nursing some forty or fifty years ago. Thus, it is evident that concepts and theories have been with us for some time.

In reviewing the literature in several fields such as social science, education, and philosophy, one finds a variety of uses of these terms, only adding to our confusion. In addition to this variety within specific disciplines, there appears little evidence of a standard use of these words from one field to another.[5]

The need to identify the meaning of the word "concept" is evident when we read the literature concerning theory. Concepts are the basic elements and the subject matter of a theory.[6,7] Language consists of words and sentences; the words describe objects, properties, or events and constitute the descriptive terms or concepts, which are combined

[2] Lavina L. Dock and Isabel M. Stewart, *A Short History of Nursing,* 4th ed. New York: G.P. Putnam's Sons, 1938, p. 355.

[3] New York League of Nursing Education, Program Committee, Martha R. Smith, chairman, "A Concept of Nursing." *American Journal of Nursing,* 33:565, June 1933.

[4] Effie J. Taylor, "Of What Is the Nature of Nursing?" *American Journal of Nursing,* 34:473-476, May 1934.

[5] George L. Newsome, Jr., "In What Sense Is Theory a Guide to Practice in Education?" *Educational Theory,* 14:33, January 1964.

[6] Margaret E. Hardy, "Theories: Components, Development, Evaluation." *Nursing Research,* 23:100-107, March-April 1974.

[7] Ada Jacox "Theory Construction in Nursing." *Nursing Research,* 23:4-13, January-February 1974.

into sentences or statements to form the theory.[8][9] Harre[10] and King[11] identify concepts as involving images. Concepts are also thought to be word symbols, "abstract ideas that give meaning to our sense perceptions [and] permit generalizations."[12] Harre also connects concepts with language involving pictures and models.[13]

The word "construct" is frequently used in association with concepts. Both Jacox[14] and King[15] utilize a construct to mean a group of concepts descriptive of the real world. Jacox calls a construct a high-level concept. The word nursing is a high-level concept, being formed of certain different images depending on our perceptions. Our general ideas and beliefs concerning the word "nursing," which are a complex product of abstract or reflective thinking, thus give us our conception of nursing, including the *who* (all the various types of nurses) as well as the *what* (our notions about nursing care) of nursing. (It would be most difficult to specify precisely all the ideas or images one could have in relation to the concept of nursing.) "Society" is another high-level concept, composed of many "lower-level" concepts (people, relationships, cultural norms, etc.). We in baccalaureate nursing education usually give meaning to five concepts in our statements of philosophy—"man," "society," "health," "nursing," and "learning."

In light of these notions of concepts, let us look at the word *theory*. In reviewing the literature as to the definition of theory, we find some prevalent notions and some specific ideas presented. Terms frequently cited in relation to theories include hypothesis, assumptions, unifying and organized concepts, and interrelated logical propositions. A common belief is that a theory is the opposite of a fact. When an unsubstantiated hypothesis or theory concerning reality is confirmed, it becomes a fact.[16] A theory is also considered to be "an invention of concepts

---

[8] *Ibid.,* p. 5.

[9] May Brodbeck, "Logic and Scientific Method in Research in Teaching," in N.L. Gage, ed., *Handbook of Research in Teaching.* Chicago: Rand McNally & Company, 1963, pp. 44-45.

[10] Rom Harre, "The Formal Analysis of Concepts," in Herbert J. Klausmeier and Chester W. Harris, eds., *Analysis of Concept Learning.* New York: Academic Press, 1944, p. 4.

[11] Imogene M. King, *Toward a Theory for Nursing.* New York: John Wiley & Sons, 1971, pp. 11-12.

[12] *Ibid.,* p. 12.

[13] Harre, *op. cit.,* p. 4.

[14] Jacox, *op. cit.,* p. 5.

[15] King, *op. cit.,* p. 12.

[16] Calvin S. Hall and Gardner Lindzey, *Theories of Personality.* New York: John Wiley & Sons, 1957, p. 9.

in interrelation."[17] If these statements are correct, we can perhaps state that concepts and theories relate, but that the words are substantially different in their meanings. Although these words are frequently utilized in the literature, they are seldom defined and so are often, and mistakenly, used interchangeably.

Generally, we can find agreement that a theory is a set of statements. The disagreement comes with discussion of the criteria for evaluating a theory.[18] This disagreement and the vagueness in theories are what cause confusion and frustration. Yet, if we can identify those characteristics in which there is some agreement, we will be able to move toward a greater understanding of the whole notion of theories.

There is a general agreement that theories fulfill three functions: description, prediction, and explanation.[19] Kerlinger's definition identifies these three functions: "A theory is a set of interrelated constructs (concepts), definitions, and propositions that present a systematic view of phenomena by specifying relations among variables, with the purpose of explaining and predicting the phenomena."[20] While Travers[21] and Brodbeck[22] also see a theory as having a predictive component, Dickoff et al. believe it is quite possible to have theories that deal with relations among states of affairs but that are not predictive in terms of a time relationship or sequence.[23] Theory is thought to be a unifying phenomenon that should cluster relevant assumptions systematically.[24],[25] Coombs and Snygg put it rather simply in stating that a theory "...is nothing more than an organization of data, or a way of looking at data, to make them meaningful."[26]

Phenix takes a somewhat different position in emphasizing that the essence of theory is vision. He describes a theory as an illuminating perspective which yields insight. He supports this notion by reminding us that the root meaning of the word, from the Greek *theoria,* signifies

---

[17] James Dickoff, Patricia James, and Ernestine Wiedenbach, "Theory in a Practice Discipline. Part I: Practice Oriented Theory." *Nursing Research;* 17:419, Sept.-Oct. 1968

[18] Frank Logan and David Olmstead, *Behavior Theory and Social Science.* New Haven: Yale University Press, 1955, p. 4.

[19] D.J. O'Connor, *An Introduction to the Philosophy of Education.* London: Routledge and Kegan, Paul, Ltd., 1957, p. 81.

[20] Fred N. Kerlinger, *Foundations of Behavioral Research.* New York: Holt, Rinehart and Winston, 1965, p. 11.

[21] Robert M. W. Travers, *An Introduction to Educational Research,* 2nd ed. New York: The Macmillan Co., 1964, p. 16.

[22] Brodbeck, *op. cit.,* p. 70.

[23] Dickoff et. al., *op. cit.,* p. 419.

[24] Hall and Lindzey, *op. cit.,* pp. 10-11.

[25] George A. Beauchamp, *Curriculum Theory,* 2nd ed. Willmette, Ill.: The Kagg Press, 1968, p. 11.

a vision.[27] Theory, then, can be thought of as an insight into the truth about reality. If utilized, this definition could make theorists of us all.

Theory is generally thought of in terms of the pure sciences such as chemistry, physics, and biology. These fields have developed theories that are capable of explaining and predicting the phenomena with which they deal. The behavioral sciences have had shorter histories and are less well defined in relation to theories.[28] Thus, theories that apply to nursing and other health-related sciences may not be able to meet all the criteria for evaluating theories.

We might apply to nursing the ideas presented in relation to the theory of instruction formulated by the Association for Supervision and Curriculum Development of the National Education Association[29]; thus, a theory of nursing would be represented by a set of statements, based on sound and replicable research, which would permit one to predict how particular changes in the clinical environment would affect nursing care.[30] This ties research and theory development together.

A nursing theory, then, should meet the following criteria:

- **It should include a set of postulates and definitions of the terms involved in these postulates.** These premises should be based on a train of reasoning and should speak directly to nursing. We have all functioned professionally as nurses, utilizing basic postulates that have all too often been untested; we do this in education, also. Such postulates generally relate to what is obvious and familiar, and it is recognized that without them we could not proceed in the development of nursing theories. Interrelating various concepts about nursing might give us significant postulates from which to develop theories.
- **It should be explicit in its boundaries and its concerns and limitations.** Although a theory represents a set of generalizations related to various concepts, it should be fully developed or formulated and should express precise and determined limitations.
- **It must be internally consistent and its concepts must have a logical set of interrelationships** resulting from inferences that are reasonably drawn from events or circumstances. These interrelationships should be seen as inevitable or predictable.

[26] Arthur A. Coombs and Donald Snygg, *Individual Behavior*. New York: Harper and Brothers, 1959, p. 7.

[27] Philip P. Phenix, "Educational Theory and Inspiration." *Educational Theory*, 13:1, January 1963.

[28] Jacox, *op. cit.*, p. 5.

[29] National Education Association, Commission on Instructional Theory, "Theories of Instruction: A Set of Guidelines." A position paper presented at the Annual Conference of the Association for Supervision and Curriculum Development, NEA, Dallas, Texas, March 1967, p. 5.

[30] *Ibid.*, pp. 16-23.

- **It should be congruent with empirical data.** A theory should coincide with previously identified and valid principles.
- **It should be capable of generating hypotheses.** Theories should generate other theories by finding new or differing relationships between concepts. The development of new theories in nursing could be generated by reviewing older concepts and /or theories that have been at least partially validated.
- **It must contain generalizations which go beyond the data.** If theory is to be meaningful to a professional group as a whole, it should allow for the practitioner to draw additional propositions from the data.
- **It must be verifiable and must be stated in such a way that it is possible to collect data to prove or disprove it.** As we develop our theories in nursing, it is important that we constantly reconfirm or substantiate them.
- **It must explain past events and predict future ones.** As we have seen from the definitions of theory, without the capacity to explain and predict, a formulation is not truly a theory.
- **Its propositions should be properly derived from the data.**

It seems appropriate at this point to ask the question, "Does nursing presently have theories of its own?" Note that the question was not *whether nursing should or should not have theories,* for the answer to that seems rather clear, if nursing claims to be a profession. On the subject of a profession's intellectual responsibilities, Dickoff and James state, "A professional cannot just watch, cannot just do, and cannot just hope or dream."[31] They go on to state that a professional or practice discipline must provide for more than mere understanding; it must provide for "conceptualization specially intended to guide the shaping of reality to that profession's professional purpose."[32]

There is controversy over whether nursing has theories of its own other than those offered by the supporting disciplines. The literature speaks freely of concepts of nursing, and it may be said that we either don't have theories about nursing or we just seem to refrain from using the word "theory." King writes that the concepts identified by nurses indicate a movement in nursing to identify and test theories in nursing.[33] It may be that to combine and relate these *concepts* through analysis, definition, and formulation of propositions in order to give them some predictive characteristics would create *theories* of nursing.

We, as nurse educators, will vary on the issue as to whether nurs-

---

[31] James Dickoff and Patricia James, "A Theory of Theories: A Position Paper." *Nursing Research,* 17:199, May-June 1968.

[32] *Ibid.*

[33] King, *op. cit.,* p. 8.

ing has theories or not, depending on the definition of theory to which we subscribe. How often have we said to ourselves or even to others, "I have a theory about that"? What we really mean is, I have some *assumptions*. Some nurses seem to accept this rather unscientific approach to theory, which would lead one to believe that almost any assumption is a sound theory. At the other end of the continuum are those who feel that the criteria to be met in evaluating theories about nursing must be as rigorous as they are for the "pure" sciences.

We have had some "theories" about nursing, for example, which have tended to classify nursing problems.[34] Homans refers to classification as the lowest form of theory.[35] Classification as a theory-building activity can be a means of organizing and integrating concepts. Dickoff et al. discuss four levels of theory,[36] with the first or basic level being "factor-isolating" theories or *naming* theories. They see this type of theory as a verbal counterpart of creating and inventing conceptual unities. Although they urge that nursing theory be of the highest, most sophisticated level, ("situation-producing" or "prescriptive" theory), they find no objection to using the term "nursing theory" to refer to the lower-level or "naming" theory.[37] Thus, we might accept the idea that, as a young profession, nursing has at the present time only low-level or unsophisticated theories. Maybe it can be said about nursing, as it has been said about the social sciences, that for a considerable period of time we will have to settle for highly tentative theories based on propositions that are really nothing more than plausible assumptions.[38]

The relationship between theory and practice in education and nursing is frequently discussed. Theory is seen as a mental exercise, while practice denotes action. As a noted philosopher maintains, "We learn how by practice, schooled indeed by criticism and example, but often quite unaided by any lessons in theory."[39] Gertzels writes, "Theories without practices, like maps without routes, may be empty; but practices without theories, like routes without maps, are blind."[40] Theory has as one of its purposes to guide practice and research by identify-

[34] Faye G. Abdellah et al., *Patient-Centered Approaches to Nursing*. New York: The Macmillan Co., 1961.

[35] George Homans, *The Human Group*. New York: Harcourt, Brace and World, 1950, p. 5.

[36] Dickoff et al., *op. cit.*, pp. 420-423.

[37] *Ibid.*, p. 423.

[38] M.H. Blaylock, Jr., *Introduction to Social Research*. Englewood Cliffs, N.J.: Prentice-Hall, Inc., 1970, p. 11.

[39] Gilbert Ryle, *The Concept of Mind*. New York: Barnes & Noble, Inc., 1949, p. 41.

[40] Jacob W. Gertzels, "Theory and Practice in Educational Administration: An Old Question Revisited," in Roald F. Campbell and James M. Lipman, eds., *Administrative Theory As a Guide to Action*. Chicago: Midwest Administration Center, University of Chicago, 1960, *Guide to Action*. Chicago: Midwest Administration Center, University of Chicago, 1960, p. 42.

ing connections and giving insights which allow the practitioners to do things they would be unable to accomplish otherwise.[41]

The criteria for the appraisal of baccalaureate and higher degree programs, prepared by the membership of the NLN Council of Baccalaureate and Higher Degree Programs, seem to make several assumptions when they speak to curriculum on both the graduate and undergraduate level.[42] These criteria speak to a curriculum focused on the theory and practice of nursing and to a curriculum plan based on a conceptual framework. Thus, the membership of the Council, in approving these criteria, have assumed that we do indeed have theories of nursing. However, one must admit that their definition of "theory," as utilized in the criteria, is unstated.

We hope this paper has been able to make the following three important points:

- The ideas of having nursing concepts and teaching theoretical foundations as related to practice are neither new, unique, nor innovative.
- The words "concept" and "theory" have a relationship but are not identical in meaning; therefore, they should not be used interchangeably. Theories are composed of a set of related concepts which have the capacity to describe, predict, and explain phenomena. Concepts involve images and are word symbols.
- Nursing presently has at least low-level theories, which can be utilized to generate new hypotheses.

Let us, as nurse educators, accept responsibility for and encourage the development of nursing theories, to be further researched, taught, and utilized as a way of moving our profession forward. Although in a sense this paper has been an exercise in semantics in attempting to give added meaning to two very significant words, let us not throw up our hands in confusion. Let us, instead, come to grips with the essential notions about these words and begin truly to communicate on some common grounds.

---

[41] Phenix, *op. cit.*, p. 2.

[42] National League for Nursing, Council of Baccalaureate and Higher Degree Programs, *Criteria for the Appraisal of Baccalaureate and Higher Degree Programs in Nursing.* New York: The League, 1972, pp. 8-9.

170

22 EDUCATIONAL TRENDS WHICH INFLUENCED THE DEVELOPMENT OF THE CONCEPTUAL FRAMEWORK WITHIN THE CURRICULUM

Helen Yura, PhD, RN and
Gertrude J. Torres, EdD, RN

Keeping up with what is going on has been, is, and will be an important preoccupation for persons in all walks of life. The economist, the fashion designer, the engineer, the merchant, the builder, and the educator alike must be tuned in to what people need and want and then must fashion the means for satifying those needs. This entails knowing what is happening in all sectors of human endeavor, for no one area is so pure as not to be influenced by what is occurring in other areas, whether directly related or not. And knowing what is going on involves looking, listening, and feeling; we can then make judgments when all the data are accumulated.

Failure to look all around for what is going on can result in decisions and solutions that fall short in resolving problems or in producing a marketable product and having it available at the right moment. Remember the tragic fate of middy skirts, when women clearly said they would not wear them because they preferred having a choice of lengths in clothes rather than having a single mode dictated to them. Some of the widespread financial disaster that might have resulted was offset by individual merchants who got the message before the designers did and thus did not stock their stores with the ill-fated garments.

Trend refers to a general tendency of events, of opinions. Tendency means an inclination to move or act in a particular direction or way; a course toward some purpose, object, or result. A trend suggests a general direction, with neither a definite course nor goal and subject to fluctuation or change caused by some external force. It is highly probable that the direction of one trend may be influenced by another trend progressing parallel to it. The reader may remember the era a few years earlier when there was a definite trend for college admissions to increase. College construction was at an all-time high and dormitories were proliferating to accommodate the increasing numbers of students. The cement was scarcely dry on these dormitories when they began to stand empty or only partially occupied. One of the reasons was a trend for college students to prefer off-campus living accommodations. Failure to look at the broader trends influencing the patterns of living of young people may have resulted in construction decisions which were inappropriate.

In identifying a trend, one must look back a bit to determine its beginnings. The discovery and substantiation of trends can be made by historians, statisticians, economists, behaviorists, educators, and perceptive individuals in all walks of life. However, there is some measure of fragility in talking about trends or designating trends.

In selecting educational trends, I will limit myself not only to those of substance with support in a number of sectors, but further to those trends which have influenced the development of the conceptual framework within the curriculum. The conceptual framework itself may have been considered a trend at an earlier time but has come to be thought of as an important dimension in curriculum development in education generally, and in nursing education specifically.

The following influential general educational trends have been detected: (1) the focus on developing curriculums for the future; (2) the increasing quality and quantity of available knowledge; (3) the increasing pressure to cope with change and complexity; and (4) the changing goals for baccalaureate education. The following important trends are more specific in nature and flow from the general trends. These are: (1) focusing on process rather than content; (2) teaching by concepts; and (3) integrating theoretical and laboratory learning experiences with emphasis on the whole person rather than on isolated parts and on whole concepts rather than on a collection of courses containing facts and information.

172

Inherent in all these trends, and perhaps responsible for the start and continuation of them, is the call for accountability. There is a demand for the best education in the same or shorter time and for the product of the educational experience to be readily marketable. Furthermore, this product is expected to contribute solutions to the problems of society by virtue of his academic involvement.

We mentioned earlier that the development of the conceptual framework itself may be regarded as a trend. As we considered the general and specific trends listed, we came to conclude that the development of the need for a conceptual framework for the curriculum was inevitable. We believe that the conceptual framework may be the very structure to operationalize accountability and that it is an effective mechanism to influence the future, to improve the selection of knowledge needed to cope with complexity and change, and to accommodate the changing goals and expectations for baccalaureate higher education. The very process of identifying and defining what concepts are relevant to the preparation of the graduate with a baccalaureate degree in nursing is really the process of specifying the very substance of nursing. Thus, what is needed is a framework of significant concepts, with a careful selection of the theoretical formulations which describe and define concepts and which contain the hypotheses that influence practice and the practitioner's choice of behaving. A conceptual framework with the accompanying theoretical formulations is modified by the practice and research that emanates from it in the same fashion as the philosophy and terminal behavioral expectations give birth to the conceptual framework.

Let us review what educational theorists, practitioners, and philosophers are saying relative to these educational trends. The future is considered a crucial variable in education. A curriculum is never developed for the past and should not emphasize the present alone. A curriculum must focus on the future in terms of what its graduates will do and, from a practical point, it must first be designed and then be implemented over a period of time. Bell states that as change accelerates and time shortens, educators must guard against the danger of being trapped in a world of the future that we do not want or one that is hostile or threatening to human life.[1] "Freedom and responsibility to know and to choose the future we want can only come from our imaginings and anticipations of the future combined with our understanding of means and ends."[2] He goes on to say that a fundamental shift in time perspective is needed to catch up with, to get ahead of, and to obtain and keep control of the vast changes that surround us. Only in this way will we obtain the power to design the future.[3]

---

[1] Wendell Bell, "Social Science: The Future as a Missing Variable," in Alvin Toffler, ed., *Learning for Tomorrow: The Role of the Future in Education*. New York: Vintage Books, 1974, p. 100.
[2] *Ibid.*, pp. 100-101.
[3] *Ibid.*, p. 101.

Lasswell tells us that accent put on future events gives new prominence to preferred events, to value goals, since the probability is perceived that some act of selection may influence the sequence of future occurrences.[4] Nurse educators must have a grasp on the direction of and the direction for the future to prevent the preparation of practitioners obsolete shortly after graduation.

Speaking about the social studies curriculum, McDaniel states that new, future-focused and change-oriented materials are desperately needed to replace the past-oriented and static materials to which most high school students continue to be exposed. He talked with students and elicited their responses to a question about the learning materials most needed to prepare them for life in the year 2001; materials included were those which help maturing individuals cope with their society, understand themselves, understand their investment in the future, see the means of affecting the direction of change, identify roles they can take in the change process, incorporate classroom learning into their immediate environment, transfer classroom learning to future responsibilities, and help mature and maturing individuals change immature institutions.[5]

Note the implications for and applicability to nursing and nursing education. Inherent in these responses is the recognition of the role of the past in creating the future. They emphasize coping and understanding and give full recognition to power and change. Changes of this nature in elementary and high school education will have repercussions for baccalaureate education generally and for nursing education specifically.

"Overchoice" (McDaniel's word for the superabundance of available choices) is a reality for the designer of educational curricula in general education and in nursing education. There is so much that *could* be taught that it is almost impossible to decide what *should* be taught. McDaniel says, "A way must be found to narrow the choices.... We can make important choices by asking questions such as what concepts, values, ideas will help us adapt to (or intelligently resist) the future? What concepts, values, ideas have helped people in the past adapt to their future?"[6] He continues with these thoughts when he says that the educator must continue this direct attack on the problem of too many choices by deciding what to exclude and what to include. To accomplish this, the educator must select concepts that are highly generalized and of wide application for the curriculum that focuses on the future.[7] It is the broad themes and concepts, tied together with theoretical formulations, that assure a grasp on change, afford continuity, and help to identify and resolve conflict and obtain

---

[4] H. Lasswell, *The Future of Political Science*. New York: Atherton, Prentice-Hall, 1963, p. 157.
[5] Michael McDaniel, "Tomorrow's Curriculum Today," in *Learning for Tomorrow, op. cit.*, p. 105.
[6] *Ibid.*
[7] *Ibid.*, p. 106

consensus from the participants in academic exercise and the citizens who are direct recipients of the services of the graduate.

It is not the purpose of education for the future to display a wide range of data or factual material, but to encourage the student to search for the organizing concepts or generalizations. It is necessary to set these concepts in a well-defined structure, so that both student and teacher can see how they are related as a system. For the future, the student's ability to use a concept is more important and will be more important than his ability to describe it.[8]

It can be said that teachers have emphasized particular knowledge at the expense of systematic knowledge. To pursue a systematic direction, we must state our assumptions about teaching—what we think people are like and what they become—for what we do in research and what we do in teaching depends on these assumptions. The curriculum of an educational program must be capable of being changed, to provide a solid core of organized concepts while nevertheless remaining open to new facts and information from many sources, so that students can move from the basic curriculum to the real environment outside the classroom to gather facts and take significant action.[9] To quote McDaniel again, "The idea currently popular in education that diversity alone can reform the curriculum is similar to the idea of automakers that a diversity of models solves the problem of good transportation; it equates relevance with immediacy rather than with ideas and gives us an 'overchoice' of 'non choices'."[10]

The crucial question, then, is: What knowlege is of most worth? It has been estimated that more than 15,000 journals are published annually and that the body of knowledge doubles annually. In the final analysis, it is that knowledge retained for potential application that is of most worth; the student needs structure to help him in this retention of knowledge. Teachers and students must concentrate on the extraction of the crucial themes and threads from significant and persistent contemporary problems. Simultaneously, the interconnections among these problems must be envisioned. Thus, there is need for a conceptual framework.

Kirschenbaum and Simon challenge us to consider other futuristic dimensions. They point out that learning for the future must deal not merely with what is possible or probable, but more crucially, with what is preferable. They go on to say that if we believe that the future is inevitable, we have no control over our public and private destinies. Any study of the future, then, must include possible, probable, and preferable futures. "This is why the broad movement aimed at shifting education into the future tense also brings with it a heightened concern with values."[11] In a world in which the amount of knowledge

---

[8] *Ibid.*

[9] *Ibid,* pp. 107-108.

[10] *Ibid.,* 109-110.

[11] Howard Kirschenbaum and Sidney Simon, "Values and the Futures Movement in Education," in *Learning for Tomorrow, op. cit.,* p. 257.

increases dramatically, making it difficult to keep pace, it follows that there is a need to change our emphasis from *what* to learn to *how* to learn.[12]

Buchen presents his views in an eloquent manner. He reminds us that the real conflict we face now is a conflict not between the old and the new, but between the new and the futuristic, between what is known and what is emerging, between the individual and the new, emerging image of what he terms "the collectivized individual."[13]

Presently, curriculums are emphasizing the processes of a discipline—the way in which the historian, the scientist, or the artist goes about investigating his subject. This represents a shift from content to process. Learning how to learn, think, and decide has become far more important than learning specific facts and data. Kirschenbaum and Simon recommend that a similar change of orientation must take place with respect to values (i.e., how to develop values, with the processes of prizing, choosing, and acting clearly defined).

Another important dimension is related to ways in which students experience and create change. For future movement in education to succeed, it must become movement for social change as well. A prerequisite to the implementation of a futuristic curriculum is effective student participation in the decision making of the college or university. Students need to develop skill in imagining possible futures, in predicting probable futures, and in deciding preferable futures.[14] This involves deciding against certain futures.

Werdell believes that the greatest public service higher education can perform is to develop graduates who can help solve society's emerging problems, who can articulate their own needs, who can understand the needs of others, and who can go on to create new goals and develop new forms of learning and doing. It is only persons so educated that will be able to assume new roles as old ones become obsolete. "Only those who have gained confidence in their own identity and direction can create healthy future goals for society. The challenge is to develop future-oriented, self-directed learners."[15] This means that every student needs an action curriculum, with learning experiences in which he can test the implications and practicality of ideas so that he can see for himself which subjects and styles of learning are relevant, so that he can generate his own ideas, select the problems he will pursue, and examine the future consequence of present action.[16]

Woodruff, who has done considerable exploration of the use of concepts in teaching and learning, states that the most useful aspect of

---

[12] *Ibid.,* p. 267.

[13] Irving Buchen. "Humanism and Futurism: Enemies or Allies?" in *Learning for Tomorrow, op. cit.,* p. 136.

[14] Philip Werdell. "Futurism and the Reform of Higher Education," in *Learning for Tomorrow, op. cit.,* p. 273.

[15] *Ibid.,* p. 286.

[16] *Ibid.,* p. 297.

this type of development is the obvious foundation it furnishes for curriculum planning and development. "It is a relatively easy step from the description of concepts as hypothetical paths of action to the concept of education as the process of acquiring concepts, and from there to the definition of curriculum as a body of perceptual and organizing experiences with the objects and events that constitute the real world."[17]

To facilitate the application of presently accepted and tested generalizations regarding teaching and learning, to advance this knowledge, and to acknowledge the importance of these generalizations, Emans believes that a conceptual framework must be developed to give direction to the application of knowledge advanced in fields related to teaching and learning.[18] This framework would identify important elements of the curriculum and the relationships between and among these elements and would indicate the organizational principles and requirements for its operationalization.

A conceptual framework should answer questions relating to the what and the how of organizing significant knowledge to fulfill the educational objectives. The problem is to plan a curriculum, bringing together the all-important understandings of theory and practice. The decisions that ensue are based on the consideration of many issues, and a decision involving one issue may affect decisions involving many others. A conceptual framework is necessary to visualize the entire complex of decisions to assure that certain considerations are not under- or overemphasized. "What seems to be needed is a framework which is so designed as to aid in continual examination, revision, and growth."[19]

Emans suggests a useful analogy when he compares the conceptual framework to a system of lighthouses at sea. "It does not tell where to go or restrict movement, but it is necessary to guide movement and warn of the danger spots."[20] He goes on to say, "American education may be at a point where advance in practice will not come about without a conceptual framework which takes into account all the forces within the curriculum."[21] Emans feels that the major concepts and themes within a framework should be fundamental to all curricula and that the closer a conceptual framework resembles reality in terms of how curricula develop, the more likely it is that the framework will be seen to have practicality.[22] This is the case for baccalaureate nursing curriculum.

---

[17] Asakel Woodruff, "The Use of Concepts in Teaching and Learning." *Journal of Teacher Education,* 15:85, March 1964.
[18] Robert Emans, "A Proposed Conceptual Framework for Curriculum Development," *Journal of Educational Research,* 59:327, March 1966.
[19] *Ibid.*
[20] *Ibid.*
[21] *Ibid.*
[22] *Ibid.*

Brennan, a social work educator, points out that conceptual and theoretical process is generally recognized as aiding the practitioner in focusing more systematically on essential factors and variables, in expanding the scope of perspectives, in explaining underlying causal dynamics, in providing leads for practice strategies, and in formulating predictive statements about probable outcomes of various treatment modalities.[23]

A number of nurse educators have stated their views on the need for a conceptual framework for the nursing curriculum. Conley points out the importance of what knowledge to select and how to organize this knowledge.[24] She says that a conceptual frame of reference of the object and process of nursing is needed to provide a guide for the selection of content. Hodgman defines the conceptual framework as a basic structure in which a complex of ideas or concepts are united so as to portray a large general idea.[25] This structure guides the selection of nursing theory presented over a span of time and gives meaning to the learning experiences chosen to correlate with theory.

In concluding, we wish to call attention to the fact that the trends described are not in conflict with each other. In fact, they are closely related, each having an impact upon the others. It appears that the conceptual framework puts it all together and operationalizes the futuristic curriculum by focusing on concepts which organize learning to achieve a particular end. These concepts are organized into a whole to facilitate conceptualization and internalization on the part of the student—all of which is directed to prepare the generalist practitioner of nursing.

The careful spelling out of the whole curriculum framework, with all its parts put together, serves as the basis for evaluation and for our accountability to the student and to the citizens who are the recipients of care.

[23] William Brennan, "The Practitioner as Theoretician." *Education for Social Work,* Spring 1973, p. 5.
[24] Virginia Conley, *Curriculum and Instruction in Nursing.* Boston: Little, Brown and Company, 1973, pp. 276-277.
[25] Eileen Hodgman, "A Conceptual Framework to Guide Nursing Curriculum." *Nursing Forum,* 7(2):114, 1973.

23 TODAY'S CONCEPTUAL FRAMEWORKS WITHIN BACCALAUREATE NURSING PROGRAMS

Helen Yura, PhD, RN
Gertrude J. Torres, EdD, RN

In earlier presentations we considered the meaning and function of concepts in nursing and the educational trends influencing the development of the conceptual framework within the curriculum. This presentation is based on the conclusion that the conceptual framework is an essential component within the nursing curriculum.

Like educators generally, nursing educators are faced with an increasing amount of knowledge and information in the biological, physical, social, and behavioral sciences and with the need to develop a futuristic curriculum. These conditions have placed a strain on the selection of content for the curriculum of the baccalaureate degree program in nursing. It is not possible to accommodate all the increased knowledge available in disciplines related to nursing. Although to attempt to do so would be an exercise in futility, recognition must be given to the *selective utilization* of theoretical content from the biological, physical, social, and behavioral sciences. This selective utilization of theory from related academic areas is but one part of the picture, however. Emphasis must also be directed toward developing theory directly from the context of professional nursing practice.

To attempt to include all facts relevant to nursing—if this were even remotely possible—or to ask the student to accumulate an assortment of such facts would have serious effects not only on the development of the student but also on the faculty's accountability to the student. Therefore, nursing educators have to choose essential components that need to be learned by the student.

The conceptual process with theoretical formulations, as noted in the model on pp. 210-211, is needed to assist the present and the potential practitioner to focus more systematically on essential factors and variables, in expanding the scope of perspective for practice in explaining causal forces, in providing leads for practice strategies, and in formulating predictive statements and hypotheses relating to outcomes of probable nursing intervention.[1]

Dorothy Johnson, in a thoughtful presentation in *Nursing Research,* states that nursing, as an occupation created by society long ago to offer a distinctive service, stands today as a field of practice without a scientific heritage and as a profession without the theoretical base it seems to require.[2] She points out that many prospective nurse scientists have had advanced education and research preparation in one or another of the basic sciences rather than in nursing and have thereby acquired the scientific orientation of the other discipline; as a result, however, the cause of nursing is not necessarily furthered.[3] She goes on to designate three alternate routes to nursing theory development. First, the laissez-faire alternative would allow each nurse scientist to follow her own scientific orientation, permitting the future course of events to evolve as it may. The second alternative is to follow medicine's path. "Progress toward a theoretical body of *nursing knowledge* via this route is inconceivable to anyone who envisions a distinctive professional identity for nursing. And without such an identity, there is little reason to be concerned about theory development at all. If nursing represents simply an area of specialized competence in medical practice, then whatever theoretical contributions nurse scientists, who do not have a medical education, might make to *medical science* are likely to be restricted along much the same lines as would hold for the basic scientist, or to be limited to technological advances."[4] The third alternative is to accept the premise that nursing has a distinctive service to offer and that the nurse's primary concern has been and is for the person who is ill, rather than for the illness itself. "It is a concern that is expressed in the attention given to patient adjustments and adaptations under the changed circumstances

[1] William Brennan, "The Practitioner as Theoretician." *Education for Social Work,* Spring, 1973, p. 5.

[2] Dorothy E. Johnson, "Development of Theory: A Requisite for Nursing as a Primary Health Profession." *Nursing Research,* 23:373, September-October, 1974.

[3] *Ibid.,* p. 374.

[4] *Ibid.,* pp. 374-375.

of illness, to coping abilities and strategies, to personalized care and patient comfort during illness, to development of life styles and behavior patterns conducive to a sense of physical, psychological, and social well-being and the like.... Patients require precisely that which nursing ... seems uniquely qualified to give: a concern for the person and assistance in living and coping with his circumstances and his environment in such a way that illness may be prevented or recovery may be facilitated."[5] She goes on to say that nursing will make a valuable and valued difference in the lives of people. "There remains the necessity of building a focused and cohesive conceptual system of the person to be served and of deriving from that system an abstract model for practice that will allow such a purpose to be fulfilled."[6]

The graduate of the baccalaureate degree program in nursing must have some framework within which to base the theory for nursing. This theory can then develop, enlarge, and continually change to maintain its relevancy. Strategic to the enveloping framework are the beliefs the nursing faculty hold about man—man the learner, man the teacher, man the citizen and recipient of nursing service—and their beliefs about nursing—nursing education and the teaching-learning process, to mention only two. It is necessary to maintain a clear focus on the nursing graduate, keeping in mind the descriptive behavioral statements that identify the end product of the baccalaureate degree program in nursing. These statements clearly delineate what the graduate will be like, what the graduate can do and with whom.

Further, the careful selection of concepts and theories for the baccalaureate nursing curriculum based on the philosophy, objectives, and behavioral expectations can lessen the gap between theory and practice by providing the framework to guide the practitioner's continuing function of bringing order out of the sometimes chaotic proliferation of knowledge, concepts, theories, and models.[7] In addition the conceptual framework may be viewed as the *keystone* for the total curriculum framework.

Recently, baccalaureate nursing educators have focused on integrating the nursing content of the program. This is generally thought to reduce the possibility of teaching the same content in several nursing courses and thus to allow more time to give the student a greater amount of available knowledge. This supports the notion that students need to learn related concepts rather than a collection of facts.

In the last few years, there has been an ever-increasing emphasis on identifying a conceptual framework for the nursing curriculum. In March 1972, members of the NLN Council of Baccalaureate and Higher

---

[5] *Ibid.*, p. 375.
[6] *Ibid.*
[7] Brennan, *op. cit.*, p. 7.

Degree Programs approved its *Criteria for the Appraisal of Baccalaureate and Higher Degree Programs in Nursing* and included a criterion stating that curriculum should be based on a conceptual framework.[8] Nursing programs throughout the country have identified such frameworks. However, there seems to be confusion in the use of terms, especially in relation to such words and terms as "concept," "conceptual," "theoretical," "unifying threads" and "strands." Educators often use these words interchangeably, with a resulting confusion.

Thus, in order to identify concepts commonly held by nursing faculty and the terms in which they are expressed, the writers surveyed a sample of baccalaureate nursing programs accredited by the NLN Board of Review for Baccalaureate and Higher Degree Programs in 1972-73. Fifty programs articulating a conceptual framework were easily found. The majority of these had written self-evaluation reports based on the 1972 *Criteria*.

It seems necessary at this point to dwell on some of the terms discussed earlier. A *concept* is a general notion or a symbol, and it is the function of symbols to give structure to the curriculum, so that its parts can be fitted and united into the entire program. A *theory* is an hypothesis involving an interesting idea or opinion; the word "theory" is synonymous with "conjecture," "contemplation," or "guess." Theories differ significantly from principles or laws in that the latter are based on scientific or empirical data. Therefore, a *theoretical formulation* consists of an hypothesis which is either speculative, partially tested, or untested and which may give a plausible, though unproven, explanation to a concept or relationship between concepts. Since notions and symbols are different from hypotheses, which could lead to principles and laws, it seems inappropriate to use the terms "concept" and "theory," "conceptual framework" and "theoretical framework" interchangeably. Thus, if faculty were to use the term "conceptual framework" rather than "theoretical framework" in relation to curriculum and then to identify appropriate theoretical formulations *within* the conceptual framework, there would be a greater clarity in the use of terms. These definitions have been used in analyzing the conceptual frameworks in the self-evaluation reports encountered in this study.

Curriculum development involves both concepts and theories, which are mirrors of the philosophy, program objectives, and terminal behavioral expectations of the program. Let us imagine a large box (see Figure 1) which has as its outer covering the philosophy, objectives, and terminal behavioral expectations of a particular program. The middle layer is the conceptual framework, and the core is the theories identified

[8] National League for Nursing, Department of Baccalaureate and Higher Degree Programs, *Criteria for the Appraisal of Baccalaureate and Higher Degree Programs in Nursing.* New York: The League, 1972, p. 8

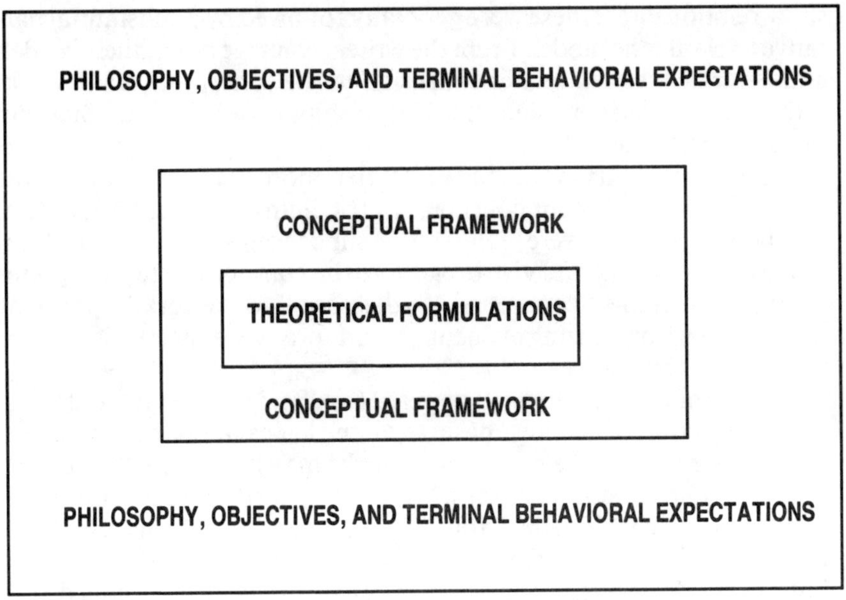

Figure 1. Theoretical formulations within the curriculum.

by faculty as most related to the outer shells. We can call this inner core the theoretical formulations, which give guidance to the entire nursing content. The notions or symbols that nursing educators believe to be intrinsic to nursing give rise to the theoretical formulations which represent their hypotheses about the concepts they have identified.

The conceptual frameworks under review covered a broad range of development. At the most primitive level was the mere statement, without any development, that a particular conceptual framework would be used. At the other end of the spectrum was the well-developed conceptual framework which clearly incorporated the program's philosophy, contributed to the ordering and selection of theoretical content for learning, and provided a rationale for learning experiences to develop, hold, and implement theory. In the latter instance, the conceptual framework could clearly be seen at every level, in every course, and in each learning experience.

Each conceptual framework in the study was analyzed for components, themes, topics, and threads. These, in turn, were grouped and organized according to similarities, commonalities, and subgroupings. Respondents frequently used a diagrammatic approach to the conceptual framework, with spirals, boxes, and straight and broken lines to

183

show relationships; these were generally followed by a substantial narrative to clarify the model. From the writers' vantage point, these models and diagrams tended to add confusion to the conceptual framework, rather than to clarify it, since the relationships between and among concepts were unclear.

Most curriculums in the study reflected more than one concept; the average was three to four concepts. Curriculums which utilized greater numbers of concepts were really stating subconcepts and theoretical formulations to clarify and give breadth to the concepts. A few programs attempted to define "conceptual," "theoretical framework," "unifying threads," or "organizing elements," and some gave their rationale for using these approaches.

The major concepts identified were Man, Society, Health, and Nursing. These concepts seemed basic to all the baccalaureate nursing programs reviewed. While some frameworks may have focused more intensity on one or another of these concepts, the fifty frameworks in this study generally included all four. Thus, it can be said that *most* baccalaureate nursing programs identify a common conceptual framework, but the development, emphasis, and priority of these concepts differ. The identification, clarification, and development of the subconcepts and/or theoretical formulations related to the major concept for a particular curriculum establish the uniqueness of the particular baccalaureate nursing curriculum.

Concepts and Subconcepts

Man. Many subconcepts were identified by nursing educators in the study under the larger concept "man," thus giving greater meaning to the whole. "Man" was basically seen as a bio-psycho-social-spiritual being, holistic and unique. Theoretical formulations most frequently identified in relation to "Man," related to man and his needs (especially Maslow's Hierarchy of Needs); man as developmental; man and change; man as learner; man as a system; and man and his relationships with others.

Society. The subconcepts related to "Society" focused on man's environment, on the family, the community, the nation, and the universe. Theoretical formulations involved man in a changing society; man as a member of a family; man as a system; and man communicating.

Health. The subconcepts related to "Health" were wellness and illness. These were used in relation to words such as continuum, level, spectrum, and cycle. Theoretical formulations included stress, crisis, homeostasis, promotion, and prevention.

Nursing. The major subconcept under "Nursing" was the nursing process; almost all respondents included this subconcept. Other subconcepts included role and functions. Theoretical formulations were drawn from communication, decision making, leadership, and systems.

Figure 2 summarizes the concepts, subconcepts, and theoretical formulations found in the survey and analysis. It should be noted that some theoretical formulations frequently related to more than one major concept.

While one or two concepts, subconcepts, or theories might have been listed by the nursing faculty, frameworks that were sufficiently developed to be subjected to analysis revealed all four major concepts, even though these were not designated as such or were subordinated to a specific theory.

The analysis seemed to substantiate a difference in meaning between concept and theory, emphasizing that while they are not interchangeable, they are closely related, complementary to each other, and necessary to give explanation and focus to the specific content selected for learning in nursing.

Brennan, a social work educator, tells us that many concepts, theories, and ideas borrowed from other fields still exist in an overly abstract, untested, and untestable form and emanate from a mulitiplicity of contexts quite different from those in which the professional practitioner actually functions.[9] No constellation of concepts nor any one theory can possibly exhaust the infinite variability of human behaviors found in the practice setting. However, there appears to be some agreement that certain concepts and theoretical formulations have more support and popularity than others, based on the beliefs about professional nursing practice at this point in time. It would be expected that modification of theory—really *theoretical formulations*—would be necessary to accommodate the area of nursing practice. Practice, being a concrete expression of abstract theory, necessarily presses toward a clarification of the scope and meaning of concepts and aids the expansion of theory by incorporating into it new concepts and new elements resulting from the insights gained in professional practice.[10]

Dorothy Johnson emphasizes that ". . . as long as the conceptual system for understanding is reasonably sound scientifically, the question of 'truth' plays no part in judging a model for nursing practice, education, and research based on that conceptual system. The question of whether any model is right or wrong *for nursing* is a social decision, and criteria extrinsic to the substance of the model must be utilized."[11]

---

[9] Brennan, *op. cit.*, p. 8.
[10] *Ibid.*
[11] Johnson, *op. cit.*, p. 376.

Major Concepts	MAN	SOCIETY	HEALTH	NURSING
Subconcepts	Bio-psycho Social Spiritual being	Family Community Nation Universe	Illness Wellness	Nursing Process Role Function
Theoretical Formulations	Communication Theory Need Theory Developmental Theory Change Theory Learning Theory Behavior Theory Systems Theory Interpersonal Theory	Communication Theory Family Theory Role Theory Change Theory Systems Theory	Stress Theory Adaptation Theory Crises Theory Change Theory Systems Theory	Communication Theory Decision Theory Role Theory Change Theory Learning Theory Leadership Theory Systems Theory Interpersonal Theory

Figure 2. Major concepts identified within baccalaureate nursing programs. *

*Source: Gertrude Torres and Helen Yura, *Today's Conceptual Framework: Its Relationship to the Curriculum Process.* New York: National League for Nursing, 1974, p. 6.

Thus, the identification of the specific concepts and the designation of selected theories from other disciplines most appropriate for the delivery of nursing services and the precise identification of the nursing process show the greatest promise for the development of substantive nursing theory.

The survey and analysis reported here support the need for a conceptual framework and acknowledge the vision of the nursing faculty members who sanctioned the importance of the conceptual framework when they voted its acceptance as one of the accreditation criteria. Support is seen for some of the convictions held by nursing faculty about man, society, health, and nursing. The uniqueness and individuality of the nursing program were seen in the selection, focus, relation-combinations, emphasis, and definitions of concepts, subconcepts, and theoretical formulations utilized. Hopefully, these were then incorporated by the students, who continued to develop the concepts, subconcepts, and theoretical formulations with the ideas, processes, and events basic to the baccalaureate degree program in nursing and possibly to their life style.

BIBLIOGRAPHY

Brennan, William, "The Practitioner as Theoretician," *Education for Social Work,* Spring, 1973.

Copi, Irving, *Introduction to Logic.* New York: The Macmillan Co., 1961.

Johnson, Dorothy E., "Development of Theory: A Requisite for Nursing As a Primary Health Profession," *Nursing Research,* 23:372-377, September-October 1974.

Lackman, Sheldon, *The Foundations of Science.* New York: Vintage Press, 1960.

Smith, Vincent E., *The Elements of Logic.* Milwaukee: The Bruce Publishing Co., 1957.

24 THE CONCEPTUAL FRAMEWORK AND ITS INFLUENCE ON LEARNING EXPERIENCES

Gertrude J. Torres, EdD, RN
Helen Yura, PhD, RN

It seems essential to start this paper with a workable definition of a learning experience. Broadly conceived, a learning experience could represent any activity, within or outside the institution of higher learning, in which the student engages and which has an effect on his or her meeting both college and program objectives. This approach sees the college as a total community and life experiences as having a significant impact on learning.

We, as nurse educators in curriculum development, tend to identify learning experiences in a more narrowly conceived context. Viewed in this manner, learning experiences are those planned activities that are provided by the faculty both inside and outside the classroom and that support the meeting of specific course objectives. The greatest impact in support of the conceptual framework can be made in the classroom, where the content is either presented or reinforced by a variety of teaching methods, and where the student is often given the base on which other learning experiences can be built. All too often in nursing the major focus in the classroom is on science content and on offering concepts of medical science rather than on nursing and its related concepts and theories. Without an emphasis on the conceptual framework in the classroom, students will have difficulties utilizing concepts and theories outside the classroom.

Learning experiences outside the classroom include activities in the clinical laboratory as well as those activities frequently carried out independently by the student, such as term papers, group projects, research studies, community analysis activities, case studies, reading activities, and learning laboratories with audio-visual aids. All have become significant aspects of the total learning activity.

Out-of-class activities represent a significant investment in time and effort on the part of both faculty and student and are viewed as an essential component of all nursing courses. Our beliefs that nursing is both a science and an art and that it consists of cognitive, interactive, and technical skills support our commitment that learning experiences must take place beyond the college and beyond the classroom. It is through these learning experiences that we truly communicate to the students our beliefs about learning, man, society, health, and nursing. The selection of experiences in terms of frequency and priorities, as well as the tools we use to evaluate the learning that has occurred, gives strong clues as to the faculty's real beliefs.

The ways in which the conceptual framework affects learning experiences is an essential measure of its effectiveness within the curriculum. For if the faculty do not utilize the conceptual framework in making decisions about the types and amounts of specific learning experiences, its development may have served no useful purpose.

Behavioral level and course objectives, as noted in Model I (pp. 210-211), dictate course content and learning experiences. Yet, special efforts are needed, even with well-developed objectives, to ensure that the concepts and theories identified within the conceptual framework become an integral part of each learning experience.

Let us once again review Figure 2, p. 186, which represents the major concepts identified within baccalaureate nursing programs. Assuming that the students have been well grounded in the theories identified in their general education, science, and nursing courses, the question is how to ensure that these theories are implemented in all learning experiences. Out-of-class written projects and assignments, which frequently represent a significant effort on the part of students and faculty, especially in terms of time, should be oriented around specific theoretical formulations. For example, term papers done early in the student's educational program could have as their emphasis a thorough search of the literature as related to specific theories and their implications for nursing in general. Later papers developed by the students could require an incorporation of theories into the nursing process as practiced in the clincal setting. For example, in the care of the child, the student would incorporate various developmental theories in her assessment, intervention,

190

and care of the child. In a family study, the assessment could include adaptation, change, and interpersonal theories, if such are identified within the conceptual framework. In a community health study, many social and behavioral theories could be utilized as a frame of reference. Thus, all types of independent written activities could clearly support the conceptual framework.

Other out-of-class activities that may also be considered learning experiences include the use of audio-visual equipment, usually within some type of learning center. The selection of the software, such as cassettes and film strips, should be done in full recognition of the need to implement the conceptual framework. If the student spends hours reviewing filmstrips related to specific technical skills, but with no scientific involvement of the related theories, how can we later expect her to utilize the conceptual framework as she practices? We must keep in mind that conceptual framework in essence represents the faculty's beliefs about nursing in its totality.

Textbooks and references can be two of the most significant factors in either implementing or failing to implement the conceptual framework. Nursing texts should be selected which will assist the professional student in identifying basic scientific principles and theories which support the conceptual framework. The use of any single text within a given period of time seems self-limiting, since no one author or group of authors would incorporate the concepts and theories identified within a specific curriculum. It would seem that a variety of texts and references would be needed and that these should be identified at the time the conceptual framework is developed.

If the conceptual framework is to be implemented, one of the most important learning experiences where it must be reflected is the clinical laboratory experience. As an extension of the classroom essential if course objectives are to be met, laboratory experiences are selected in terms of the course objectives and generally reflect a variety of settings throughout the program. Two aspects need to be considered in the selection of the specific clinical environments to be utilized by the students. These are the type of agency or setting and the specific types of experiences within each setting. Without serious consideration to the type of setting, it would be difficult, if not impossible, to obtain the specific experiences that are essential in meeting objectives. Furthermore, although the setting may be appropriate, the experiences selected may be inappropriate.

The frequency with which a setting is utilized relates not only to the number of students to be accomodated, but also to the types of concepts and theories being stressed. For example, if the conceptual framework strongly emphasizes health and its promotion, the majority of the health agencies utilized as settings within the program should have similar objectives—the maintenance and promotion of health. This would contraindicate the use of the acute care setting as a base for most experiences in such a program. Approaching laboratory experiences with a defined conceptual framework in mind frees us from the rigidity of seeing the acute care setting as the most significant environment for meeting objectives. We might add that, when service agencies and educational programs share similar philosophies and objectives, both groups are better able to meet health care needs.

None of the theories identified in Figure 2, p. 186, is specifically oriented toward any one setting. Many theories can best be understood and applied to practice outside the crisis setting. Even crisis theory can be implemented in settings other than hospitals. If we utilize the nursing process in relation to change and communication theories, for example, we can identify unlimited environments in which the student can reinforce her learning.

Clinical learning experiences can also include a variety of observer activities to reinforce concepts and theories. For example, attending an Alcoholics Anonymous meeting, or an ileostomy group meeting can reinforce theories such as adaptation, change, and stress. Visiting hotels that cater to the aged can reinforce communication, interactive, and developmental theories. Observing an industrial setting for an understanding of its health and safety policies can give the student a deeper understanding of need and organization theories. Although there are many different types of observational and participant-observer approaches that can be used in a multitude of settings, what is truly important is that the student understand why she is in the particular setting and which concepts and theories she should be most concerned about. These experiences require preparation of the student by faculty prior to the experience and an opportunity for the student in a group to synthesize her learning. Since not all students have identical experiences, faculty need not be present during these observations, thus giving the student an opportunity for more independence.

At times faculty will need to create learning experiences when a particular community does not offer the type of setting needed. For instance, if a conceptual framework includes concepts and theories related to *healthy* families and the available community agencies focus only on families where there is an *ill* component, methods will have to be identified to find well families for pertinent clinical experiences. One method could be to present a Health Fair at the college, where citizens could obtain health screening; families attending could then be requested to allow students to visit them. Faculty can also contact local physicians and clergy about obtaining such families. In rural areas, faculty might suggest to local mayors that students offer a store-front nursing service to focus on health maintenance. The concept of creating learning experiences is rather new to nursing. Although many may feel this will require funds which are unavailable, costs can be minimized. Since colleges have long supported science laboratories for students, why not a nursing laboratory within or outside the campus community?

Let us summarize the major points made about learning experiences as related to a conceptual framework:

- Learning experiences represent activities within and outside the classroom that are organized in order to assist the student to meet course objectives.
- Decisions related to the type and frequency of all experiences should support the specific concepts and/or theories identified as most significant to nursing by the faculty.
- Differing approaches to identifying more diverse types of experiences should be utilized to support the conceptual framework.

25 THE CONCEPTUAL FRAMEWORK AS A COMPONENT OF CURRICULUM DEVELOPMENT

Rose P. McKay, EdD, RN

The identification of a conceptual framework is based on the implicit assumption that the highly complex decisions required in designing and implementing a nursing curriculum are made more effective when this requirement is an integral part of the process. The framework defines the relationships among the factors involved in the program. It identifies priority concepts, indicates logical sequence for course progression, and implies the method of inquiry, the nature of the support required, and the format of the evaluation. The value of these operations, which provide structure for the selection of learning experiences and teaching strategies, is that while the resulting pattern may fall short of the standards for a theoretical framework it provides an absolutely essential component for program development in nursing.

The need for a logical design on which to base curriculum decisions is more crucial than the extent to which it is theoretical (i.e., empirically based, cumulative, nonethical, parsimonious, systematic, and explanatory). Theory is characterized by a deductively connected set of assumptions from which additional generalizations may be derived and by which a variety of seemingly unrelated empirical phenomena are explained. Concepts describe a characteristic that is the same in different individuals or objects. To be most useful, a concept should be defined so that instances can be identified and the relationships between this particular characteristic and others can be postulated. A conceptual framework is not necessarily at the level of a theoretical model but it does provide a logical boundary for decisions.

Bruner,[1] in discussing the nature of the educative process, identified the following points: structure, rather than facts or techniques, is important in the teaching-learning process; the basic ideas from science and the humanities are as simple as they are powerful and can be identified and used (an important point in career ladder programs) in increasingly complex situations; the intellectual technique of arriving at plausible but tentative formulations is a part of productive thinking; and interest in learning must be stimulated. Of these four—structure, readiness, intuition, and interest—the one of most concern to us is structure. If we agree that understanding fundamentals makes a subject more comprehensible, that we remember facts when they are integrated into a pattern, that knowledge of fundamental principles and ideas serves as a model for understanding other like things, and that this type of emphasis reduces the problem of becoming rapidly outdated as knowledge advances, we must agree that the nursing curriculum should be determined by understanding the underlying principles that give structure to that subject.

Well-established fields of knowledge have the following characteristics: well-defined central methods of inquiry; clearly stated princples, generalizations, and theories; a hierarchy of concepts; a constantly growing body of knowledge; and a group of workers who are in agreement about the nature of the process of investigation and who have become experts in the application of these methods in a variety of situations. It might be said that nursing has at least the following components as a subject-matter field:

1. A substantial body of time-tested ideas.

2. A technique suitable for dealing with these concepts.

3. A defensible claim to being an intimate link with basic human activities and aspirations.

4. A tradition that links the present with the past and provides inspiration and sustenance for the future.

---

[1] Jerome Bruner, *The Process of Education*. New York: Vintage Press, 1963.

Even if a field is not yet recognized as scientific, it can become more so as it builds up its dependable generalizations. If we can accept this approach, then, it is necessary to develop tools to deal with the subject matter at hand. These tools are not the facts or techniques of the field but the generalizations and concepts which result from asking, "What is essential content?"

We have, then made the following points:

1. Knowledge is acquired as it is integrated into some structure or pattern.

2. Teaching is effective when the subject matter is related to the essential structure of a field of knowledge.

3. A conceptual structure can be identified from which the appropriate concepts and generalizations develop.

4. There is a recognized mode of inquiry within nursing which is used by practitioners in the application of knowledge to presenting problems.

This approach—trying to identify the essential content, the key concepts, and the methods of inquiry—would seem to be an important step for nursing in this time of rapid growth in scientific knowledge, change in health services, transition in educational preparation for the profession, and in particular our interest in development of our knowledge base. The identification of this framework seems to be a necessary effort before we as educators can talk about the competencies required for professional practice.

As long as a field has a strong theoretical component that provides a base accepted by all, there is no problem. We see this clearly illustrated in fields like mathematics or physics. In other, less sophisticated disciplines, where the theoretical structure is not so clearly defined, it may be more difficult to organize instruction around the conceptual approach (e.g., anthropology). In a profession like nursing, where we are concerned with human interactions, it is even more difficult to delineate.

The figure below presents a Model for Process of Curriculum Development which reviews where the conceptual framework is located in regard to the other components of the process.

We have usually started the process of curriculum development by making a statement of our beliefs and values. While such an effort may be an essential step, it does not, by itself, add to the conceptual validity of our framework. Such a statement of philosophy may influence the choice of which concepts become part of our framework,

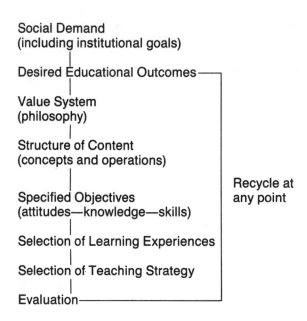

Figure 1. Model for process of curriculum development.

but it is not itself an integral part of the conceptual structure.

The basis for building a conceptual framework, then, is the structure of nursing knowledge and the methods of inquiry used in practice. It requires an explicit definition of nursing and of the nursing process. Analysis of various definitions of nursing clearly outline its knowledge base. Practice depends not only on knowledge from the physical, biological, social, and behavioral sciences, but on the results of clinical nursing research which are becoming more available to us. The importance of defining the scope, outcomes, and methods of practice is that, once these statements have been made, the arrangement of knowledge needed to operationalize them will lead not only to new insights but to the pattern or design which will guide curriculum development.

A well-developed framework does not merely provide a list of high priority concepts: it makes a serious attempt to explicate the relationships among the components and project the design into the nature of presenting patient and family problems encountered in clinical practice.

The following kinds of questions can assist faculty to formulate a systematic design which will support curriculum decision making about the priorities, categories, scope, language, and process of nursing knowledge (it might also be helpful in interdisciplinary efforts to define common courses or programs):

1. What is scope? What limits or boundaries prevail? What is the subject matter of the field? (For nursing, is it illness, wellness, interpersonal relations, maintenance and/or support of system adaptations to environmental stress?)

2. What are the methods of inquiry? Observation, application of projected estimates, refining and recycling, cooperative planning, assessment, instruction.

3. What are the key concepts which characterize the field? Probability, open system, ecology, steady state, perception, ethnic group, disease, patient.

4. How are these key concepts organized?
   a)   Priority of order. Life, education, adjustment. Is the value system reflected?
   b)   Interrelationships or patterns.
   c)   Hierarchical arrangements. Are they the same for all areas—maternal-child nursing, medical-surgical, psychiatric, community health?

5. How are principles defined in the field?
   a)   What are the generalizations—scientific, ethical, technological?
   b)   What is the place of laws—scientific, evolutionary, hereditary?
   c)   What is the nature of the theories—predictive, prescriptive, or hortatory?

6. What are the nature and classification of presenting problems? These may be defined by utilizing a combination of priority concepts and methods of inquiry to define the nature and scope.

Examples of Concept Development

I would like first to present an example of concept development from physical science. One aspect of physics is concerned with how motion occurs or with the metrical (measurable) aspects of the world—particularly with change. It is dependent on sense data (i.e., observation). Several derivative concepts are based on the three central concepts at the most general level—mass, distance, time.

At the second level, speed is derived from distance and time:

$$\frac{\text{distance}}{\text{time}} = \text{speed}$$

At the third level, we can identify another instance of relationship between concepts:

$$\frac{\text{difference in speed}}{\text{time}} = \text{acceleration}$$

In nursing, general concepts are health, man, society. At the secondary level, we can define other concepts:

$$\frac{\text{man}}{\text{society}} = \text{individual differences}$$

$$\frac{\text{society}}{\text{man}} = \text{cultural groups}$$

$$\frac{\text{society}}{\text{health}} = \text{norms for health behavior in different conditions}$$

At the third level, we can project as follows:

$$\frac{\text{norms for health behavior in different conditions}}{\text{individual differences}} = \text{assessment}$$

The characteristics of scientific knowledge are that it is: (1) empirical, (2) theoretical, (3) cumulative, (4) nonethical, (5) controlled, and (6) systematic. The advantages for nursing when knowledge is scientific are too obvious to explain in detail. Its contribution to research teaching and practice is extremely desirable. But what other characteristics of nursing knowledge exist? It is always best to conceptualize it only in the mode of science? Is nursing knowledge ever intuitive, applied, specific, moral?

There are limitations of scientific content as the only base for nursing curriculum:

1. Scientific content does not include that nursing knowledge which is specific, concrete, and skill-oriented. Knowing "what" is the specific base; but much of nursing is based on knowing "how," which is not essentially scientific. In the same sense, information and performance are different.

2. It does not include value-oriented requirements for professional behavior (e.g., ethical concepts of right–wrong, ought, should, better). Statements of this sort are *prescriptions*. Given an ethical dilemma for a nurse—a value conflict—what knowledge guides her action? Is it scientific or ethical?

200

3. Scientific knowledge minimizes the importance of intuitive clinical judgments based on non-theory-oriented experience (but it does lead to more sophisticated insights). The fact that practitioners must act even when there is little scientific support for decision emphasizes the utility of the intuitive approach mentioned here.

4. Scientific knowledge challenges tradition, history, and ritual as a source for empirical evaluation of nursing care. Yet, what percentage of current evaluation in nursing relies on a predictable theoretical basis? To differentiate between science and tradition may be more important as research efforts give a broader base for predictable interventions. The Quality Assurance Program, even if retrospective, may also affect this point. Meanwhile many activities in practice reflect the nonscientific basis for practice decisions. Students must learn some of these activities as our efforts to insure performance competence according to employer standards increasingly affect curricular decisions.

5. Scientific knowledge is abstract and general, while practice is specific and individual. How is the application made?

6. Scientific knowledge includes probability statements as accepted generalizations; these alone cannot guide practice. The specific instance may be the exception.

7. Legal knowledge also directs and guides practice.

8. Science is but one form of knowledge. As we have shown, there are others that may be important in nursing and that probably should be a part of the framework.

Nursing includes believing, knowing, and doing. A nurse acts with:

- Integrity, when she acts according to professional values.
- Understanding—with knowledge when she knows the rationale for and the probable results of actions.
- Skill—high correlation between intentions and results of actions.

Sources of knowledge may then include:

- Values from philosophy, religion, ethics (this learning may even be based on observation of role models).
- Knowledge from science.
- Methods of practice (at least partly from subtleties of interpersonal relations and mastery of techniques, both technological and cognitive).

Once the major concepts are identified, additional actions to clarify the structure, as considered in light of the conceptual framework, might be:

1. Define the life process or other selected processes.
2. Identify the goals of nursing regarding these processes.
3. Describe the nature of the nurse-patient interaction.
4. Describe the process of nursing intervention (i.e., the methodology of nursing):
   a) the classification of types of stages of nursing action;
   b) sequence or cycle of stages of action.

5. Classify the types of patient problems according to this conceptual formulation—define health, illness, disease, death, recovery, disability.

6. Develop a category system for dealing with health, illness, or deviations, kinds of disequilibrium, a taxonomy of nursing diagnostic conditions.

7. Develop a category system for dealing with the components of a particular clinical problem area (i.e., taxonomy of nursing diagnostic labels for a specialized area—different health behaviors for different health conditions, such as pregnancy).

8. Define the nursing process according to this formulation (i.e., method of inquiry).

9. Identify the most important concepts in your current courses—describe them according to language of the conceptualization.

10. Describe the relationship to other health professionals or the way this formulation views nursing in relationship to medicine or social work.

11. Consider implications for the curriculum patterns. What kind of courses do you visualize? Design plan for program.

12. Identify the system boundaries for your course (sequential, conceptual, methodological).

13. What outcomes do you expect from each course? Describe content of courses.

The development of the conceptual framework, though crucial, is only one part of curriculum process. The most characteristic activity in program development seems to be the series of options about which choices have to be made. As the definition of the professional values and goals is influenced by the constraints of the current social environment and the institutional setting (e.g., affirmative action programs and budget), so the selection of the learning experiences is affected not only by the average abilities and interests of students, but also by the variety and location of clinical learning opportunities. For example, if intrapartal and ill-child experiences are limited, what variations are developed—simulation, group assignments, eliminate completely for some sudents, alternative experiences planned? If student language abilities or cultural norms are divergent, what strategies are developed to handle these issues? It has been suggested by Chater[2] that the concepts and theories related to both students and setting (e.g., selection of a particular learning theory or the nature of administrative organization) are an integral part of the conceptual framework itself. An alternative approach is to consider the options and constraints related to these components as input variables that significantly affect the total program. The critical point is that these are factors that cannot be overlooked in the process of curriculum development.

We could say, perhaps, that the structure of nursing knowledge includes the key concepts and generalizations around which content is organized and that the methods of inquiry are to be found in the nature of the professional practice. In this way we may even see that we have an advantage over some other fields. For example, instead of debating the relative merits of the problem-centered vs. the subject-matter approach, we may take the position that the scientific, abstract, and possibly ethical content of nursing is organized as a part of the framework and that problem solving (or, as we define it, the nursing process) is a generally agreed upon method of inquiry. We might also say that we have had an extensive trial of the broad-areas approach (e.g., Medical-Surgical Nursing, which developed from the integration of separate subjects such as Orthopedic, Gynecological, Ear, Nose and Throat, and Emergency Nursing). This pattern, which resulted from transplanting medical specialties into the nursing functions related to them, has been recently considered inadequate as the nursing profession assumes more distinctive and independent functions.

Attempts to define an "integrated" approach to the organization of the subject matter of nursing have had great popularity. However, I believe we are not at a recycle point, where for various reasons we may be returning to a more traditional subject area format, at least for the last part of the nursing program. Even if this is true, the need to define the priority concepts, generalizations, and operational modes of knowledge application within these historical divisions of subject matter in nursing still exists, and the need for adequate concepts to formulate statements of nursing care outcomes is crucial. Whether the

---

[2] Shirley Chater, "A Conceptual Framework as a Basis for Decisions about Teaching Strategies," in *Exploring Nontraditional Study: Changing Strategies for Changing Times,* COGEN Workshop Proceedings, Burlingame, California, 1973.

primary divisions are stress, developmental stages, nursing process, hospital geography, or medical diagnostic categories, the major structural organization must be expanded by defining priority concepts, relationships, clinical instances, and performance strategies according to terms operationally defined for nursing in areas where it can control access and intervention.

Summary

Nursing as a subject area (or profession) is based on the claim of a social need for our specialized *knowledge*. This knowledge has structure and process or method of inquiry which require consistent efforts to outline and organize. The identification of this structure and process is central to the question of what is the composition of a nursing curriculum. Curriculum has been defined by Johnson[3] as a structural series of intended learning outcomes. These outcomes can be categorized as knowledge, skills, and values; they can be classified as cognitive, psychomotor, and affective; and they may be described behaviorally and evaluated in that way.

Selection is basic to the development of a curriculum and this is determined by :(1) values which define the worth of the knowledge chosen for inclusion; (2) structure of scientific knowledge in the field, which defines priority of concept; (3) agreed upon process of practice; (4) professional norms for right behavior; (5) expected levels of technical competence and speed; and (6) institutional norms and goals, which affect the scope and balance of the selection. Evaluation and recycling are required continuously.

Efforts to include application of curriculum theory and nursing theory are not easy since both are relatively undeveloped. Slogans are generalizations with emotional appeal that offer implications but are not prediction as theories.[4] They may be useful, however, as long as the nature of the generalization is clear (e.g., primary care, leadership role, practitioner). Defining connections between the conceptual and the abstract and their application in practice is the reason for selecting learning experiences and designing instructional strategy as integral parts of curriculum process. The structure and priority of concepts defines the objectives and design of the program. The processes of practice and the relationship of these to the concepts define the clinical experiences. Content in nursing includes both conceptual forms and applications in practice; otherwise, there is abstract learning with no reality or rote practice with no prediction.

[3] Mauritz Johnson, "Definitions and Models in Curriculum Theory." *Educational Theory*, 17:127-140, April 1967.

[4] Komisar, Paul and McClellan, "The Logic of Slogans," in B.D. Smith and R.H. Emmes, eds., *Language and Concepts in Education*. Chicago: Rand McNally, 1961.

BIBLIOGRAPHY

Harms, Mary, *Development of a Conceptual Framework for a Nursing Curriculum.* Atlanta: Southern Regional Education Board, 1969.

King, Arthur, and Brownwell, John, *The Curriculum on the Disciplines of Knowledge.* New York: John Wiley and Sons, 1966.

Phenix, Philip, *Realms of Meaning.* New York: McGraw-Hill, 1964.
Schwab, Joseph, "The Concept of the Structure of a Discipline," *The Educational Record,* July 1962, pp. 197-205.

26 THE CONCEPTUAL FRAMEWORK AS PART OF THE CURRICULUM PROCESS

Gertrude J. Torres, EdD, RN
Helen Yura, PhD, RN

This paper will discuss the place and influence of the conceptual framework, with its theoretical formulations, in the entire curriculum process. Certain assumptions have been made to insure that the conceptual framework is truly functional within the curriculum, for if it is not functional, we are engaging in needless rhetoric. These assumptions are:

- That the curriculum process is an effective guide to the development and maintenance of a sound nursing program on both the undergraduate and graduate levels.
- That theories in nursing, the arts, and the sciences are fundamental to all baccalaureate and master's nursing programs, but that the emphasis and selection of certain theories give uniqueness to each program.
- That professional nursing has a unique body of knowledge, as do other health care disciplines, through its combinations and use of certain theories.
- That the further clarification of the conceptual framework within the nursing program can assist the profession of nursing in organizing its body of knowledge and can give greater direction to research.

- That the core of nursing programs might be identified as man in society as related to the health care system and the contribution of nursing to man, to society, and to the health care system.

In looking at Model I, we can see the philosophy of the institution and the nursing program, as well as the characteristics of the graduates, gives direction to the conceptual framework and theoretical formulations. The horizontal and vertical strands, the level behavioral objectives, then the course behavioral statements and descriptions must take into account the conceptual framework. Thus, the conceptual framework, through its identification of concepts and theories, gives increased clarity and direction to the program's philosophy so that it can be clearly developed into courses and learning experiences. We might think of the curriculum process as representing a continuum going frm the philosophy all the way to the identification of specific learning experiences, with the conceptual framework in the middle. This notion demonstrates that clarity in relation to the conceptual framework is essential if faculty are effectively to incorporate the philosophy into all learning experiences.

The model also demonstrates an appropriate method of developing the curriculum components and design. After the completion of the program's philosophy, the curriculum components can be identified in relation to the general education and supporting courses. It is not until the behavioral level objectives are developed that the most appropriate sequence of course requirements can be identified and descriptions of the nursing courses can be developed.

The philosophy of the nursing programs, which was developed within the framework of the university's philosophy, should give strong clues as to the types of concepts and theoretical formulations a particualr faculty will identify as the essence of their program. Their particular and unique way of looking at man, society, health, nursing, and learning will assist others, as well as themselves, in identifying the curriculum components and approaches that will follow. These components include those general education courses that relate to the college core requirements for all students, as well as those identified by the nursing faculty as essential in terms of the stated philosophy. For example, if the faculty were to identify the understanding of research as a component of the nursing process and as an essential part of the nurse's leadership role, a statistics course might be required.

Another component of the curriculum relates to the supporting courses that will be required. If the philosophy speaks to Man as a bio-psycho-social being who is unique in nature, then course requirements need to include biology, chemistry, anatomy and physiology, psychology, and sociology. Within certain private religious institutions where there is a strong emphasis on man as a spiritual being, course requirements might also include religion and philosophy. The number of course requirements within any area depends on the faculty's concepts in terms of the breadth and depth they feel are needed to support the philosophy they have developed.

The measure of emphasis on each particular science will be influenced by the faculty's frame of reference. For example, if faculty identify man as having the greatest commitment to his physical and/or basic needs and as constantly striving for physiological adaptation, the curriculum design would focus on the biological sciences. On the other hand, man can also be approached as basically a social being, with theoretical formulations related to his relationship to himself and society; this would dictate a greater number of course offerings in psychology and sociology. If faculty identified the need for the nurse to relate to man as he acts within his culture, course offerings in anthropology would be indicated.

What becomes evident, as the curriculum components are identified in terms of the philosophy, is how truly committed the faculty are to their concepts; this commitment will assist them in developing the concepts which will, in turn, aid them in developing the conceptual framework. For example, if faculty identify man as basically developmental, but do not really see the need to require a course in developmental psychology, it would seem unlikely that developmental theories would be stressed as an important theoretical formulation. If the philosophy speaks to "Society," emphasizing the family and change process, then theories specifically related to the family and the change process need to be strongly incorporated into the conceptual framework. If the philosophy emphasizes health maintenance through adaptation and/or coping, the theoretical formulations need to emphasize wellness, not illness. If the philosophy identifies the unique role of the professional nurse as that of leadership through the utilization of the nursing process in relation to man, theoretical formulations to be emphasized are interpersonal theories, leadership theories, and decision theories.

Thus, if we take a very close look at a program's philosophy, we can identify the faculty's incorporated concepts or notions about man, society, health, and nursing and identify the theoretical formulations that those concepts emphasize.

In moving along the curriculum process, we must often return to the philosophy to see if we truly are incorporating its ideas. Of course, if the philosophy of the nursing program has weaknesses in its development, identifying appropriate concepts and theories may present a problem to the faculty. For example, a philosophy might seem nonoperational and idealistic rather than a realistic statement of beliefs. It is sometimes created as a masterpiece of verbiage that looks beautiful on paper, but is merely placed in a drawer for occasional review. Sometimes

MODEL I

CONCEPTUAL FRAMEWORK WITHIN THE TOTAL CURRICULUM PROCESS
(Sample approach)

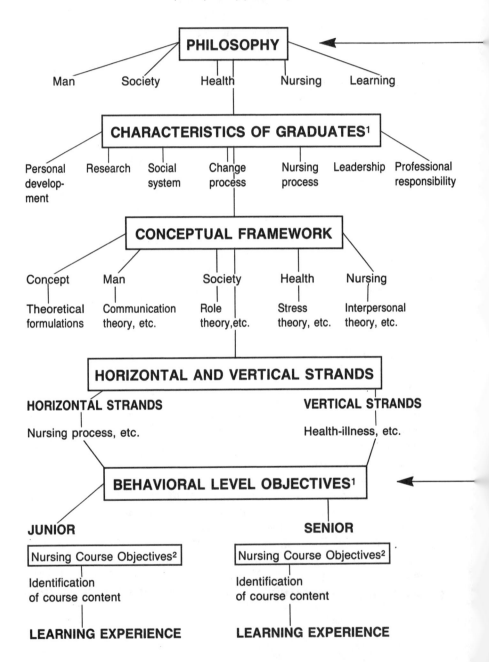

CURRICULUM COMPONENTS

┌General education requirements
├Supporting course requirements
└Placement of nursing major

CURRICULUM DESIGN

┌Sequence of course requirements
└Development of nursing course
  descriptions

─────────

[1] Utilized for program and total curriculum evaluation.
[2] Objectives utilized for students' theoretical and clinical evaluation.

a philosophy is so "sophisticated" that few can claim to comprehend its meaning. Also, it may reflect various beliefs about the concepts held by nursing "leaders" but not by the faculty and so may be difficult to utilize.

The program's objectives and the characteristics of the graduates or terminal behavioral objectives can be viewed as giving the philosophy a structure that can be implemented and later used for total curriculum evaluation. As with the philosophy, the objectives give direction to the conceptual framework and theoretical formulations. In reviewing many programs and/or terminal behavioral objectives, one finds major areas identified by most baccalaureate programs. These are: professional nursing within the social system, the change process, the nursing process, leadership, professional responsibilities and development, and research. Of course, programs vary widely in how the objectives are stated and which objective is emphasized over others. This emphasis supports the philosophy and also gives strong clues as to the devlopment of revision of the conceptual framework. Since the conceptual framework in and of itself cannot be evaluated and program objectives can, it is essential that the framework speak to the objectives and that it be seen as a way of meeting the objectives. Here again, if the program and/or behavioral objectives of graduates are not succinctly and clearly stated—possibly with a glossary of terms to add clarity to the terminology—they will be of little assistance to the faculty in developing the conceptual framework and appropriate theories.

Let us assume for the moment that a faculty, in their efforts to develop or revise a quality nursing program, have a sound philosophy, program, and/or terminal objectives and a conceptual framework with theoretical formulations and that all these components of the curriculum are closely linked and support one another; what then follows in the curriculum development process should be quite uncomplicated and fairly easy. This is especially true if the faculty utilize their accomplishments fully to make each of the decisions that will follow—decisions relating to curriculum design and the development of level behavioral and course objectives and learning experiences.

It is often helpful, after the development of the conceptual framework and prior to the development of the level behavioral objectives, to identify the horizontal and vertical threads within the curriculum. This is demonstrated in Model II. Sample beliefs were written so that the appropriate concepts, subconcepts, and theories could be identified. These beliefs were also utilized to develop several strands within the curriculum. These strands, within Levels I and II of the nursing component, are built upon the foundational components, which are generally prerequisite to the nursing courses. They are dependent on the concepts and/or theories taught in both the supporting and general educational requirements. For example, concepts and theories related to adaptation and stress taught in the pure and behavioral sciences are prerequisite to the vertical strand, the health-illness continuum. Concepts and theories related to the family and community are prerequisite to the vertical strand, individual-family community.

The more highly developed the concepts, subconcepts, and theoretical formulations, the greater will be the dependence on general education and liberal arts learning to provide not only the base for, but also continuing support for the curriculum throughout the nursing major. This approach also supports the need for the nursing major to be concentrated in the upper division, allowing the nursing student fully to transfer the learning supportive of man, society, and health to the nursing major. Nursing content then truly becomes nursing content, and the selection of course requirements, especially the supporting courses, has a clear rationale that can be identified within the conceptual framework.

In Model II, the nursing process is a horizontal strand and the vertical strands are the individual-family-community and the health-illness continuum. The identification of strands as either horizontal or vertical will depend on the faculty's philosophy of education and nursing and may easily differ from those on the model presented, which were selected arbitrarily as a means of discussing the curriculum process.

In the development of behavioral level objectives from Model II, Level I objectives will reflect the use of the nursing process in a one-to-one relationship with a client/family and in relation to health promotion and maintenance. It is later, at Level II, that students will deal with illness and the community as a whole, since this is at the end of the vertical strand. Here again, the conceptual framework, with its theoretical formulations, provides faculty with a basis for the identification of vertical and horizontal strands and assists them in the development of the level behavioral objectives which give meaning to the course objectives.

The relationships between the conceptual framework and the course descriptions, objectives, learning experiences, and methods of evaluation become crucial in the development of the program. For if the entire curriculum process results in learning experiences that have little or no relationship to the concepts and theoretical formulations identified, all the faculty's efforts are wasted and the students are left confused as to what the nursing curriculum is all about and what the rationale was for their course requirements. We can engage in all the discussions in the world and have beautifully written philosophies and objectives, but we fail as nurse educators if these philosophies and objectives do not make an impact on each learning experience of the nursing student.

Let us now present some possible approaches to nursing courses that might be implemented, granted that we as nurse educators believe that the selection of theories within the conceptual framework is a valid approach. Since we have said that content throughout the nursing courses is built on scientific principles and theories as well as on the arts and humanities, it would seem logical that prior to the first clinical course in nursing we give the student some theoretical background in nursing.

MODEL II

THEORETICAL FORMULATIONS AND THE UTILIZATION OF VERTICAL AND HORIZONTAL STRANDS WITHIN A CURRICULUM
(Utilizing sample beliefs and theoretical formulations)

SAMPLE BELIEFS

- Man varies in his state of well-being within the *health-illness* continuum

Theoretical formulations

- Adaptation theory
  Stress theory
  Crisis theory
  Change theory

- Man as an *individual* is part of the total environment which includes *family and community*

Theoretical formulations

- Communication theory
  Family theory
  Role theory

- Professional nursing involves the utilization of the nursing process in a variety of settings

Theoretical formulations

- Communication theory
  Decision theory
  Role theory
  Leadership theory
  Interpersonal theory

THEORETICAL FORMULATIONS AND THE UTILIZATION OF VERTICAL AND HORIZONTAL STRANDS WITHIN A CURRICULUM
(Utilizing sample beliefs and theoretical formulations)

CHARACTERISTICS OF GRADUATES

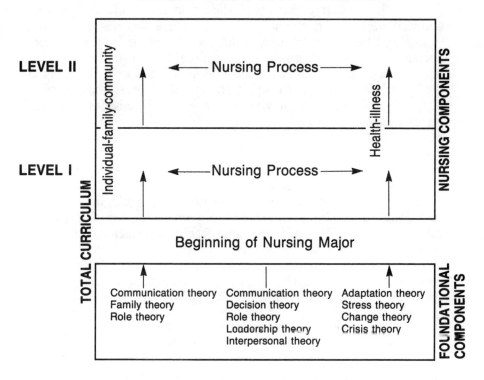

HORIZONTAL STRANDS
- Nursing Process

VERTICAL STRANDS
- Individual-family-community
- Health-illness continuum

This would involve offering a nonlaboratory nursing course assimilating the theories, laws, and principles already learned in the supporting courses and further relating these to various nursing theories. Nursing theories have been developed by some nursing leaders; faculty would also offer the student their own particular theory of nursing as seen in the program's framework.

We in baccalaureate education seem to ignore our own nursing theories. If we shared these with the student as a kind of base of knowledge, the student could then test these theories of nursing throughout her clinical nursing courses and could more easily incorporate the educational program's conceptual framework into her professional practice. It would seem that an emphasis on such theories would further orient the student to perceive herself as a professional, utilizing her profession's body of knowledge in her everyday activities. Learning experiences would emphasize the nursing process through the utilization of theories which can be learned and practiced in any setting, for no nursing theory presented to date speaks to any particular specialization or environment, but applies wherever the client and/or patient is found.

In structuring nursing courses, differing concepts and/or theories can be utilized for course descriptions. For example, faculty may identify such concepts as adaptation, stress, body image, or oxygenation and utilize them to develop each of the specific courses, teaching one or two concepts each semester and focusing on the horizontal and vertical strands. Nursing content and theories are then placed under the most appropriate concept. Nursing courses can also be totally oriented around specific concepts like Maslow's Hierarchy of Needs, Abdellah's 21 Nursing Problems, or Erickson's developmental approach. Whatever structure is given to the nursing courses is not significant. What is important is that each nursing course truly reflect the components of the conceptual framework. All too often the student is oriented toward a particular framework in her first nursing course but is not reinforced in this framework later in the curriculum.

Let us repeat that the conceptual framework and theoretical formulations reflect the philosophy, objectives, and behavioral expectations of the nursing program. This framework permeates every aspect of the curriculum design, every learning experience. It gives the nursing faculty a common and specific meaning for the incorporation of content at every level of the curriculum. And let us close by saying that if every baccalaureate program would identify the theoretical formulations that relate to its conceptual framework, we would then be able to identify those theories that educators find most appropriate to the profession of nursing. This information would have implications for graduate education in nursing and for the types of continuing education programs that could be offered and would encourage nursing research in relation to the theories identified.

216

BIBLIOGRAPHY

Abdellah, Faye G., et al., *Patient-Centered Approaches to Nursing.* New York: The Macmillan Co., 1961.

Beauchamp, George, *Curriculum Theory,* 2nd edition. Willmette, Ill.: The Kagg Press, 1968.

Brennan, William, "The Practitioner as Theoretician," *Education for Social Work,* Spring 1973.

Brodbeck, May, "Logic and Scientific Method in Research in Teaching," in N.L. Gage, ed., *Handbook of Research in Teaching.* Chicago: Rand McNally and Company, 1963.

_____. "Models, Meanings, and Theories," in Llewellyn Gross, ed., *Symposium on Sociological Theory.* Evanston: Row Peterson and Company, 1959.

Bruner, Jerome S., "A Theory of Instruction," *Educational Leadership,* 20:523-532, May 1963.

Coladarci, Arthur P., and Gertzels, Jacob, *The Use of Theory in Educational Administration.* Pal Alto, Calif.: Standford University School of Education, 1955.

Conley, Virginia, *Curriculum and Instruction in Nursing.* Boston: Little, Brown and Company, 1973.

Coombs, Arthur W., and Snygg, Donald, *Individual Behavior.* New York: Harper and Brothers, 1959.

Dickoff, James; James, Patricia; and Wiedenback, Ernestine, "Theory in a Practice Discipline. Part I: Practice Oriented Theory," *Nursing Research,* 17:415-435, September-October 1968.

Di Renzo, G.J. (ed.) *Concepts, Theory and Explanation in the Behavioral Sciences.* New York: Random House, 1966.

Emans, Robert, "A Proposed Conceptual Framework for Curriculum Development," *Journal of Educational Research,* March 1966.

Gertzels, Jacob W., "Theory and Practice in Educational Administration: An Old Question Revisited," in Ronald F. Campbell and James M. Lipman, eds., *Administrative Theory as a Guide to Action.* Chicago: Midwest Administration Center, University of Chicago, 1960.

Gowin, D.B., "Can Educational Theory Guide Practice?" *Educational Theory,* 13:8:6-12, January 1963.

Hage, Jerald, *Techniques and Problems of Theory Construction in Sociology.* New York: John Wiley & Sons, 1972.

Hall, Calvin S., and Lindzey, Gardner, *Theories of Personality,* 2nd ed. New York: The Macmillan Co., 1965.

Hardy, Margaret, "Theories: Components, Development, Evaluation," *Nursing Research,* 23:100-107, March-April 1974.

Harre, Rom, "The Formal Analysis of Concepts," in Herbert J. Klausmeier and Chester W. Harris, eds., *Analysis of Concept Learning*. New York: Academic Press, 1966.

Hodgman, Eileen, "A Conceptual Framework to Guide Nursing Curriculum," *Nursing Forum,* Vol. VII, No. 2, 1973.

Homans, George, *The Human Group*. New York: Harcourt, Brace and World, 1950.

Jacox, Ada, "Theory Construction in Nursing." *Nursing Research,* 23:4-13, January-February 1974.

Kerlinger, Fred N., *Foundations of Behavioral Research*. New York: Holt, Rinehart and Winston, 1965.

Logan, Frank, and Olmstead, David, *Behavior Theory and Social Science*. New Haven: Yale University Press, 1955.

Mouly, George S., *The Science of Educational Research*. New York: American Book Company, 1963.

National Education Association, Commission on Instructional Theory, *Theories of Instruction: A Set of Guidelines*. A position paper presented at the Annual Conference of the Association for Supervision and Curriculum Development, NEA, Dallas, Texas, March 1967.

National League for Nursing, Department of Baccalaureate and Higher Degree Programs, *Criteria for the Appraisal of Baccalaureate and Higher Degree Programs in Nursing*. New York: The League, 1972.

Newsome, George L., Jr., "In What Sense Is Theory a Guide to Practice in Education?" *Educational Theory*. 14:36: 31-39, January 1964.

New York League of Nursing Education, Program Committee, Martha R. Smith, Chairman, "A Concept of Nursing," *American Journal of Nursing,* 33:565, June 1933.

O'Connor, D.J., *An Introduction to the Philosophy of Education*. London: Routledge and Kegan, Paul, 1957.

Phenix, Philip P., "Educational Theory and Inspiration," *Educational Theory,* January 1963.

Reynolds, P.D., *A Primer in Theory Construction*. Indianapolis: Bobbs-Merrill Company, 1971.

Ryle, Gilbert, *The Concept of Mind*. New York: Barnes and Noble, Inc., 1949.

Taylor, Effie, "Of What is the Nature of Nursing?" *American Journal of Nursing,* 34:473-476, May 1934.

Toffler, Alvin, ed., *Learning for Tomorrow: The Role of the Future in Education*. New York: Vintage Books, 1974.

Torres, Gertrude, and Yura, Helen, *Today's Conceptual Framework: Its Relationship to the Curriculum Development Process*. New York: National League for Nursing, 1974.

Travers, Robert N.W., *An Introduction to Educational Research,* 2nd ed. New York: The Macmillan Co., 1964.

Woodruff, Isabel, "The Use of Concepts in Teaching and Learning," *Journal of Teacher Education,* March 1964.

4 UNIFYING THE CURRICULUM—THE INTEGRATED APPROACH

27 EDUCATIONAL TRENDS AND THE INTEGRATED CURRICULUM APPROACH IN NURSING

Gertrude J. Torres, EdD, RN

Since the beginning of organized education, curriculum has been the subject of much study and the focus of much effort toward innovation. Yet schools have shown in the past an infinite capacity to absorb change without really changing at all.[1] Beckerman believes it takes thirty to fifty years for an idea to gain wide acceptance in American schools.[2] In spite of this apparent past resistance on the part of education to change, an accelerated movement to change some aspects of the educational process has appeared in the last decade. The ideas for change and the need for it are by no means new, as this paper will later demonstrate, but the educators' readiness to accept differing concepts of education and learning and to implement them does seem to be a new trend.

Today, we have a questioning of values related to the purposes of education, we have increasing amounts of technology being utilized within education, we have a greater emphasis on remediation and assisting minority goups, and we have governmental agencies mandating differing educational policies. Thus, it appears that, whether we like it or

---

[1] James R. O'Brien, "The Most Important Force for Change," *School and Community.* 58:44, April 1972.
[2] Marvin M. Beckerman, "Are Teachers Against Innovations?" *School and Community,* 58:14, December 1971.

not, we must change the way we educate to some degree.

A review of over fifty baccalaureate nursing programs, carried out by the NLN Department of Baccalaureate and Higher Degree Programs, showed that the shift in focus in the nursing curriculum from the medical model to an integrated approach is the most dynamic change in nursing education in the last ten years. Programs are either currently engaged in the revision of their curriculum to create an integrated approach or are already utilizing that curriculum method. Nursing educators seem to have jumped on the integrated approach bandwagon without, however, any specific identifiable rationale or concensus as to why.

This paper is not meant to be an exhaustive review, but rather a highlighting of what seem to me to be the major forces that support the integrating of the nursing curriculum. As trends and issues are discussed, it might be helpful for the reader to take a position as to their validity from his or her individual frame of reference.

Before proceeding, however, it is essential that we concern ourselves with some definitions. In nursing and nursing education, we frequently use words or terms without any agreement as to their specific meanings. Some believe it is futile to discuss the specific meanings of words, since agreement is unlikely. However, it seems essential to me that, before we engage in rhetoric about integration, we have some common idea as to how we are using the word today. Otherwise, we cannot know whether we are truly engaging in integration or not. Since my review of the literature revealed much use of the word "integration," but no definition of it, let me offer my thinking on this subject.

Words that come to mind when we think of the word or the concept *integration* include "completeness," "whole," "unity," "mix," "integrity," and "blend." This last word, "blend," seems to offer the most appropriate synonym for "integration" in reference to curriculum. What we really seem to be doing, or attempting to do, is combining or associating scientific and nursing content in such a way that the separate constituents or lines of demarcation cannot be distinguished. In blending the curriculum, we promote an undivided total effect so that the parts (as utilized in the medical-model approach) cannot be distinguished. Bringing many parts together to sit side by side and presenting them as a whole is *not* integration, it is merely sorting out the parts differently. Thus, for the purpose of this paper, unifying the nursing curriculum by means of the integrated approach means *blending the nursing content in such a way that the parts or specialties are no longer distinguishable.* This involves concentrating on the generalizations relating to nursing rather than the specifics.

Few ideas in education are truly innovative, as the following short historical review of the literature will demonstrate.

In the 1930s and 1940s, progressive reformers proposed a new approach to curriculum, one oriented toward personal and social problems. This was an attempt to escape from the time-honored subject-matter approach which offered bits and pieces of information in the hope that somehow or other these would be useful in the lives of the students.[3] Social scientists, recognizing that their content was organized into separate and isolated divisions, encouraged that the organization of their instruction be more closely integrated with other activities and subjects.[4] Dewey's voice was heard at that time loudly calling for greater concern for the internal relationships of subject matter.[5] Beard felt that there was a disintegration of higher education into thousands of courses, without any center of gravity in intellectual or moral purpose.[6] In 1929, Alfred North Whitehead urged that "we eradicate the fatal disconnection of subjects which kills the vitality of our modern curriculum."[7] Thus, we can see that some forty years ago educators were encouraging the development of curriculums that were oriented away from the acquisition by the student of bits of information—the subject-centered approach. It is significant to note that, although they were not suffering from the effects of the modern explosion of information as we are, these thinkers recognized the need for subjects to be interactive.

One of the most widely quoted leaders in the curriculum literature is Jerome Bruner. He contends that there is a "structure of knowledge—its connectedness and its deviations that make one idea follow another—[which] is the proper emphasis in education."[8] He speaks of organizing ideas by inventing concepts and feels that it is these concepts which generally permit us to understand and at times even to predict or change the world. The structure of the discipline, as related to principles and concepts, can be thought of as a way of understanding and knowing how a nurse thinks about nursing through the utilization of concepts of nursing. For the present, might we think of the nursing process as the structure of the discipline of nursing? Also, Bruner feels that details are rapidly forgotten unless placed into some structural pattern; learning general or fundamental principles thus helps us to minimize memory loss and permits us to reconstruct the details when needed.[9] Learning principles

[3] Arno A. Bellack, "The Structure of Knowledge and the Structure of the Curriculum," *A Reassessment of the Curriculum,* ed. Dwayne Huebner (New York: Teachers College, Columbia University, 1964), pp. 25-26.

[4] Commission on the Social Studies, American Historical Association, *Conclusions and Recommendations* (New York: Scribner's, 1934), p. 49.

[5] Hollis L. Caswell, "Difficulties in Defining the Structure of the Curriculum," *Curriculum Crossroads,* ed. A. Harry Passow (New York: Teachers College, Columbia University, 1965), p. 105.

[6] Charles A. Beard, *The Nature of the Social Sciences* (New York: Scribner's, 1934), pp. 137-138.

[7] Alfred North Whitehead, *The Aims of Education* (New York: The Free Press, 1929), p. 6.

[8] Jerome Bruner, *On Knowing* (Cambridge, Mass.: Harvard University Press, 1962), p. 120.

[9] Jerome Bruner, *The Process of Education* (Cambridge, Mass.: Harvard University Press, 1960).

also gives what Bruner calls "a sense of excitement about discovery with a resulting sense of self-confidence in one's ability."[10] It is also generally agreed that the half-life of knowledge in a profession has shrunk to perhaps five years.[11]

In education, there is an ever-increasing emphasis on relationships among allied disciplines, such as the relationship between the literary world and the scientific world or the relationship between the intellectual and aesthetic resources of a culture. In nursing education, this involves finding relationships between the behavioral and physical sciences, between the concepts of man held by nursing and by the humanities, and between nursing and scientific knowledge and values.

Searching for relationships often leads to interdisciplinary approaches to education. All too frequently, this has been restricted to honors programs of study. Educators in the humanities, the sciences, and the health professions—including nursing—are all seeking newer ways of offering interdisciplinary approaches to modern education.

Educators are becoming increasingly concerned with the modes of thought—the analytic, the empirical, the aesthetic, and the moral— that transcend the boundaries of individual fields. Today's living requires that the student become a thinker who can solve problems, formulate concepts, make judgments, analyze, summarize, and form valid conclusions,[12] attributes which are frequently identified in NLN's *Characteristics of the Baccalaureate Graduate in Nursing* as essential not only for the personal enrichment of the student, but also for her professional development. These behaviors will not develop solely by the information-oriented or subject-oriented curriculum approach.

Although many educators, including nurses, claim their goal is to create thinkers, yet the written examinations they give often clearly show that what the learner is expected to accomplish is knowledge as related to facts. This is not to say that curriculum should exclude information or facts, but that these should become only the means to achieve the greater goal of teaching problem-solving skills. This approach is sometimes called the problem-centered or process-centered approach to education.

The process-centered approach requires a different type of teaching to produce different kinds of behavior. Involved are new patterns of study, different ways of organizing reading materials, and different cognitive different ways of organizing reading materials, and different cognitive

---

[10] Bellack, *op. cit.,* pp. 28-38.

[11] *Ibid.,* p. 35.

[12] Richard W. Burns and Gary D. Brooks, "Process, Problem Solving, and Curriculum Reform," *Curriculum Design in a Changing Society,* Burns and Brooks, eds. (Englewood Cliffs, N.J.: Educational Technology Publications, 1970), p. 56.

operations. There is now ample evidence that lectures and discussion-type classes yield different results. Lectures are superior for the transmission of information, while discussion classes provoke more active thinking.[13] Group discussion allows the learner to gain experience in integrating facts, formulating hypotheses, and amassing relevant evidence with others.[14] Independent study and tutorials are also useful with the process-centered curriculum. In this approach, the instructor helps maintain coherence and direction and questions fallacious reasoning and distorted interpretations. Comparison and integration of knowledge enable students to comprehend relationships. Also, in the unifying of the curriculum, faculty tend to become an intellectual community with insights and information from various disciplines.[15]

Educators are also becoming more interested in using the knowledge already at hand more effectively than in continually increasing present amounts of knowledge. They seek to bring together and connect the concepts of different disciplines as a way of using present knowledge more effectively. Samford writes that a high level of personality development is involved in dealing with complexities and wholeness, which relate to differentiation and integration; differentiation is seen as having specialized functions, integration as representing a state in which communication among the parts is sufficient to allow them, without losing their identity, to become larger wholes.[16] This emphasis is not new, in a sense, since Dewey emphasized in 1938 increasing perceptions of the connections and continuities of our activities.[17] Education brings imperceptible connections together, which is integration of the highest order.

Phenix tells us that the special purpose of education is to widen one's view of life and to deepen one's insights into relationships—concepts which are part of the integrated outlook. Conceiving of a person as essentially an organized totality and not just a collection of separate parts, Phenix feels that a course of study can best contribute to the person's growth if it is oriented by a goal of wholeness. He states, "The value of any subject is enhanced by an understanding of its relationship with other subjects."[18]

In the selection of content, one needs to choose those items which are particularly representative of the field as a whole and are the characteristic features of the discipline. Thus, a relatively small volume of knowledge may be sufficient for an understanding of a larger body

---

[13] *Education and Identity* (San Francisco: Jossey-Bass, Inc., 1972), p. 207.

[14] W.J. McKeachie, "Procedures and Techniques of Teaching: A Survey of Experimental Studies," *The American College,* ed. N. Sanford (New York: John Wiley and Sons, 1972), p. 326.

[15] *Education and Identity, loc. cit.*

[16] N. Sanford, "The Developmental Status of the Entering Freshman," *The American College,* ed. N. Sanford (New York: John Wiley and Sons, 1962), pp. 253-282.

[17] John Dewey, *Democracy and Education* (New York: Macmillan, 1938), pp. 89-90.

[18] Phillip Phenix, *Realms of Meaning* (New York: McGraw-Hill, 1961), p.11.

of material. This approach is essential today with the vast proliferation of knowledge and can best be achieved by utilizing key concepts.[19]

I do not want to convey the notion that all educators have supported the idea of integration of curriculum. Those who have attempted to integrate knowledge through core course have frequently been accused of offering content that was superficial and vague and of having failed to educate for disciplined thinking. Although many might feel that such criticisms by specialists are an attempt to maintain the integrity of their own field, some of the criticisms are well-founded. Merely combining topics into a course of study rather than truly unifying and integrating concepts and ideas is bound to result in superficiality.

Aside from the emphasis on the teaching structure of the discipline and on interdisciplinary courses in education, other movements in higher education have strongly encouraged the integrated approach to nursing education. The following are but a few:

- Increasing interest in preparing for the future at a time of rapid change, with the development of "futuristic" courses. Since the future is questionable, many feel that teaching principles or structure of the discipline rather than outmoded facts will better equip the student for the future.
- Increasing interest in learning theories, especially as related to concept formulation.
- Increasing interest in higher education's being more accountable to the learner and the society which encourages change in general.

Educators today are looking at education in a different way, with an interest in finding the structure of a discipline; in dealing with overreaching facts and relationships, rather than separating content; and in developing students who can discover, create, express meaning, and think, rather than merely accumulate facts. If I may indulge in a metaphor: the integrated curriculum is similar to a symphony orchestra—all the instruments are represented and each is vital to the total sound, yet except for occasional movements of emphasis, no one instrument can be clearly heard alone. The differences in sound are minimized to create a unifying whole that is exciting and dramatic.

Let me close with a quote:

> If you give man a fish he will have a single meal;
> If you teach him how to fish he will eat all his life.
>
> Kuan-tzu

---

[19] Hilda Taba, *Curriculum Development Theory and Practice* (New York: Harcourt, Brace and World, Inc., 1962), p. 191.

28 THE INTEGRATED CURRICULUM AND NURSING EDUCATION

Gertrude J. Torres, EdD, RN

To prove that the emphasis on thinking, judging, systematizing, and classifying is not new in nursing education, I offer the following quote from the 1917 *Standard Curriculum for Schools of Nursing:*

> The quality of teaching can be measured by a few fundamental lists. . . The pupils are doing real live thinking for themselves and not simply memorizing facts. They are observing, comparing and judging things and learning to seek out reasons and weigh conclusions. . . . The pupils show the clearness and thoroughness of their knowledge by their ability to systematize and classify their ideas and to find them when needed. . . . and their ability to adapt and apply their knowledge in new situations.[1]

One would have to admit on reading further in this book, however, that the general scheme of practical instruction or course of study suggested was not very supportive of the concept of teaching; as is so often true today, the ideas are good but the implementation of them is quite another matter. Courses at that time represented the medical model rather than the structure of the discipline of nursing, as is frequently true even today.

---

[1] Committee on Education, National League of Nursing Education, *Standard Curriculum for Schools of Nursing* (Baltimore: Waverly Press, 1917), pp. 27-28.

Some ten years later, the title, *Standard Curriculum for Schools of Nursing,* was changed to *A Curriculum for Schools for Nursing* in an apparent attempt to imply that what was offered was not to be viewed as a "model" curriculum. This text emphasized that undergraduate nursing should be considered a basic course, general (as opposed to specialized) in nature. It was to be considered a foundation on which all additional training and experience should be built.[2] The authors treated of the differences between undergraduate and graduate education (as we understand those terms) and confirmed the general nature of bedside nursing.

The 1927 curriculum guide gave a stronger anticipation of the ideas of integration, spoke of bringing the parts of the program of studies into a whole, and discouraged the splitting up of materials into compartments or subjects of study.[3] Since the emphasis was on teaching in such a way that integration could readily take place in the student's mind and personality, here again the student did the integrating of materials, while the curriculum focused on specifics. Except for an additional introductory course in nursing arts, the medical model persisted. History speaks to us in various ways: it tells us how far we have progressed; it tells us how long change often takes; it tells us that ideas are generally not new, and it tells us that the traditionalists often outnumber the futurists.

One of the most significant factors, historical and present, that influences nursing education is the definition of what nursing really involves. According to Dock and Stewart, the word "nursing" was originally used to mean the nurture and care of the well child; only later did it come to mean care of the sick and infirm. They noted in 1920 that nursing was becoming involved to a greater extent in the promotion and conservation of health and prevention of disease, the protection and care of people's environment, and the care of the whole patient.[4] The history of nursing seems to be cyclic, swinging back and forth between emphasis on health and emphasis on illness. It is significant to note, however, that, with all the variety of our interpretations of nursing through the years, none speaks to the medical model approach; rather, our concepts of nursing involve all people in all places. Even in 1927, the first two classifications of what should be taught to nursing students spoke to nurses caring for the widest variety of human beings, as classified by age, sex, intelligence, and social status, as well as by stages of health from normal to acutely ill.[5]

If our concept of nursing continues to reflect the past emphasis on

---

[2] Committee on Education, National League of Nursing Education, *A Curriculum for Schools of Nursing* (6th ed.; New York: The League, 1927).

[3] Commission on Curriculum, National League of Nursing Education, *A Curriculum Guide for Schools of Nursing* (New York: The League, 1937), p. 69.

[4] Lavinia Dock and Isabel Stewart, *A Short History of Nursing* (New York: G.P. Putnam's Sons, 1920), p. 355.

[5] Committee on Education, NLN, *op. cit.,* 1927, p. 44.

the whole patient in sickness and in health, we should at no time in our teaching divide the whole human being into parts. Many would say that just because they teach via the medical model and relate to a specific environment, it does not mean they educate in terms of parts of people. Maybe these people should look carefully at how specialization in medicine has created a piecemeal approach to patient care; let them also examine their own nursing curriculums to see how often the mind and body are taught without true relationship.

One of the characteristics of a profession is that it has a body of knowledge and skill that is unique and transmissible.[6] The word to be emphasized here is *unique*. If this is so, we must not approach nursing content as though it were a subsidiary of medicine or any other health care discipline, and we must continue to identify content related to our concepts of nursing. What we need to understand is that there are a number of concepts of nursing, but that none of them is related to specialization or to the medical model. Let us look at a few of these concepts as presented by nurse leaders.

Rogers sees nursing as related to our fundamental postulates about man, with man as a dynamic organism moving on a continuum of life from minimum to maximum states of well-being.[7] Peplau, Brown, and Fowler conceptualize nursing as a process of interaction applying to all recipients of nursing care.[8] Nordmark and Rohweder apply scientific principles to nursing to cut across specialties; Abdellah's and Matheney's ideas on nursing problems as fundamental to the practice of nursing also cut across all areas of specialization and the medical model approach.[9] McCain's concept includes the belief that the primary goal of nursing is to assist patients in attaining and maintaining a state of equilibrium.[10] This is by no means meant to represent an all-inclusive list of the concepts of nursing, but it does show that many nursing leaders hold concepts of nursing that cut across specialties and deal with man as a whole. King says that one of the major problems facing our profession today is the organization of our body of knowledge.[11] This organization should be in keeping with our concepts of nursing and should affect, if not dictate, the way we educate for the profession.

An issue that comes up more and more frequently among nurses is the question of the nature of practice—are we specialists or are we generalists? Is nursing primarily a generalized profession, or are we a

---

[6] Dan W. Anderson, "Toward an Unambiguous Profession? A Review of Nursing," *Health Administration Perspectives,* No. A6 (1968), p. 10.

[7] Martha Rogers, *Educational Revolution and Nursing* (New York: Macmillan Co., 1961), pp. 16-22.

[8] Imogene M. King, *Toward A Theory for Nursing. General Concepts of Human Behavior* (New York: John Wiley and Sons, 1971), pp. 4-5.

[9] *Ibid.,* pp. 5-6.

[10] Faye McCain, "Nursing by Assessment—Not by Intuition," *American Journal of Nursing,* 65: 82-84, April 1965.

[11] King, *op. cit.,* p. 7.

group of specialists with only a few concepts in common? These questions may, on the surface at least, appear rather simplistic or obvious to some. We can take the position, for instance, that nursing is a generalized profession and that the more specialized we become, the harder it is to identify a unique body of nursing knowledge. For example, pediatric specialists frequently tend to be greater experts in medical pediatrics than in pediatric nursing. Thus, the more specialized we become, the greater the chance that we will lose the essence of our broad concepts of nursing. This approach would not negate the need for specific information relative to specialization or to medicine, but such information would be only supportive data, rather than a major focus.

On the other hand, one can believe that nursing is not totally generalized, but a combination of different specialty areas. Graduate programs have identified new specializations, such as rehabilitation, adult nursing, and family care nursing. Clinical specialization is becoming even narrower in some areas (e.g., cardiovascular nursing and respiratory nursing). To illustrate the confusion, there has been at the same time an increasing combination of clinical specialties. For instance, obstetrics and pediatrics, once separate specialties, are now offered as maternal-child nursing; this is also true of medical-surgical nursing. Graduate schools now offer a major in community-mental health nursing, which is another effort to decompartmentalize the specialties.

Whether we call ourselves generalists or specialists, however, we need to change the way we educate to relate more effectively to our concepts. It would seem that the only basis for teaching via the medical model is the belief that there is basically little real nursing content that does not relate to medical and other health sciences. Think about the answers to these questions for a moment:

- How much time do we spend in a typical class emphasizing medical or other science content, rather than showing how such content relates to nursing and the concepts of nursing?
- In developing examinations, are our questions frequently medical or science in nature, rather than related to the process or essence of nursing?
- How often have we thought to ourselves, "If only I had more time to teach, I could emphasize nursing more!"?
- Do the textbooks I use, even though identified as nursing texts, truly speak to the essence of nursing, or do they emphasize medicine with only a mention of the implications for nursing? (Just a thought here—how about a nursing text which emphasizes nursing, with an occasional area directed to the implications for medicine?)

As we focus more and more on nursing concepts, processes, and dimensions and attempt to divorce ourselves (or maybe only separate ourselves) from medicine, we become increasingly aware of our need to unify the curriculum, especially at the baccalaureate level. As we become more sophisticated in our theories, this need will become even more evident.

I would like to mention other changes taking place in nursing and nursing education that support this movement toward integration.

The use of the nursing process, which is similar to the old problem-solving approach, in the practice of nursing is a core concept which cuts across all specialties. In utilizing the nursing process and its components (assessment, diagnosis, intervention, and evaluation), we can more easily focus on the whole patient. Nursing diagnoses, as they are being developed today, relate to such things as alterations in comfort level, impairment in regulatory functions, integrity of the skin, and ineffective sleep or rest patterns.[12] Although these are only a beginning in the development of a system of nursing diagnostic categories, they do reflect a nonmedical concept of nursing and should influence nursing education. The integrated curriculum is very useful in helping the student to understand the nursing process in greater depth. Although for years nursing philosophy has held that man should be viewed holistically, we have not given serious thought to how this might influence the design of our curriculum. Although nursing educators have always identified broad categories rather than narrow specialties in developing program objectives, increased sophistication in curriculum theory has allowed us to incorporate into our teaching more effectively our beliefs about man and nursing. This apparent change has influenced the way we think about students and learning. One might even say we have become educators and theorists first and nurses second. We now teach the holistic concept of man as a bio-psycho-social, and often spiritual, being to the student in every course at each level, thus avoiding specialized courses, such as psychiatric nursing and public health nursing.

Another trend in nursing education with great impact on baccalaureate educators is the rapid development of associate degree programs. Many of the early AD programs (in 1958-59) had integrated curriculums, and many still do. The success of associate degree educators in defining and describing their product—the nursing technician—with clarity has spurred baccalaureate educators to move ahead in their struggle to identify their product as unique and different from the technician. As we further developed the charateristics of baccalaureate graduates, identifying their unique functions in the care of clients/patients, we have been forced to look at the effectiveness of our curriculum designs in producing this type of professional. A review of the characteristics of the baccalaureate

[12] Kristine Gebbie and Mary Ann Lavin, "Classifying Nursing Diagnoses," *American Journal of Nursing*, 74: 250-253, February 1974.

graduate, as enunciated by the NLN Department of Baccalaureate and Higher Degree Programs, will show an indifference to the specialties within nursing and an emphasis on the nursing process, on concepts and/or theories, on decision making, and on interdisciplinary activities.

Probably one of the most dramatic changes to affect nursing in this decade has been the increasing interest in the development of new and better methods of delivering health care. Meeting the health and nursing care needs of all citizens—especially in the inner cities and in rural areas—is gaining greater attention, especially from legislatures. As a result, nurse educators are realizing that the professional nurse of the future will function in many different settings and possibly only minimally in the settings in which health and illness care takes place today. This leads the educator to be less concerned, in developing nursing education courses, with the *where* of nursing as a way of developing courses in nursing and more interested in identifying the *what*—the structure—of the discipline.

Due to the present job market, with its oversupply of workers in certain fields (e.g., teaching), interest in nursing has increased. Today there are over 82,000 students in baccalaureate programs, over 79,000 students in associate degree programs, and over 70,000 students in diploma programs—a total of over 232,000 nursing students. There are also over 57,000 practical nursing students. As a result, there has been increased concern about the number of clinical agencies that can be utilized for clinical learning experiences by these students. In many areas, schools compete for time in choice agencies. Furthermore, obtaining obstetrical experiences for students in acute settings is becoming more and more difficult, due to the reduction in the birth rate; pediatric experiences within hospitals are a problem, due to the limited number of acute care facilities for children. Since hospitals and public health agencies are becoming increasingly concerned over the large number of students they are being asked to accept, baccalaureate educators are having to find other ways of meeting their clinical objectives; one way has been to offer integrated nursing programs with broad objectives rather than with objectives specifically oriented to specialty settings. This approach to objectives does not require that all students have the same type or amount of clinical experiences.

Closely related to the large numbers of students in nursing today is the fact that most authorities recognize that we no longer have a nursing shortage, but an oversupply. Leaders in nursing believe we are creating too many nursing technicians and not enough professional nurses. Baccalaureate nursing programs are being pushed to create a new type of practitioner, a pressure which has almost forced curriculum change. For if, in the eyes of the society and other health care professionals, all nursing programs are basically producing technicians, then baccalaureate students will have to compete in the oversupplied job market with "true" nursing technicians.

232

Let me summarize at this point the major ideas of this paper:

- The idea of integrating nursing curriculum is not new; in essence, we have been moving in that direction since the early 1900s. What is new is the impetus toward implementation of the concept.
- Changes in our concepts of nursing have supported the integrative approach.
- Increasing interest in the development and utilization of concepts and/or theories as a basis for nursing practice, and the realization that these concepts do not speak to areas of specialization, has encouraged us to reevaluate our curriculums.
- The increasing recognition that nursing is an independent discipline, and not dependent on medical science for its content, has supported the need for curriculum change.
- The identification of the need to teach nursing process has made us examine more specifically what we should teach.
- Faculty are becoming increasingly sophisticated in curriculum theories and can therefore better implement their beliefs about man and learning.
- There is a growing need to identify the uniqueness of the baccalureate graduate with greater clarity, resulting in a greater interest in educating differently.
- The increasing number of students within baccalaureate nursing programs requires different types of clinical learning experiences which are less oriented toward the medical model.

Let me close by admitting my bias toward the concept of unifying the curriculum in nursing. I must admit that problems arise from this type of curriculum model (these will be discussed in a later chapter), but let me cite here the advantages, as I see them, of unifying the curriculum through the integrated approach:

- Supports the student's ability to integrate ideas and concepts.
- Focuses on nursing's unique functions rather than on other health sciences.
- Stresses the generalizations and core concepts we have about nursing which will be useful throughout the life of the practitioner as she practices her profession, rather than offering her facts which change and are quickly forgotten.
- Emphasizes the *what* of nursing, rather than the *where*.
- Reduces the amount of time it takes to meet program objectives, since redundancy of specific content is reduced to a minimum or eliminated.
- Supports our beliefs about man, nursing, and learning.
- Challenges faculty to be creative in the development of a dynamic curriculum that will facilitate the education of nurses for the present and future.

29 CURRICULUM PROCESS AND THE INTEGRATED CURRICULUM

Gertrude J. Torres, EdD, RN

The curriculum development process is a valuable mechanism for reviewing, revising, or evaluating a curriculum. The development of an integrated nursing program offers nursing educators an opportunity to revise or change their curriculums.

Before we proceed to a discussion of the use of the curriculum process in relation to unifying the nursing curriculum, certain assumptions need to be made:

- That there should be educational changes in programs in nursing to meet the changing demands of society in terms of health care and that these changes should be evolutionary. The present trend toward integration of the curriculum reflects an evolutionary trend, rather than a dramatic change.
- That baccalaureate nursing programs do in fact produce generalists who are able to hypothesize, think critically, and integrate knowledge best when the knowledge and skills they are taught are presented by means of a unifying curriculum method.
- That professional nursing as practiced by the baccalaureate nursing graduate is *unique*, possessing a distinct body of knowledge which has components from other physical and behavioral sciences, medical science, and some aspects of technical nursing. Its methods of conceptualizing and/or generalizing and using the various com-

ponents to create its own body of knowledge are different and unique.
• That professional nursing is a science, with its own concepts and developing theories, and an art, as reflected in its skills of analysis, interaction, and intervention.
• That, due to the vast, accumulation of knowledge, the newer concepts of learning, and the differing emphasis in baccalaureate programs from content to process, it is essential to teach students using different approaches than we have in the past.

Philosophy

The philosophy of a baccalaureate nursing program supports the institution's philosophy, especially its beliefs about the purposes of education and its concepts of learning. These are usually stated in global terms and are expected to be guidelines to all the faculty and students in relation to curriculum structure and appproaches to teaching. These beliefs do not speak to a particular department or course of study but reflect a recognition that among specialists from all fields of study there are certain common denominators. For example, colleges often recognize their responsibility to prepare the student for work, as well as to cultivate, refine, and inform him or her for the most rewarding possible individual life. Inherent here is a strong belief in the totality of the individual similar to the ideas about man as a patient expressed in most nursing program philosophies.

Most of us view man as holistic, with his bio-psycho-social, and often spiritual, aspects inseparable. As a social being, we frequently view man as part of a family, culture, and community. These beliefs in the nature of man should have a compelling influence on how we teach students about themselves and those who will be the recipients of their care.

Generally, baccalaureate nursing programs speak to society, health, nursing, and learning, as well as man, in their written philosophies. If we view society as involving individuals, families, and communities, and man as holistic and affected by total environment, then our curriculum should reflect these views. For example, if we teach around the concept of adaptation or stress or body image, we need to identify the whole of man with the whole of his environment. This is not to deny that at any given moment the student may need to focus on one particular aspect of man or his environment, but the emphasis in teaching should relate to the whole concept. By deductive and inductive reasoning, the student is able to move back and forth from the parts to the whole with a dignified comfort.

236

Concepts related to the health-illness continuum (as stated in the philosophy) tend to be more generalized than specific; for example, we speak of levels of wellness, equilibrium-disequilibrium, and maximizing man's potential in relation to a state of health. This, in essence, represents nursing's total commitment to man as he moves back and forth along the health-illness continuum and gives us a broad responsibility within the health care system. Thus, by necessity, we must approach our content in such a manner as to offer the student the basis for generalized nursing through conceptualization and focusing on the structure of the discipline.

The nursing process is inevitably identified within our philosophy as the essence of our role, both present and future—even though sometimes it is not specifically identified as such, but rather as nursing through the problem-solving method, and so forth. Understanding of the nursing process in depth means the ability to utilize it in any setting with individuals and/or families, whether healthy or not. The student who can effectively utilize the process need not relearn it in different settings, but needs to gain increasing sophistication in its use as it is related to such things as research, leadership, change, and concepts. If a student can effectively make a developmental assessment, she can apply Erickson's concepts of learning in any setting with any age group.

We frequently express beliefs about learning, such as "Students can transfer learning from one situation to another," and "Students learn best when there is intellectual excitement taking place, especially through discovery, and when they are challenged."

Learning through the use of critical thinking, principles, and concepts is a focus frequently expressed in nursing philosophies. This approach assumes a meaningful grasp and reorganization of much separate learning into a higher level of cognition.

Thus, the philosophy of a nursing program, which is the foundation on which the entire curriculum rests, is written by nurse educators to support the unification of the curriculum. Presently, I am not aware of any statements of philosophy for baccalaureate nursing programs that support the medical-model approach, with its emphasis on illness and the acute care setting, or that support the notion that nursing differs in any one setting in which the professional nurse gives care.

Objectives

Terminal behavioral objectives are, by necessity, broad in scope in identifying common core concepts. As such, they do not truly dictate the curriculum model that must be followed. It is possible to give the student the "specialty" parts to help her meet the terminal objectives. Yet, it makes more curriculum sense to develop level objectives and course descriptions and objectives from these broad terminal objectives. Under the integrated approach, it is more appropriate to emphasize the nursing process in terms of leadership, change, and utilization of research findings than in terms of each specialty area, which does little to increase depth and much to support repetition.

The characteristics expected of baccalaureate graduates have traditionally emphasized objectives which cut across all areas of specialization. As we continue to identify more clearly the functions of the professional nurse, we move toward concepts of nursing care, leadership, quality control, utilization of theories, professional and personal development, and research. Unification of the baccalaureate curriculum around these kinds of concepts seems essential to the development of today's professional practitioner.

Bloom, in his *Taxonomy of Educational Objectives*, designates the cognitive domain as identifying the knowledge of specific facts or bits of information as related to a specialty area;[1] another capacity of the cognitive domain is knowledge of theories and structures emphasizing a body of principles and generalizations which are interrelated.[2] The latter reflects more complex and abstract ideas, which focus on the concepts we as nurse educators are attempting to give our students. The more complex the student's intellectual abilities, the more likely she is to be able to give a complete report on her attack on a problem. Thus, it is essential that course objectives emphasize a high level of handling knowledge rather than a vast framework of specifics relating to specialty areas.

Conceptual Framework

The development of a conceptual framework within the nursing curriculum has been one of the strongest forces to support the integrated curriculum approach. A program's conceptual framework, which stems from the components of its philosophy, represents the faculty's notions about nursing and nursing education and gives structure to the curriculum, so that its parts can be fitted and united into the entire program.[3] The process of developing a conceptual framework brings specialists together to create "core" concepts about nursing. These "core" concepts generally speak to man, society, health, nursing, and their interrelatedness. Once these concepts are identified, generalizations about nursing taken from the specialties can be the essence of the theoretical and clinical content taught within the program. The greater the identification of knowledge included in the generalizations about nursing, as related to the theory and practice of professional nursing, the more the curriculum will be integrated. Thus, if one closely examines a program's conceptual framework and how it is implemented, one can identify the extent of integration within the program. Specialties related to content may be mixed within the courses so that the parts are identifiable or, they can be totally blended so that the parts are not identifiable. Thus, it is essential that, when we talk about integration of a specific program, we recognize the extent to which it is mixed or blended; programs vary widely in the amount of integration within the curriculum.

Since the conceptual framework is probably one of the most important steps within the curriculum process and transmits the faculty's beliefs from the philosophy into the course description and objectives, it is essential that it be functional and clearly understood by faculty and students. Frequently, one finds conceptual frameworks that are complex, unclear, and diagrammed with circles, spaces, and boxes which only add to the confusion. This creates a kind of nonfunctional conceptual framework, causing a break in the curriculum process and an unimplemented philosophy. If a diagram is to be utilized, it should be followed by an explanation and should show clear relationships. We need to keep in mind that the conceptual framework represents the faculty's beliefs about the discipline of professional nursing; its clarity, simplicity, and health will do much to make a curriculum dynamic.

Horizontal and Vertical Strands

After the development of the philosophy, the characteristics of the graduate, and the conceptual framework, it is most helpful for a faculty to identify the horizontal and vertical strands so that the essence of the philosophy can be incorporated more easily into the behavioral level objectives. These strands reflect the essence of the nursing curriculum. In reviewing Model I, (see pp. 246-247), which speaks to the utilization of vertical and horizontal strands, one can identify how beliefs can be diagrammatically presented. The major components of the beliefs include the nursing process in all settings, which is frequently considered a horizontal strand, and the individual-family-community component, the health-illness continuum, leadership, concepts and theories in simple-complex situations, and research, which are vertical strands.

Faculty need to make decisions about how they conceptualize each strand and whether it is vertical or horizontal. The health-illness continuum, for example, could be identified as horizontal. That would mean that the student would be given theory and practice as related to healthy and ill clients and patients during each level. As it is now identified on the model (as a horizontal strand), the student would be given the theory and practice related to basically healthy persons at Level I and to ill persons at Level II. (By the way, a glossary of terms would be most helpful as part of any nursing program, so that words like simple-complex, health-illness would be clearly understood by all involved in the program.) The faculty's beliefs about learning and the purpose of education may have implications for decisions about which strands are to be taught vertically and which horizontally.

One of the major purposes for identifying curriculum strands diagrammatically is that it assists faculty in the development of level objectives which stem from the philosophy and objectives of the program. Using Model I, the following are a few sample objectives that would be appropriate:

Level I

- Utilizes the nursing process in the care of healthy individuals in all settings.
- Recognizes the need for research in her nursing practice.

Level II

- Utilizes the nursing process in complex situations in the care of patients, families, and the community.
- Participates in collecting research data.

Of course, these objectives would need to be developed further, for example, to include the components of the nursing process for each level. These represent only some of the possibilities.

The diagrammatic approach also gives direction as to what would be inappropriate. Thus, it would not be correct to have a Level I objective which stresses illness, coordination within the health team, or participation in research, for these are the components of Level II.

Let me add that the medical model, as it is often taught, contains the specialties as vertical strands. By this method, if students are rotated differently in and out of specialties, a program could have dozens of vertical strands, depending on the number of students. Frequently, the sequence is medical-surgical nursing, maternal-child nursing, psychiatric nursing, and public health nursing. This approach, as you know, creates level and course objectives oriented to specialized facts and a particular setting.

Let us now look at the components of the curriculum process in relation to the unified or integrated approach. Model II (see pp. 248-249) represents a follow-through sample of beliefs as frequently seen in baccalaureate nursing programs.

A review of the model as a total gives us the following:

- The essential components of the curriculum process that need to be considered in curriculum change or revision. This is a kind of total package with a definite sequence. One cannot change any component without looking at it in its entirety.

- A sense of direction as to how the parts relate to one another. Central to the process are the conceptual framework and the horizontal and vertical strands.
- A demonstration of how beliefs can be incorporated into all the other aspects of the curriculum.
- The significant points in which total curriculum and student evaluation should occur.

The model does not speak of the total curriculum design of a program, general education or science requirements, or methods of approaching the nursing content.

Total Curriculum Design

Let us now focus on the total curriculum design, structuring nursing courses, and identifying content and learning experiences within an integrated curriculum.

The total curriculum design represents a mechanism for carrying out the philosophy and the objectives of both the institution and the nursing program. The core requirements, as spelled out for all students within the university or college, represent the institution's way of meeting its goal as stated in the catalog. Thus, the nursing curriculum represents requirements spelled out by the total institution, as well as those identified as essential to the nursing program. Generally, in relation to the total requirements, it is helpful to require one-third general education courses, one-third supporting courses, and one-third nursing courses. Thus, if 120 credits are required for a Bachelor of Science degree in nursing, approximately 40 to 45 credits would be in nursing. The number of credits allocated for electives within and outside nursing strongly depends on the faculty's beliefs about learning. If the faculty have strong commitments to individualized curriculum patterns, independent learning activities, and individual self-fulfillment and development, the curriculum design must afford the student opportunities which support such beliefs.

In terms of specific requirements, as related to the supporting courses, these must, above all, reflect the philosophy and objectives of the nursing program. We all know the typical requirements in biology, anatomy, physiology, chemistry, microbiology, psychology, and sociology. The depth and breadth of each should be based on how the faculty view man and nursing. If the faculty, for example, require many courses in chemistry and physiology, it is evident that they view man as more basically biological than behavioral. If the faculty stress man as cultural and holistic, it would seem appropriate to require a course in anthropology. Also, if faculty identify research as an essential component in the practice of nursing, then a course in statistics may be essential. The significant point here is that course requirements are not selected merely because they might be helpful in supporting the nursing courses, but because of the specific beliefs of the faculty. If we were to approach course requirements from the position of what is helpful, we might easily end up with a six- to eight-year nursing program. Priorities and a rationale must be established for all course requirements, and these must be based on the philosophy and objectives of the program.

After developing the behavioral level objectives, whether there be three levels (with nursing starting at the sophomore year) or two levels (with nursing starting at the junior year), we need to identify how these objectives can best be met through a sequence of nursing courses. Let me add here that there is a built-in danger in beginning nursing courses during the sophomore year. Since the student has not had sufficient time to complete all her science courses prior to the first clinical nursing course, the nurse educator frequently has to teach the science superficially before she teaches nursing; the students then learn that nursing is not truly based on scientific theories or concepts, but can be practiced without an adequate base.

With the utilization of the conceptual framework, horizontal and vertical strands, and behavioral level objectives, the integrated approach to the nursing content can be identified. Generally, nursing courses in this approach must be sequenced to support the framework and strands and must have a greater allocation of credit hours than in the medical model approach. Since the emphasis is on generalizations, concepts, and theories rather than on specialties, there seems little value to students' taking two or more nursing courses at one time. Thus, some kind of structure is usually developed to offer these as seven- to ten-credit nursing courses. The following are but a few possibilities:

- Utilize the concepts and theories identified within the conceptual framework. For example, the faculty may identify such concepts as adaptation, stress, body image, immobility, and oxygenation and utilize them to develop each of the specific courses, teaching one or two concepts each semester and focusing on the horizontal and vertical strands. Nursing content is placed under the most appropriate concept.
- Utilize the case method of presentation and study. Here the faculty develop specific cases which include clients/patients and/or families involving health/illness in a variety of settings, depending on the strands identified within the curriculum. The emphasis is placed on the nursing process as related to such cases and may or may not include such things as leadership, research, or change, depending on the level of the student. One or more cases can be utilized per semester, but the faculty must keep in mind that all cases

given within a particular level must assist the student in meeting the objectives of that level. Here the emphasis is on the depth of understanding and knowledge relating to each case. The student is later expected to transfer her learning to other situations as she does during her laboratory experiences.

• Utilize the various broad nursing diagnostic categories as the major emphasis for each nursing course. For example, in reviewing the tentative nursing diagnoses that were identified by the participants in the First National Conference on the Classification of Nursing Diagnoses,[4] one could develop certain diagnostic categories as related to a conceptual framework and use these to give the nursing courses some structure.

• Nursing courses could be totally oriented around specific concepts like Maslow's Hierarchy of Needs, Abdellah's Twenty-One Nursing Problems, Erickson's developmental approach, etc.

With the utilization of any of these approaches, the emphasis is on generalizations, concepts, or theories and away from the medical model. Faculty become concerned with these approaches, especially in their attempts to integrate such areas as pharmacology, interactive and technical skills, and nutrition or diet therapy. Once again, these are incorporated into all the nursing courses as they relate to a concept, the case method, or a specific theory. Faculty often express concern about the student's learning about specific diseases. If we identify the nursing process as the essential structure of the discipline of nursing and realize that assessment and gathering data is only one part of the entire process, we then acknowledge that the patient's medical diagnosis is only one small part of the entire nursing assessment and nursing process. It is valuable data (who could deny that?), but is is not the major component of the nursing process nor a major component of the knowledge given to students in nursing. Ways need to be identified that will assist the student to conceptualize and classify nursing and medical diagnoses differently so they become useful to the practitioner. The physician and the professional nurse must utilize the medical diagnosis of a particular patient or client differently since their roles are not identical.

In developing each nursing course, we must constantly be aware of the total nursing curriculum to see how the parts fit to make a unified whole. Specific course content should be offered with a sense of the priority of knowledge and skills needed to meet the objectives. The content should also support the transfer of learning from one situation to another. Unless the course content truly reflects the philosophy, objectives, and conceptual framework, the faculty's efforts to create a dynamic curriculum is all in vain. Little is achieved if on paper the philosophy speaks to the professional role of the nurse in health care,

[4] Kristine Gebbie and Mary Ann Lavin, "Classifying Nursing Diagnoses," *American Journal of Nursing,* 74: 250-253, February 1974.

the characteristics of the graduate stress the nursing process, and the conceptual framework emphasizes theories and/or concepts in nursing, while the content of the nursing courses speaks mostly to medical diagnosis and medical science. In reviewing course outlines across the country, I have generally noted that when the faculty spell out the specific approaches to content within each class, the integrated curriculum disappears and the medical model reappears.

Let me now focus on learning experiences as related to the integrated nursing curriculum. If one can identify the greatest reward for developing an integrated curriculum, it is the flexibility that it creates in terms of laboratory experiences within all settings—no longer do students need to be rotated every four to eight weeks within every specialty area in a tight clinical schedule. With increasing enrollments and the development of new programs, clinical facilities cannot be utilized as previously. Since the emphasis is placed on the process in relation to nursing concepts and theories, learning experiences can be found in many new and different types of environments. The number and types are limited only by the ability and inability of the faculty to be creative. If we focus on the *what* of nursing and not the *where*, the potential for clincial laboratory experiences becomes enormous. Utilizing the health-illness continuum allows us to offer the student initial learning experiences in settings which focus on the healthiest part of our population. Nursing schools, newborn nurseries, schools, industry, and health maintenance organizations are settings which allow the student to focus on the nursing process in depth in nonthreatening and noncrisis environments. All students would not need to have identical experiences, but could share their experiences in conferences. For example, if the emphasis is on assessment of a healthy family, students could have laboratory experiences in the home, in nursery schools, or in clinics and then all come together to discuss the similarities among and differences between their experiences. If the emphasis is on crisis intervention in terms of oxygenation, students could care for patients in ICU, CCU, allergy clinics, or chest clinics, again sharing experiences with each other. What becomes most evident as the curriculum develops is that the faculty do become increasingly aware of the many experiences available to meet specific objectives which are oriented to the essence of nursing rather than to medical diagnosis. Some would say that this is much too loose, that students must all care for cardiac patients, or cancer patients, and so forth. Since these two categories are among the two major health care problems in this country, it seems impossible that, if she is offered a variety of experiences, the student could complete her program without a substantial number of experiences with both types of problems.

If we are to educate for the future as well as the present, we need to create different types of experiences and settings for the student. Look at the possibilities of the following examples:

- Utilizing a small mobile trailer, move from community to community to offer programs in health promotion. Allow students to practice the nursing process, especially with all its components of assessment, with members of the community, free-of-charge at regularly scheduled times. Imagine how many families could be picked up for home visits and how many referrals could be made by students to other health care workers and agencies. Here the integrated approach allows the student to care for all patients of all ages, since the emphasis is not on a specialty.
- Get funds, if possible, to support a store-front nursing center and employ a nurse practitioner. Here again, the emphasis is on nursing as a generalized profession.
- Give students a 24-hour caseload within long-term settings and allow them to be responsible for quality nursing care. They could utilize the nursing process in depth with a stable client population and through leadership skills create changes within the environment. A 24-hour caseload could also be done in an acute care setting. With the integrated approach, students could select any setting in which they would like to practice.

These types of experiences take time and effort and are initially more difficult to plan, yet they support our concepts of the emerging unique functions of the professional nurse.

A balance in clincial experiences is needed so that the student does not develop a narrow concept of the health care system. This balance should reflect the faculty's beliefs about where professional nursing will be practiced in the near and distant future. If the faculty believe that as the health care system changes—especially with the possible impact of National Health Insurance—the professional nurse will function less and less within acute care settings, then priority needs to be given to affording students experiences in other types of settings. Given such a belief, it would be inappropriate for 80 percent of students' clinical laboratory experiences to take place in an acute care setting. Faculty must select, from the available settings, the most appropriate setting in which the objectives can be met. Since the objectives in an integrated curriculum are broad in scope, emphasizing concepts and/or theories, laboratory experiences are also broader in nature rather than narrowly oriented to an acute care institution or community public health agency.

In looking at a totally integrated nursing curriculum and its different approachs to content, one becomes aware of the need to revise some teaching methods and approaches. Any teaching method must be con-

MODEL I

UTILIZATION OF VERTICAL AND HORIZONTAL STRANDS WITHIN AN INTEGRATED CURRICULUM
(Utilizing sample beliefs)

SAMPLE BELIEFS:

- Man as an *individual* is part of total environment which includes *family* and *community.*
- Man varies in his state of well-being to a *health-illness* continuum.
- Professional nursing involves the utilization of the nursing process in a variety of settings.
- Learning takes place by the utilization of *concepts and theories* that can be applied initially in *"simple"* situations, followed by "complex" situations. (Simple involves a limited number of priorities and/or problems, while complex involves a multitude of problems.)
- Identifies *research* as an essential part of nursing practice.
- Nursing involves *collaboration* and *coordination* as well as *dependent-independent-interdepedent* types of functions.
- Utilizes decision making and other *leadership skills* to improve nursing care.

HORIZONTAL STRANDS
- Nursing process in a variety of settings.

VERTICAL STRANDS
- Individual-family-community.
- Health-illness continuum.
- Utilization of concepts and theories, simple to complex.
- Appreciation-utilization-participation in research.
- Dependent-independent-interdependent functions.
- Collaboration-coordination.
- Leadership skills.

MODEL I (Continued)

UTILIZATION OF VERTICAL AND HORIZONTAL STRANDS WITHIN AN INTEGRATED CURRICULUM
(Utilizing sample beliefs)

CHARACTERISTICS OF GRADUATES

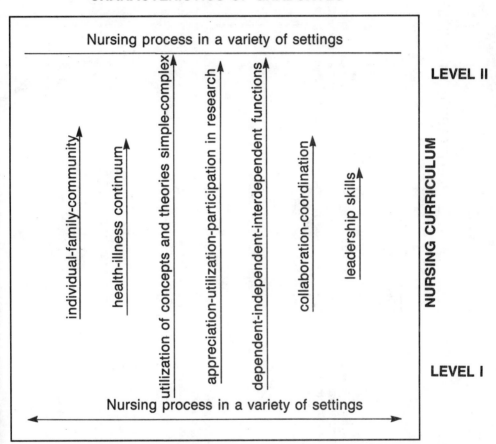

BEGINNING OF NURSING CURRICULUM

MODEL II

THE CURRICULUM PROCESS AND THE INTEGRATED CURRICULUM
(Follow-through of sample beliefs)

COMPONENTS OF A PHILOSOPHY

Professional nursing involves helping man to maintain a state of well-being.

Identifies the present and emerging role of the professional nurse as involving the nursing process, critical thinking, independent and interdependent functions.

Beliefs about the holistic view of man as a bio-psycho-social spiritual being. Identifies the patient/client as a member of a family, community and culture.

Recognizes the influence of physical, social and cultural forces in health care. Utilizes biological and psycho-social principles in giving nursing care.

CHARACTERISTICS OF GRADUATES[1]

Practices nursing to promote and/or maintain optimum health of individuals, families, and the community.

Utilizes the nursing process, assessment, diagnoses, planning, intervention and evaluation in caring for all patients/clients in all settings.

CONCEPTUAL FRAMEWORK

Stress theory, adaptation theory, crisis theory, etc.

Communication theory, decision theory, leadership theory, inerpersonal theory, etc.

Man relation to need theory, developmental theory, interpersonal theory, etc.

HORIZONTAL AND VERTICAL STRANDS

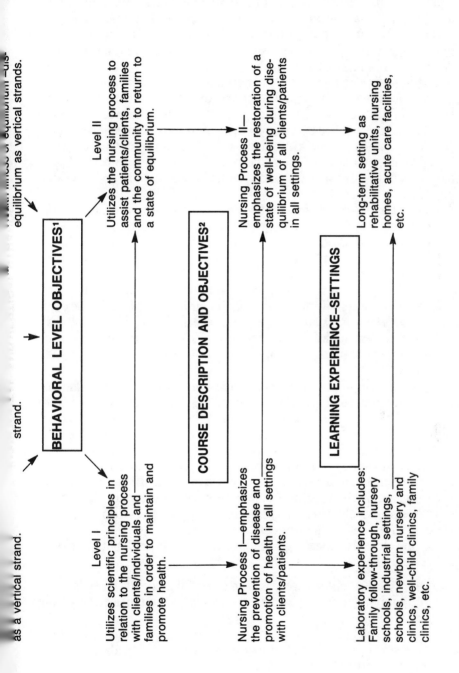

as a vertical strand.

strand.

equilibrium as vertical strands.

BEHAVIORAL LEVEL OBJECTIVES¹

Level I

Utilizes scientific principles in relation to the nursing process with clients/individuals and families in order to maintain and promote health.

Level II

Utilizes the nursing process to assist patients/clients, families and the community to return to a state of equilibrium.

COURSE DESCRIPTION AND OBJECTIVES²

Nursing Process I—emphasizes the prevention of disease and promotion of health in all settings with clients/patients.

Nursing Process II—emphasizes the restoration of a state of well-being during disequilibrium of all clients/patients in all settings.

LEARNING EXPERIENCE–SETTINGS

Laboratory experience includes: Family follow-through, nursery schools, industrial settings, schools, newborn nursery and clinics, well-child clinics, family clinics, etc.

Long-term setting as rehabilitative units, nursing homes, acute care facilities, etc.

¹ Utilized for program and total curriculum evaluation
² Objectives utilized for student's theoretical and clinical evaluation

sidered in relation to the specific course objectives that are to be met. We have utilized a wide variety of teaching methods in nursing; for example, the small group and/or large group discussion method, audiovisual teaching tools, programmed instruction, independent study, term projects or papers, panel presentations, conferences, and so forth. All of these can be utilized within a given curriculum, but their selection should reflect the faculty's beliefs about the student and learning.

The selection of audiovisual software, or other self-learning devices, should reflect the nursing content presented. Films on specific disease entities and the medical care involved, programmed instruction oriented toward technical skills without an emphasis on a strong scientific background, or a series of extensive independent study projects oriented toward a particular specialty may not be appropriate in an integrated curriculum.

Due to the development of integrated nursing programs, one of the major recent changes in teaching methods is the utilization of the team-teaching method. Simply stated, team teaching is the reorganization of teaching personnel so that two or more teachers have a responsibility to work together with the same group of students in teaching a specific course. Their responsibilities include planning, actual teaching, and evaluation. In nursing education in an integrated curriculum, the composition of the team is mixed in terms of specialty areas. Generally, an effective team includes four or five specialists, one for each area. One member of the team is either appointed as a leader or voted in by the members.

One of the major aspects of team teaching is communication. The success of the team will depend on the members' ability and willingness to communicate with one another. Decisions relating to specific approaches are no longer made alone, but by the group. Differing personalities, expertise, and teaching talent have a strong effect on group dynamics. The presumed advantage to this approach is that it allows the more committed, experienced, and competent to play a more significant role within the program by their influence on others within the team. It also encourages peer evaluation, and in a sense team members help to educate each other as well as the students.

Let me close by repeating some of the major points that have been expressed:

- The curriculum process is an essential guide to the revision of any nursing curriculum and especially in the unification of the curriculum.
- The blending and unifying of a nursing curriculum requires a revision of the faculty's previous ways of thinking about nursing and education.
- The extent to which a nursing program will integrate its curricu-

lum depends on the faculty's ability to generalize about nursing rather than seek specifics.

- The integrated approach sets us apart from the medical model and medical science and helps us concentrate on the theory and practice of nursing, especially as related to the nursing process.

If we, nurse educators, view the role of the professional nurse as evolutionary in a changing health care system and recognize the changing educational trends, we then become committed to a careful examination of our curriculums. Whether this moves us toward an integrated curriculum, or causes us to continue support of the medical model, is not as significant as our continuing to examine and identify what we are about as nurses and educators.

30 IMPLICATIONS FOR EVALUATION IN AN INTEGRATED CURRICULUM

Eleanor A. Lynch, MA, RN

One's viewpoint on the nature of the integrated curriculum in nursing affects significantly one's plan for the evaluation of the outcomes of such a curriculum. Evaluation is an integral part of the curriculum development process and functions reciprocally with the other major components of the process—educational objectives and learning experiences. Because of this interrelatedness, the purpose of evaluation can best be achieved if evaluation procedures are adapted to reflect the structural approaches and methodology of the curriculum.

Dr. Torres, in her first paper in this volume, "Educational Trends and the Integrated Curriculum Approach in Nursing,"[1] identifies the integrated nursing curriculum as a blending of content pertinent to the practice of professional nursing in such a way that each component contributes to the development of larger and more meaningful wholes, representing the unification and melding of relevant concepts and ideas. She further refers to criticisms of the integrated curriculum that stem from the belief that coordination of nursing content into core courses would lead to vagueness and lack of precision for disciplined thinking. These two concepts of integration in the nursing curriculum are somewhat analagous to the two definitions of an alloy.

Webster defines an alloy as: "1. a substance composed of two or more

---

[1] Above, pp. 221-226.

metals, intimately mixed and united, usually by being fused together by dissolving in each other when molten; and 2. to lower or debase by mixture.''[2] If bronze and steel are used as examples of the first definition, disagreement about the value of admixing the tin and zinc with copper to form steel, would be hard to come by. The end products would generally be viewed primarily in light of their greater usefulness, without value judgments being attached to the constituents of the alloys. If, however, gold or silver is admixed with copper to make a product such as coins, no one would deny the necessity of alloying the metals to provide a more durable product, but someone could certainly say that the gold or silver had been debased by the combination, thus illustrating the second Webster definition.

Both the intrinsic and extrinsic values of each structural component of the curriculum should be assessed as it relates and contributes to the implementation of the process of nursing. However, a curriculum in which major consideration is given to the value of each separate component part, with little or no focus on the whole process of nursing, is not likely to prepare nurses who can solve the wide variety of problems related to health care. Integration, representing a fusion of content which cuts across clinical entities and binds courses together by concepts, is more likely to produce nurses capable of achieving quality results through the nursing process. An integrated curriculum need not represent a thinning-out of content, limiting coverage to the more common health deviations, nor should it represent an expansion of content to incorporate many courses under a broader heading. The establishment of an articulated relationship between course content would serve only the purpose of correlation, but not that of integration.

In what ways does evaluation in an integrated nursing curriculum differ from that in an unintegrated curriculum—that is, one focused on a systematic building of parts, brick-upon-brick, with emphasis on the parts rather than on the whole? The response to the question is, ''The differences are in terms of degree rather than kind.'' The narrow and broad definitions of evaluation in education commonly found in evaluation and measurement texts are applicable; the steps in the evaluation process are essentially the same, but greater stringency must be established and maintained for the process if the goals of the integrated curriculum are to be met.

The more the curriculum is integrated, the greater the need for the program developed for evaluation to be focused on the analysis of objectives and content so that meaningful segments can be delineated for evaluation. Evaluation, unlike teaching, is a process of analysis. The determination of qualitative and quantitative aspects of educational

---

[2] *Webster's Third New International Dictionary* (Springfield, Mass.: G. & C. Merriam Company, 1961).

254

outcomes involves the separation of a whole into its constituent or essential parts. Synthesis serves the purposes of teaching, whereas analysis serves the purposes of evaluation.

Yura and Walsh state that dividing the nursing process into phases is an artificial separation of actions which cannot, in actual practice, be separated. They state further that the nursing process can be divided into its components or phases—assessing, planning, implementing, and evaluating—to facilitate the performance of nursing.[3] If the purposes of evaluation are to be served, artificial or not, one must separate out the phases of the nursing process to assess the progress being made by students in achieving objectives pertinent to the nursing process. It is true that if a nursing student demonstrates a high level of competence and skill in the assessment phase of the nursing process and utilizes the scientific method effectively in gathering data about the health needs of clients and patients, these abilities would provide good bases for other phases of the nursing process. However, since the practice of nursing involves complex behaviors, is it not possible that the same nursing student might *not* demonstrate a comparable level of competence in the implementation and evaluation phases of the nursing process? Since this is a possibility, is it not incumbent on faculty to utilize measures to provide data referrable to the student's abilities at each phase of the nursing process? A global account of a nursing student's ability to utilize the nursing process would be meaningless in terms of both formative and summative evaluation. Specific data pertaining to a student's knowledge and performance are necessary to assess strengths and areas for growth and improvement and the degree to which objectives are met for grading and certification.

"The bigger the educational strands, the more carefully evaluation must be planned to take sample 'slices' of student attainment in both horizontal and vertical planes throughout the curriculum."[4] Plans for each stage of the curriculum process should include specific ways in which the vertical and horizontal components are to be assessed in terms of sequentially arranged objectives—from the least to the most specific and from the lowest to the highest degree of depth and complexity.

An effective plan for the evaluation of an integrated curriculum is comprehensive: all objectives and strands are included, with attention given to specificity. The specificity of the evaluation plan need not connote or denote inflexibility and inevitable obsolescence, nor should the attention given to achieving specificity contribute to fragmentation of the curriculum strands. Such fragmentation would be diametrically opposed to the purposes of the integrated curriculum.

---

[3] Helen Yura and Mary B. Walsh, *The Nursing Process* (New York: Appleton-Century-Crofts, 1973), p. 25.

[4] "Let's Examine. . .The Measurement of Over-All Competence And of Discrete Abilities," *Nursing Outlook,* 12:42, February 1964.

There certainly is a need to measure, by testing, students' levels of knowledge of basic concepts. If, however, measures are not included in the plan to assess the application of these concepts or to assess the students' utilization of these concepts in a variety of settings, it would be unlikely that the purposes of the integrated curriculum would be met. Effective evaluation of desired outcomes of the integrated nursing curriculum requires the use of familiar and unfamiliar experiences or situations and direct and indirect approaches that will elicit behaviors indicated by the objectives.

The development of an integrated curriculum involves the incorporation of heterogeneous elements to produce courses with broad content areas, reflecting many abilities. Factors which are unique to the health care of patients and clients of a specific age group with a specific health deviation are synthesized with factors which cut across age groups and a variety of health deviations. Because of this, faculty need to consider the degree to which unique and common factors are to be measured and appraised. Pulling apart content to analyze student achievement in relation to discrete factors is not a violation in terms of the purpose of evaluation. It is a defensible act, grounded on the idea that data obtained from such an assessment would add a significant dimension to the overall evaluation process.

Some of the points made so far can be summarized as follows:

1. Evaluation procedures should reflect the structural approaches and methodology of the curriculum.

2. Evaluation in an integrated nursing curriculum differs from the evaluation of a subject matter-oriented curriculum in degree rather than kind.

3. Evaluation is essentially a process of analysis.

4. Plans for the evaluation of the integrated curriculum should include ways in which vertical and horizontal components can be assessed in terms of sequentially arranged objectives.

5. The evaluation plan should provide for the assessment of common and unique factors.

I would like to refer now to Figure 1, "A Blueprint for Evaluation in an Integrated Curriculum, Reflecting Objectives, Vertical and Horizontal Strands, and Evaluation Methods," which was developed to demonstrate a possible method of incorporating the evaluation process into the curriculum development process in an integrated nursing curriculum. In the figure, three main aspects are identified: Objectives, Conceptual Framework, and Evaluation Methods. The Objectives, at

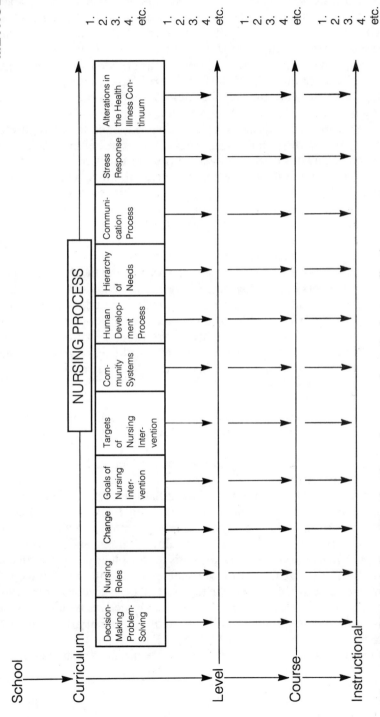

Figure 1. A blueprint for evaluation in an integrated curriculum, reflecting objectives, vertical and horizontal strands, and evaluation methods.

the left side of the figure, from least to most specific, include: School, Curriculum, Level, Course, and Instructional. The Conceptual Framework shows a major concept, the Nursing Process, as the horizontal strand and subconcepts and theoretical formulations (Decision-making, Nursing Roles, etc.) as vertical strands. These vertical strands represent possible samples of those which might be delineated by many faculties, and do not represent those of a single program. The Evaluation Methods, at the right of the figure, are blank; faculty must choose these as necessary for each level of development of the Objectives and for each aspect of the curriculum evaluated.

The School (Institutional) Objectives would, of course, be expressed in very general or global terms, identifying the behavioral changes expected as a result of the total educational program.

The Curriculum Objectives would be general, but less global than the School Objectives; they would relate to the competencies expected of graduates of the educational program. They would reflect faculty's ideas about man, society, health, and nursing. The Curriculum Objectives would serve as an overall framework for developing Level Objectives, Course Objectives, and Instructional Objectives.

Level Objectives would represent goals set by the faculty for students at various points in the program. Expressed in behavioral terms, Level Objectives would describe expected degrees of competence, and would reflect progress in terms of depth and sequence from one level to another. Since the Level Objectives are behaviors expected of all students at predetermined points in the program, they would bear a greater likeness to School and Curriculum Objectives than to Course and Instructional Objectives. Level Objectives would determine Course Objectives, and course placement.

Course Objectives, also stated in behavioral terms, would define goals of instruction in the various course or units, and they should reflect the Level Objectives.

Instructional Objectives would relate to student achievement of unit or lesson objectives.

Sample concepts and theoretical formulations are included under the Conceptual Framework. The Conceptual Framework would reflect the philosophy of the school and the nursing program and would be used as a guide for decisions about curriculum content and instructional strategies. It also would serve as the basis for the blueprint for curriculum evaluation. Horizontal and vertical strands of the Conceptual Framework would be assessed in terms of all objectives established for the program as far as possible. The Level Objectives would provide a basis for determining depth and degree of complexity in terms of the strands.

A wide variety of evaluation methods would need to be delineated.

258

Decisions about the methods would reflect consideration of the behavior indicated by the objectives, the nature of the concepts and/or theoretical formulations, and the capability of the evaluation method to elicit measurable behavior congruent with that indicated by the objective. It is necessary for faculty to distinguish those aspects of objectives which can be economically and effectively assessed by written tests from those needing some other means of evaluation.

Major advantages of such a model blueprint include:

1. A greater likelihood that plans for formative and summative evaluation would reflect cross-fertilization of vertical and horizontal components of the conceptual framework and the sequentially developed objectives.

2. A greater likelihood that plans for the evaluation process would represent a continuum, providing for the assessment of students' progress in meeting objectives pertinent to the major concepts, the subconcepts, and the theoretical formulations basic to the conceptual framework throughout the curriculum.

3. A greater likelihood of harmony between the evaluation process and the curriculum development process.

In conclusion, educators in nursing programs cannot afford to leave the assessment of outcomes to happenstance. Plans for the evaluation of the educational process should be instituted to provide data for determining the effectiveness or ineffectiveness of the approaches and methodology of the curriculum of every nursing program.

BIBLIOGRAPHY

Abdellah, Faye G., *et al. New Directions in Patient-Centered Nursing.* New York: Macmillan Co., 1973.
Bevis, Em Olivia. *Curriculum Building in Nursing.* Saint Louis: C.V. Mosby Co., 1973.
"Let's Examine...Specificity of Test Content." *Nursing Outlook* 11:348, May 1963.
"Let's Examine... The Measurement of Common and Unique Factors." *Nursing Outlook* 9:705, December 1961.
Ozimek, Dorothy. *The Baccalaureate Graduate in Nursing: What Does Society Expect?* New York: National League for Nursing, 1974.
Stevens, Barbara J. "Analysis of Structural Forms Used in Nursing Curricula." *Nursing Research* 20:388-397, Sept.-Oct. 1971.
Torres, Gertrude, and Yura, Helen, *Today's Conceptual Framework: Its Relationship to the Curriculum Development Process.* New York: National League for Nursing, 1974.

31 THE INTEGRATED CURRICULUM—PROBLEMS AND CONCERNS IN THE WORLD OF SPECIALIZATION

Gertrude J. Torres, EdD, RN

The concept of change, with the forces for it and the resistances to it, is at the very heart of many of the problems and concerns related to the development of an integrated curriculum. In moving toward curriculum change of this nature, we become aware of other changes, both outside and inside the institution of higher learning, needed to support the new curriculum approach. Within the institution, these changes involve faculty and students; on the outside, they involve the clinical settings utilized by the students.

In discussing the integrated curriculum approach, it is helpful to examine both the forces that encourage change and those that resist change. Nursing and other educators are strongly aware of the social and educational pressures to accept change, to be innovative, to create unique programs, and to get on untested educational bandwagons. To resist change is to be inevitable and essential, and change for change's sake seems to be gaining impetus in education today. Yet, in truth, we often think we are changing more than we really are. This is due to resistors functioning within our educational institutions.

The faculty is one of the strongest forces in an institution having an effect on the type and amount of change that will occur. Both faculty who resist change and those who encourage it are essential to give balance to any institution. Faculty who resist change have a strong tendency to want to teach the way they have been taught; for the most part, they feel comfortable maintaining their specialist role. Their graduate education has, for the most part, reinforced their need to support specialization. They are generally committed to society's present concept of illness care involving a limited number of settings—a concept which supports their present curriculum approach—and have difficulty generalizing and theorizing about newer nursing concepts. Faculty in nursing are often new to the environment of institutions of higher learning and, since they are still orienting and adapting themselves to this setting, have little time to think about change. As specialists, nurse educators are not often able to identify the advantages of curriculum change. Although they express a "futuristic" philosophy about education and nursing, they basically support the status quo in their concepts of nursing practice. These characteristics are present to some extent in all of us: there seem to be forces within us that, on the one hand, support change, and, on the other, resist it. Thus, we are often left with an inner conflict, and the direction we finally take is often dependent on how others react to, resist, or accept the change. We must recognize that change produces insecurity in all of us, and that we need to help each other in making objective critical decisions about the validity of any change.

Assuming that a faculty is committed to changing the curriculum and developing an integrated approach, we will now identify the problems and concerns that tend to develop. One of the problems is a lack of understanding as to the exact nature of the change involved. Some may perceive it to be a dynamic, exciting, challenging experience, creating a totally different approach, while others may see it as an upsetting, impossible, time-consuming task, with very little real improvement occurring. It seems to me that those in the middle are probably correct. Although there may be changes in approaches to content, integration of knowledge and skills basically involves no change of content. Our philosophy of man, health, and nursing is not really different, just our way of educating about these components of nursing.

As nurse educators, we have continuously changed and revised our curriculums. One only needs to look at the curriculum guides written 30 to 50 years ago to recognize that we have moved forward rather slowly. But we have changed. The move toward integration is no more dramatic than previous changes. Actually, we tend to overreact and become rather dramatic about changes. Sister John Gabriel, in her concern over what was occurring in nursing education in 1929, reminds her readers of the great changes which had taken place in just ten years.[1]

---

[1] Sister John Gabriel, *Principles of Teaching in Schools of Nursing* (New York: Macmillan Company, 1928).

Sarason believes that the more things change, the more they stay the same, which gives us much food for thought.[2]

Faculty, as specialists, are often concerned that, in the development of an integrated curriculum, they will have a less significant part in the program. The opposite is true. They have a vital responsibility to see that their field of nursing is appropriately treated and integrated, and that it is taught accurately and updated as new knowledge is found. In blending, one must start out with distinct parts that are of high quality before putting the parts together. Thus, in integrating the curriculum, faculty who are well-qualified experts in their field are essential.

Specialists are also concerned that the specific content of their fields will not be given sufficient emphasis. Since we can never educate in depth in relation to any one field and do not aim to do so when we produce a generalist at the undergraduate level, it becomes a matter of generalizing our content and establishing priorities. Specialists can be most helpful in identifying priorities and finding the relationships between their fields and others, thus assisting in structuring the curriculum so that redundancy is minimized.

Generalists can also contribute much to be development of an integrated curriculum. Although we produce few real generalists at the present (the community health "specialist" being probably the only exception), some graduate programs are moving in that direction. A nurse educator who has concentrated her efforts in a graduate program in increasing her depth in the nursing process, in research, in leadership, or in scientific and nursing theories and/or concepts can be a valuable asset in the development of an integrated curriculum.

Faculty are frequently overwhelmed initially by the work that seems to be required in curriculum change. Their concerns revolve around the seeming administrative failure to grant them adequate time to develop the new curriculum. Primarily committed to teaching their present student population, utilizing their present curriculum, faculty often cannot find the additional time or energy for change without additional support. This support can be given by reducing certain faculty responsibilities so that members can concentrate on curriculum revision. Or additional funds can be allocated for use in obtaining expert assistance. It should also be recognized that faculty can do much to reduce their own commitments to afford themselves more time for curriculum revision. It is often a matter of giving curriculum change the proper priority.

Faculty, as clinical specialists, tend to use "nursing" textbooks which emphasize the medical model. In an integrated curriculum, such texts offer little assistance to the student in identifying relationships. More recent nursing texts have moved in the direction of looking at concepts and/or theories in nursing.

[2] Seymour B. Sarason, *The Culture of the Schools and the Problems of Change* (Boston: Allyn and Bacon, Inc., 1971).

One of the major problems in *implementing* the integrated curriculum is the often-recognized necessity for team teaching. (Although team teaching does sometimes occur under the medical model, it is less frequent.) Let me admit that a totally integrated curriculum, which has been carefully planned by specialists, could be taught by individual faculty members. This would mean that faculty specialists, for the most part, would be teaching generalized concepts and the core of nursing and not their specialty. This can be a difficult task for nursing educators, and faculty tend to employ team teaching under the integrated curriculum approach.

For years, faculty have been alone in the classroom with their students, for the most part making their own decisions about approaches to content. Their need to communicate with other faculty has been at a minimum, and their methods of evaluation have been decided mostly by themselves and have reflected their philosophy in terms of what students needed to achieve. Thus, the life of the educator was not too complex and was, for the most part, independent in nature.

In team teaching, much of this independence is lost and a sense of togetherness prevails. For educators who prefer to function alone, this is quite a change. On the other hand, there are many benefits that can accrue when team teaching is practiced effectively: faculty can learn from one another, they can share concerns, and they can support each other's strengths and weaknesses.

Team teaching problems often relate to the faculty's inability to communicate, to compromise, to share leadership responsibilities, to identify and accept strengths and weaknesses within the group, to accept peer evaluation and analysis, and to interact from a positive position.

In order to improve the situation, some schools have gone so far as to institute faculty group therapy on a weekly basis. This is not mentioned to encourage such an activity, but only to emphasize that real problems, not related simply to change, occur when a program moves from the individual to the team teaching approach.

The issue of the effectiveness of team teaching has not been resolved through research. It is possible to teach on an individual basis in an integrated nursing course only if each faculty member is sufficiently informed of the content and approach and can therefore assist the student in applying theory to practice in the clinical area.

Problems in relation to students frequently occur during curriculum change. Their lack of understanding as to how this change may affect them is often at the heart of the problem. To combat this, students should not only be kept informed, but should be made an essential part of the decision-making process. Although they do not have the same expertise in nursing or education as the faculty, students can often be useful in identifying the directions for change.

Student resistance tends to be greater when there is great conflict within the faculty and can be reduced substantially as faculty themselves move more positively toward the change. Thus, when students resist curriculum change, it can be helpful to examine the position of the total faculty in relation to the change.

The integrated curriculum also sometimes necessitates significant changes in the utilization of outside agencies. No longer is it appropriate to rotate the students through a clinical specialty setting for 10 to 12 weeks at a time. Faculty no longer have "their" students for long periods of time, and the clinical setting no longer needs to receive lists of students who will be on a particular unit for a semester at a time. Instead, greater flexibility in the utilization of agencies is essential. A particular clinical setting may be used by different students weekly, or even daily, when their studies require a different orientation. The unit's particular idiosyncrasies and policies are not really significant. The student is able to focus on the objectives she must meet in terms of herself and the patient and learns to reorient herself as she moves from setting to setting. However, faculty's responsibilities are frequently increased; since a student might be in five to ten different settings in a semester, a great deal of planning is required. In the integrated approach, the concept that all students must have the same experiences is given up in favor of the belief that the same broad objectives can be met just as well in many settings.

Faculty often fear that they will be required to function in a setting different from their clinical specialty. The thought of a maternal specialist functioning in an intensive care unit can be frightening not only to the individual faculty member but to the students as well. Intelligent nursing educators must be capable of recognizing each other's strengths and weaknesses. Here reasonable judgment and flexibility must prevail. Since we are preparing beginning practitioners to be generalists, we should approach each clinical laboratory experience with that in mind.

Team teaching also sometimes creates greater problems for administrators in terms of faculty load, student credit hours, faculty assignments, and other personnel policies. These may involve policy changes which may themselves encourage resistance.

With an integrated approach, it may be more difficult to explain the curriculum to others outside the institution. Parents, advisory groups, other nurse leaders, and administrators of clinical agencies will need to have a clear understanding of the rationale for change, as well as the implications of the change for them. Faculty should take the opportunity of such a change to become community leaders, to inform and guide others in regard to the present and emerging trends in education and nursing.

These are but a few of the problems incurred by a curriculum change of this nature, and this list is by no means all-inclusive. Change involves people and their perceptions of what it will mean to them and to their profession. It involves decision making based on critical analysis. And most of all it (hopefully) involves objectivity. May we as nurse educators and leaders in nursing carefully weigh all our decisions about change!

5 THE CHANGING ROLE OF THE PROFESSIONAL NURSE— IMPLICATIONS FOR NURSING EDUCATION

32 THREE FACTORS OF SIGNIFICANCE TO BACCALAUREATE NURSING EDUCATION

Marjorie Stanton, EdD, RN

Any discussion of changes in the health care system needs to begin with a consideration of several vital points. We talk about health care delivery but, in fact, most of our efforts in this nation are given to delivery of *illness* care. The majority of insurance protection is provided for hospital care and for major medical reasons. Coverage for dental care is generally a luxury, although dental care continues to be the most common health problem. None of us cares to discuss the infant mortality rate in this country of affluence, especially that in disadvantaged areas. The largest monetary rewards among health care professionals, and I use the term advisedly, go to physicians, who focus on diagnosing and prescribing for illness. Most nurses in this country continue to work in acute-care settings. Nursing homes are conspicuous for the absence of nursing, as witness the recent nursing home scandal in New York State. And last but not least, the medical model is still a favorite with some baccalaureate nursing educators.

It has been said that in the U.S. we pay more for "health care" and get less than in any other of the developed nations. We do not now have a system of health care, but rather a non-system of fragmented illness care, with minor attention given to health. The problems are the lack availability, the inaccessibility and the discontinuity of health care services. To restate the problem, it is the inability of Americans to receive health care, *where* they want it, *when* they need it, *how* they need it, and from *whom* they need it.

A viable health care system must have aims and goals that take into account all of the above, with all health professionals and consumers having input into the design and implementation of such a system. For, as George Wald says in his Foreword to Allan Chase's *Biological Imperatives: Health, Politics and Human Survival* (New York: Holt, Rinehart & Winston, 1972), "The national health is not only a medical problem; it involves the entire operation of our society and its goals. It is much more than the business of caring for the sick. It has to be concerned with minimal incomes, nutrition, clean air and water, sewage disposal, adequate public transportation, better schools, and better housing."

Nursing started out by concerning itself with more than just the care of the sick; we were *the* health professionals, but somewhere along the way we narrowed our view and perhaps our vision. We became, like the physician, primarily concerned with taking care of sick people who come to us in the hospital where we help people to get well and from which we dismiss them, neither knowing nor caring where they come from or where they return.

Of course, we all recognize that there are many things which must be taken into account when discussing a health care system, such as population growth, increased technology, economics, and supply and demand. In my view, however, there are three major phenomena related to health care which will have significance for baccalaureate nursing education—National Health Insurance, third-party reimbursement for professional nursing care and a full realization of the potential of nurses with the first professional degree, the baccalaureate degree in nursing. All of these are interrelated, and the success or failure of one aspect affects the other two.

National Health Insurance

It is generally conceded that some form of National Health Insurance (NHI) will become a reality within the very near future. In fact, this promises to be a major political concern. There are two questions which need to be asked, however. Will it meet the *health* needs of the public? And will it acknowledge the importance of *all* health professionals in a viable health care system? Up to this point, no National Health Insurance proposal meets these qualifications, although some do touch on health care. In testimony before the House Ways and Means Committee in August, 1974, the American Association of Colleges of Nursing noted that all plans reflected the traditional concepts of insuring for the inpatient costs of sickness rather than the maintenance of health. They urged recognition of professional nurses and other qualified health professionals in terms of their ability to practice and their right to receive just fees without the permission of physicians. The testimoy went on to declare, "Health is the umbrella under which all must practice; medicine is not. Therefore any National Health Insurance Plan must allow more than medicine to practice at its optimal level."[1] Testimony by the American Nurses' Association supported this by stating, "Health insurance should guarantee access to the health care systems through the series of health care practitioners that are available and appropriate for the clients' health needs."[2] It is interesting to note that testimony by the American Medical Association indicated that the public is not concerned over NHI. They cited an opinion poll which indicated a lack of public concern over NHI and a general satisfaction with the present system and suggested that the public didn't really want Congress to aggravate its primary concern—inflation.[3]

When a National Health Insurance plan is enacted into law, the practice of all health professionals should change for the better. This, of course, will occur if the practice of medicine in a health care delivery system is viewed in proper perspective. Yes, I mean the practice of medicine. For only when medicine is considered as just one of many disciplines necessary to preserve the health of the public will we truly have a system of health care.

Third Party Payment for Reimbursement

Individual nurses have received payment from clients for direct nursing care since modern nursing was initiated. However, at this point in time, in a society where most people carry some kind of health or medical insurance plan, there is no provision for professional nurses to be paid by clients for nursing care except as an out-of-pocket expense, unless a physician or a health care administrator authorizes such care. Unless professional nurses can receive just payment for nursing care rendered under any health insurance plan conceived, the concept of professional nursing practice will be relegated to myth. The New York State Nurses' Association is actively involved in efforts to secure changes in New York State insurance laws; other state organizations are also working toward this end. They believe that the "deficiency in the law not only discriminates against the largest single group of independent health professionals in New York State [i.e., nurses], but more significantly it deprives people who desperately need and seek nursing care services."[4]

[1] *National Health Insurance,* Bulletin No. 21, August 30, 1974, p. 1.
[2] *National Health Insurance,* Bulletin No. 18, July 29, 1974, pp. 3-4.
[3] *Ibid.*
[4] NYSNA Statement on Third Party Reimbursement, *Journal NYSNA,* 5(3):5, November 1974.

Full Recognition of the Potential of Nurses
With the First Professional Degree

The baccalaureate degree in nursing is the first professional degree in nursing. However, the full potential of this graduate has never been realized. Think what we could do to health care delivery in this country if these graduates were permitted to practice at their optimum level. Have we ever considered the waste of this talent and the resulting deprivation of the public? The fact that we have failed to help these graduates attain their full potential in practice must weigh heavily on our consciences—in both education and service. We are, however, beginning to see a shift in the utilization of these graduates—a shift which we must nurture and encourage.

To reiterate: there are three major changes which will affect baccalaureate nursing education and of which we must be aware—National Health Insurance, third-party reimbursement for nurses (a necessary part of any NHI plan), and full recognition of the potential of the graduate of baccalaureate nursing programs.

Let us consider briefly how we need to prepare students in our baccalaureate programs so that they can function in a true health care delivery system. We need to remind ourselves that some of our thoughts are not so new. In 1927, a paper on curriculum prepared by the Committee on Education of the National League for Nursing Education stated, "Health nursing is just as fundamental as sick nursing and the prevention of disease at least as important a function of the nurse as the care and treatment of the sick."[5] That was forty-eight years ago. More recently, Storlie has devoted a whole unit to the concept that nursing is not for the sick alone in her book *Nursing and the Social Conscience.*[6] When will we catch up with ourselves?

I would now like to offer some thoughts on how the phenomena I have identified might affect baccalaureate education.

When NHI becomes a fact, and if it is a viable plan, professional nursing should assume a vital position in the health care system. I would follow, then, that our curriculum design must emphasize health nursing should assume a vital position in the health care system. It would learning experiences must take place outside of acute-care settings to a *much* greater degree than is now the case. It must be remembered that the acute-care setting is just one of the community agencies used by clients.

If third-party reimbursement becomes a reality, the opportunities for

---

[5] National League of Nursing Education, Committee on Education, *A Curriculum for Schools of Nursing* (New York: The League, 1927), p. 11.

[6] Frances Storlie, *Nursing and the Social Conscience* (New York: Appleton-Century-Crofts, 1970), pp. 1-29.

professional nursing practice will become unlimited. It follows, then, that recognition of accountability, continuing education, and innovation will become very important in the educational process. Where and how we will provide opportunities for students to practice independently, interdependently, and collaboratively will become matters of great significance. The usual hospital setting may not be the area of choice, nor may any other structural agency. We will need to look at private-practice settings, storefront clinics, Indian health stations, and others. Educational institutions may need to provide their own settings if appropriate ones are not available, as is being done by Adelphi University and Molloy College, both on Long Island in New York.

If we begin to see the full potential of our graduates, then our philosophical positions on health nursing and illness nursing may need a shift. Students will need experiences where they can stretch their minds and their skills. Faculty and service people will need to use their imagination and be ready to let students take the lead. Students will need to be free from the confines of time and structure at certain periods in order to learn how it feels to be a professional nurse, while still within the safety of the educational program. Research will become an important component of learning. We will also need to provide course content and opportunities for students that will make them aware of and utilize political action to improve the social condition and therefore the health of the citizens of the country.

We need to prepare nurses who are confident, cognizant, and competent. To do this, nursing educators and nursing service personnel must work collaboratively in providing the most meaningful learning experiences for the future practitioners of nursing. For as Plato said, "The direction in which education starts a man will determine his future life."

33 CHANGES IN NURSING SERVICE THAT AFFECT BACCALAUREATE NURSING PROGRAMS

Sylvia Carlson, PhD, RN

It is difficult to discuss the effects of changes in nursing service on bacccalaureate nursing programs because I don't believe that the relationship between nursing service and nursing education can really be viewed as flowing in only one direction. I believe that we are operating in an open system and that what is happening in the delivery of health care in the country affects both nursing education and nursing service *together*, and that simultaneously nursing education and nursing service affect each other in a reciprocal relationship of mutual interaction.

The main objective of nursing education is to prepare students as a source of supply for the health care delivery system in all areas of practice where a nurse's education and skills can be utilized for the benefit of the client. The purpose of the employing agency is to utilize the product of the educational system to deliver that expertise to the client. It seems to me that the former motto of NLN—"So that nursing needs of the people will be met"—encompasses the overall objectives of both nursing education and nursing practice.

Although I believe that the long-range objectives of education and service are the same, the individual responsibilities differ. One group focuses on the education of students and the other on the delivery of nursing care to clients and patients. Yet our interdependence and mutual interactions are constant. One cannot exist without the other, and that is why I am heartened by opportunities for nursing educators and nursing administrators to come together to discuss mutual concerns.

Sociologists refer to the bouncing newborn baby as a replacement unit; without such "replacement units" society would no longer exist. The socialization of these replacement units takes place within the family and in the schools. The nursing profession must also provide and nurture its own replacement units, and part of the socialization of these nursing replacement units takes place in the hospital setting.

But it is here that the frequent and unpleasant finger-pointing takes place. Nursing service personnel state that nursing education is not realistic in that what is taught to the student does not reflect the actual practice required in the service agency. On the other side, the nursing educator sees the hospital as a clinical laboratory which is needed to help the student put into practice what has been taught in theory. Yet there are few professional role models for students to follow in that clinical laboratory, and the instructor finds it difficult to teach in theory. I myself, as a clinical instructor ten years ago, admonished students not to model themselves after the nursing activity on the unit, but to do what I had taught them, since I felt that I was the role model.

The reason for this discrepancy is that the clinical laboratories (i.e., hospitals) are still functioning on the industrial model in providing patient care (i.e., tasks delegated to various levels of workers), which results, as we all know, in fragmented care. Sometimes this functional method is given the name "Team Nursing." But as Delores Little once said, "Show me a hosptial doing Team Nursing and I'll award them the Nobel Prize in Nursing." By whatever name it is called, the functional approach still results in a medication nurse, an I.V. nurse, a blood pressure nurse, a bath-giver, and a dressing changer. Differences in the basic philosophies and objectives of the nursing educator and the hospital service delivery system have caused conflict, and the so-called gap between nursing education and nursing service has resulted in a disruption within our profession. What is taught in our baccalaureate programs is not translated into service agencies.

Not only does the student nurse have no role model, but also the graduate nurse often leaves nursing because of what Marlene Kramer has called professional-bureaucratic role conflict. To quote Kramer:

> The newcomer is considered to have adjusted when she has fused her values with those of the working community. Rather than growth, fusion or absorption as a method of conflict resolution produces stagnation, apathy, and perhaps most important, continued intolerance... The work gets done, but does nursing practice and the health care system improve?[1]

The discrepancies between role theory and role practice add up to role deprivation and either a dissatisfied or conformist worker or a dropout

---

[1] Marlene Kramer, *Reality Shock* (St. Louis: C.V. Mosby Co., 1974), p. 32.

from the profession. Of course, many of our present problems are rooted in our history of so-called apprenticeship education. Moving into the university setting has created this gap: no longer are nursing education and service wedded, bedded, and dined in one setting, but they are in a state of divorce. Indeed, each parent is socializing the child with a different set of norms and values.

Yet we are confronted with the need to define the minimum requirement for a professional nurse as education in the collegiate setting, culminating in the baccalaureate degree in nursing. The need for development in this area was noted as long ago as 1923 in the Goldmark Report[2] and is discussed by Bridgman in *Collegiate Education for Nursing.*[3] Fifty years later we are nearer to our goal, but have not reached it—either actually or philosophically.

What are the responsibilities of the *educators* to service? And on the other side of the coin: how can nursing service know that the student is truly a safe practitioner (e.g., can pour medications accurately and safely for 40 to 50 patients) when education continues to use the case method assignment? How can we be sure that the new graduate is capable of accepting responsibility for evening or night shifts? What assurance does nursing service have, other than the fact of graduation, that the new graduate is at least a beginning-level, safe practitioner? The doubts are so great that some inservice departments give pharmacology exams to their new nurse employees as part of the orientation process; the nurse cannot be assigned to medications unless she passes the exam. If she cannot pass the exam, the service personnel proceed to give remedial classes, and she remains an outcast or in effect works as an aide.

I personally deplore this practice. What kind of situation can this possibly create except to continue to widen the gap between nursing education and nursing service? It results in neither feeling the other is competent in their respective roles. *Trust* is the beginning of closing the gap.

Those changes in the acute-care setting that affect baccalaureate curriculum are not changes in the acute care setting itself, but, in the words of what is now a cliche, in "the vast scientific and technological advances of the 20th century." Scientific knowledge now doubles every two years. Ingeborg Mauksch, speaking on this subject, said:

> A book I have found extremely helpful is *The Year 2000,* by Herman Kahn, of the Hudson Institute. Kahn tells us that the institute forsees roughly 1,400 technological and scientific inventions that will occur between now and then. Fourteen hundred! That's a tremendous amount. These inventions cover the entire breadth of our matrix of living; they affect the social, the economic, the professional, the spiritual components, and certainly, the care of all citizens in health and illness.[4]

[2] Committee for the Study of Nursing Education, *Nursing and Nursing Education,* Josephine Goldmark, secretary to the Committee (New York: Macmillan Co., 1923).
[3] Margaret Bridgman, *Collegiate Education for Nursing* (New York: Russell Sage Foundation, 1953), pp. 85-86.
[4] Ingeborg Mauksch, "The Future is Now," in *The Future is Now* (New York: National League for Nursing, 1974), p. 3.

Educators are as aware of this as agency people; we are all exposed to the same literature and media. The new student is exposed to more theoretically advanced knowledge every year. As an inservice educator, I found I needed to take a speed-reading course. My job description lists as hazards of the job: "keeping abreast of the literature and current trends in nursing education, nursing theory, and nursing practice."

Green writes, "As the health needs of society become complex, the educational programs of professionals prepared to meet those needs must keep pace."[5] So is this true for the hospital. One of the responsibilities of the inservice department is to set up programs for the nursing staff almost on the spot. A recent example of this in my experience occurred when the interaortic balloon was introduced at our hospital. I know this isn't being taught in the universities, and I don't expect the nurse to be able to use this equipment upon graduation. But students who are knowledgeable in theory should be able to understand how it works, why it works, and when necessary learn the skills to monitor a patient on this machine. Perhaps in the next couple of years the use of this equipment will be incorporated in nursing texts and will become just one more of the many procedures in the nursing repertoire. (Last month the *American Journal of Nursing* already had its first article on this new technological advance.)

I was taught to make linseed poultices and turpentine stupes and set up sterile intravenous tubing; I'm sure these things are no longer in the curriculum. Roughly eight years ago the ABC's of the EKG were a necessary orientation, since most nurses didn't know an R wave from a PR interval. Now this information is a part of the nursing curriculum and advanced CCU courses are given only for those who will be working in that area. This is an example of how we are mutually interdependent and how changes of curriculum can come about through technological advances.

However, my interest runs deeper. I am more concerned with the basic philosophy of nursing practice in the acute-care setting than the ability of certain graduates to understand and perform certain skills. I have had to go from turpentine stupes to the interaortic balloon pump machine. The younger generation may be practicing space nursing on the moon, on Mars, or on a satellite! (I wonder if the nursing education curriculum includes the effect of gravity on the physical and psychological well-being of man or the sociological or anthropological aspects of living on a spaceship?)

Perhaps the best way to illustrate concretely my thoughts concerning the effect of changes in the acute-care setting on baccalaureate curriculum is through a specific case study, which will demonstrate how

[5] Joan Green, "Accreditation in Nursing Education: New Trends and Responsibilities," *Nursing Forum* 8(1):9, 1974.

this simultaneous mutual interaction has occurred and has wrought changes in the nursing education curriculum and the delivery of nursing service.

Eight years ago, the nursing service at our hospital was using the industrial model of delivery of nursing care. The affiliating schools using the agency included an LPN program, an associate degree program, and a diploma program. There was no orientation for new nursing employees, whether they were recent graduates or experienced nurses. A great deal of the time of the RN staff was spent in maintaining the supply system of the units or in secretarial or clerial activities for the physician. The "highest" professional activity, next to discharging the traditional duties of head or charge nurse, was the role of the medication nurse. However, since the conceptual model of professional nursing practice was constantly being published in the nursing journals and taught in the universities, the practice in our hospital was a perfect example of the incongruence that causes the Reality Shock Syndrome.

With the coming of a new nursing director, additional schools of nursing were encouraged to utilize the agency as their clinical laboratory. (Today we have generic students from three associate degree programs, three baccalaureate programs, graduate master's students from three colleges, and occasionally doctoral nursing students.) In addition, nursing service began to plan a change from the *industrial* model to the *professional* model of delivering nursing service.

One of the changes was the introduction of the Unit Service Management concept, to free the professional nurse from non-nursing activities. This shifted responsibility for transcription of physicians' orders to a Unit Receptionist and responsibility for unit supplies to a Unit Service Coordinator.

Another facet of the change was a pilot study to introduce the professional model. This was begun in 1968 and proved so successful that it is now the modus operandi of the entire medical center.[6] On the pilot unit RNs were assigned to a group of patients for which the nurse gave total care, including medications, treatment, blood pressures, health teaching, etc. The nurse was accountable and responsible for the total care of her patients, including the recording of her nursing activities and the patient's responses. How did this affect the affiliating schools? Since we were practicing what is now being termed Primary Nursing, affiliating schools could no longer assign their students to functional tasks such as "medications"—that is, students could no longer practice delivering medications to half a unit or even a whole unit in preparation for going out into the real world. In the orientation of instructors from the affiliating schools, they were told that they could no longer make such

---

[6] Sylvia Carlson *et al.,* "An Experiment in Self-Determined Patient Care," *Nursing Clinics of North America* 4:495-507, September 1969.

assignments to their students. We did not want our nursing staff to see the functional role model being encouraged by nursing educators, while we were trying to encourage a primary care model. Nursing service had thus turned the tables; we were demanding that the clinical instructors follow hospital philosophy in the theory they taught. However, we still looked upon the clinical instructor as a role model to our nursing staff, and wished her to remain in that capacity. Team nursing experience was subsequently eliminated from the baccalaureate programs affiliating at LIJ; since we did not practice it, students could not experience it.

We had developed a practical approach to the theory of nursing process and hoped that the instructors would follow our model, which they were delighted to do. Now students who are assigned a case method approach find it no different from the primary nurse model and they fit right into the unit setting. They are able to function smoothly with the regular nursing staff, since they are working not only under the direction of their instructor but also along with a primary nurse who is responsible for the ultimate care of the patient. This encourages a dialogue among staff nurse, instructor, and student. Rather than students being a burden on the unit, they become integral members of the nursing staff. During the time they are on the unit and when they leave it, students are expected to report to the primary nurse. Conflicts between instructor and the nursing care coordinator are few, since the basic philosophy of nursing education and nursing service are similar. Students do not chart on the nursing notes, since we do not have them.

Our staff chart on the Progress Notes with the admonishment that the recording of such things as "bath," "good or comfortable day," "OOB" are not considered professional notes. We therefore do not expect nursing students to write such notes either, but rather to make professional observations, pertinent to the patient's condition. They observe our *nursing staff* (not nursing *aides*) interviewing the patient on admission and recording a nursing history. They note that our staff then make a nursing diagnosis.

The Nursing Care Plans that students are expected and required to write for their instructors are no longer a student exercise. Students see on the medical record a form called Nursing Order Sheet, on which a permanent record of nursing intervention (i.e., nursing care planning) is recorded and which becomes part of the permanent record in the patient's chart. The importance of nursing intervention is thus emphasized to the student—not as an exercise that only the student is required to do, but as an integral part of graduate professional nursing competencies and nursing service expectations.

Students observe that our staff are not expected to wear nursing caps and that they frequently wear pastel-colored uniforms (which, by the way, we encourage). It is felt that the professional role is enhanced when uniformity of dress code (i.e., everyone in full white uniform) is discouraged. We want creative, independent thinking on the part of the graduate nurse, as well as from the student.

Are we perfect? Do students see a perfect model? Of course not, but where we have deficiencies, they know we encourage communication.

In place of the senior leadership experience, in which the senior baccalaureate student is expected to practice being a team leader, there is a new program for the senior student nurse. Each baccalaureate program has modified this to conform to its individual curriculum, but basically, for a stated number of hours, the senior functions under the preceptorship of one of our nursing care coordinators. The student selects her area of interest, such as surgery, medicine, obstetrics, or pediatrics and begins to test out the theory she has been learning for the past three and one-half years, without the direct supervision of an instructor. This culminating senior experience helps the student to test herself in a working situation while still a student. It's at this time that skills can be perfected, and theory that was learned can be implemented. The experiences are clinical, bedside experiences. The student is not expected to be a team leader who is so busy directing others that she has no time for direct laying on of hands. Since the schools state they are preparing a first-level practitioner, not a supervisor, I do not believe that team leading is a valid experience.

The graduate students use our clinical facilities as well. Since we have a large number of clinical specialists, they act as preceptors for the student graduate nurse.

As part of the simultaneous mutual interaction, faculty appointments are given to our nursing care coordinator preceptors, as well as to the clinical specialists.

For the past two summers I have been involved with a special program for junior students just before entering their senior year. The student nurse is hired as a nursing assistant for 35 hours a week and in addition has classes with me in the sociological aspects of the health care system. The student nurse receives three credits for the work-study program and the evaluations have at this point been very positive.

In 1973, our director of nurses stated the hospital's philosophy in a speech she gave at the 50th Anniversary celebration of Sigma Theta Tau at Adelphi University. She said, ''I am proposing a marriage not of convenience, since a marriage of convenience is based on selfish motives, but a marriage of necessity. The obligations we took upon ourselves as professional nurses necessitate that all of us, whether in education or service, focus on the one ultimate goal. The contribution nursing can make to the health and happiness of the nation.''

34 CHANGES IN COMMUNITY NURSING SERVICE THAT AFFECT BACCALAUREATE NURSING PROGRAMS

Helen J. O'Leary, MSN, RN

I am a firm believer that education and service must form a united front if we are to meet the challenges of the continuously changing methods of health care delivery. In order to assess effectively the implications of these changes on community nursing, it is necessary to review some of the highlights of the history of nursing in the community setting.

Community nursing can be described as the outgrowth of visits, sponsored by church groups or settlement houses, to the sick poor by women of the community. The primary purposes of these visits were to give alms, interspersed with a dose of religion, and some nursing care; their target group was the sick poor. Hence, the early image of community health became associated only with the poor.

The earliest recorded community nursing commenced in New York City in 1877, under the sponsorship of the Women's Board of the New York City Mission. A few years later the two first district nursing associations were begun simultaneously in Boston and Philadelphia. However, credit for many of the organized developments in community nursing belongs to Lillian Wald, who with the assistance of Mary Brewster founded a visiting nurse service as part of the Henry Street Settlement in New York City. This became the model for similar organizations. For many years Miss Wald and Miss Brewster provided the training for community nurses associated with other groups. Miss Wald influenced many to provide nursing services as part of their community responsibility.

Perhaps the most notable development was the Metropolitan Life Insurance Company's program of home nursing services for its subscribers; this program identified the need for such services to be made available to all economic levels of the community. The image of the community nurse, which had previously shown her functioning only with the poor, began to change since not all subscribers to the life insurance company were poor. Since many could afford to pay for home nursing and demanded the same services, it became evident that all economic levels within the community needed nursing services.

In 1912 the National Organization for Public Health Nursing was founded, with Miss Wald as its president. In 1952 the organization became a part of the National League for Nursing.

In the same year (1912) the American Red Cross pioneered rural community health, and shortly thereafter county health departments followed suit with the employment of full-time nurses for home visiting.

Annie W. Goodrich, the founder of the Yale School of Nursing, instituted a program for community health nursing in the basic curriculum of the school.

The beginning services of community health nursing were geared toward maternal and child health and the control of communicable diseases and encompassed primarily preventive teaching and anticipatory guidance.

Beginning in the middle 1960's, dramatic changes occurred in the health delivery field. These changes have had an impact on community nursing services. Perhaps the most effective was the Social Security Amendments Act of 1965. This act introduced Medicare to the recipients of Social Security, and under its provisions anyone 65 years of age and older was entitled to medical care in the community or in the hospital. Tied to this was the delivery of home care by certified home health agencies that offered as their primary service skilled nursing care. In conjunction with this act, the federal government also passed the Medical Act, which provided the same benefits to the indigent and those with catastrophic illnesses. Amendments to the Social Security acts in 1972 extended Medicare coverage to the physically handicapped and renal dialysis patients.

Some of the requirements of the Medicare act have had the implications for the delivery of community nursing services. Identification of the level of care delivered to the recipients is required, as is periodic auditing of the nursing care. Certification of home health agencies is renewable every two years. Proof of the qualifications of the nurses, as well as the justification for services, is mandated for each recipient receiving care. Home health agencies are required to offer other therapeutic services (e.g., physical therapy, speech therapy, occupational therapy) in conjunction with skilled nursing service.

In addition, hospitals are required to have utilization review boards to insure that patients are discharged when maximum hospital benefits are received. This results in early discharge of many patients.

The Full Disclosure Law, enacted in 1974, now makes records available for scrutiny by individuals requesting them. The full impact of this law remains to be seen, but it is now possible for patients to read the records pertaining to them.

Nursing homes are also affected by these laws. They must provide utilization review boards and also discharge plans for their patients, which often include referral for community nursing services.

Federal and state laws regarding the reporting of child abuse were enacted in the 1970's.

The Nurse Practice Act of 1972 clearly defines the role of the nurse in an ever-expanding role and makes it imperative that the nurse function as an independent practitioner.

Now let us consider the impact of these changes on the deliverance of community nursing services. The Standards of Community Health Nursing Practice, set by the American Nurses' Association, give us a broad definition of this type of nursing practice:

> Community Health Nursing practice is a synthesis of nursing practice and public health practice applied to promoting and preserving the health of populations. The nature of this practice is general and comprehensive. . . It is continuing, not episodic. The dominant responsibility is to the population as a whole.[1]

Therefore, nursing directed to individuals, families, or other groups becomes a valid component of the practice as it intrinsically relates to and contributes to the health of the total population.

In terms of the changes in the delivery of health services, this can be interpreted as meaning that the community nurse must have a broad foundation of skills built on the acquisition of skilled nursing techniques, a knowledge of the principles of the physical, biological, and social sciences, and the ability to teach.

Community nursing practice must focus on the community as a whole as well as on each component included in that community. The nurse, if effectiveness is a primary goal, must be aware of community groups that are involved in determining what and how services are to be

[1] American Nurses' Association, Congress for Nursing Practice, *Standards of Community Health Nursing Practice* (Kansas City, MO: The Association, 1973), p. 1.

delivered. This involves identifying the political make-up of the community and the political system that controls the economics of health care delivery.

The community nurse must know the principles of good mental health and must possess the theoretical knowledge to permit the identification of those factors undermining good mental health. Mandatory discharge of mental patients into an alien community, for which they have received no preparation, necessitates community nursing intervention.

The community nurse must possess current knowledge of those lifesaving procedures that enable a patient to return to his home and community, although still requiring close medical supervision. This particular knowledge will encompass the mechanics of renal dialysis, hyperalimentation, organ transplants, and extensive surgical procedures. Not only must the nurse know the physiological effects of these conditions, but also the emotional impact on the patient, family, and community of the adjustments they must make if they are to continue and maintain a high quality of life.

If the community nurse believes that good health care is the right of every individual and not merely a privilege, she must be an effective teacher in the pursuit of making good medical care available to all. Families will need to be taught to care for the patient when the nurse is not available. All will need to learn the signs of good health so that any deviation can be detected and treated early. The nurse will participate in teaching classes on prenatal care, infant care, and preschool guidance, to name a few. Teaching will involve the entire life cycle from birth to death.

Through the resources of modern medicine the life expectancy has been expanded so that more people are living longer and remaining in their homes. The elderly have more chronic illnesses and are less economically able to care for themselves. They may require more medical supervision, more skilled nursing, and more monetary assistance from social services. They may also require supplementary nutritional assistance, which in many communities is provided by nutrition sites or meals-on-wheels programs. The nutrition sites are governmentally sponsored and have as a requisite for continual funding that a community nurse be assigned to the site. The elderly may also require ancillary personnel in order to remain safely in their homes; this may be a home health aide to assist with personal care, or a homemaker. The community nurse must be responsible for the evaluation of these situations in order to justify the placing of such personnel.

More people are choosing to live out their lives in familiar surroundings, and the community nurse will have to assist the patient and the family in accepting the inevitability of death. The nurse must know the emotional stages of death and their impact on the dying and the family. The nurse must recognize the personal feelings involved with death and must be able to cope with these feelings. She must also understand the grief process and its effect on the coping mechanisms of families.

The community nurse has a vital role in the early recognition of child neglect and abuse. The guidance and understanding of the nurse can assist in enabling parents to deal with their feelings and in seeking professional services. Community action groups are a vital link in the prevention of child abuse and often seek the guidance of the community nurse in their plans of action.

Skills in the techniques of interviewing and analysis of family interaction patterns will constantly be utilized in all aspects of community nursing—in individual counseling, in the comprehensive ambulatory health care center, in the well-baby clinic, in the drug clinic, in the community mental health clinic, in schools, in teen centers, and in the home.

The community health nurse must have a knowledge of governmental legislation that affects health care as well as the requirements for receiving such care. Since nursing records are subject to audit by those not necessarily familiar with nursing care, the nurse must be skilled in recording care and justifying reasons care has been given. She must also understand the nursing process, which describes the unique role of nursing.

While the community health nurse has long been an independent practitioner, the Nurse Practice Act serves to define the areas of her accountability and emphasizes the need for the practitioner to know the limits of her practice. The nurse has to make independent decisions which affect the well-being of the patients cared for in the home. It is therefore imperative that the nurse possess all of those skills which will enable her to do so.

The community nurse must have a knowledge of community resources which can be called upon to meet the needs of the family that cannot be met by nursing alone. This includes official agencies and community agencies. The services they offer and their criteria for acceptance must be understood by the nurse.

The nurse who practices in the community must be a general practitioner whose skills enable her to deliver skilled nursing procedures and whose broad knowledge of psychosocial components, interviewing skills, teaching techniques, resources, and the biological, physical, and social sciences support her delivery of effective care. A practitioner must know the laws governing the delivery of health care and has a thorough knowledge of the cultural make-up of the community of practice.

It behooves the educational facility to be aware of the skills needed to function within the community and to provide the opportunity for the nurse to grow and learn. It is imperative that community nursing agencies and educational institutions work together to develop an effective communication system which will permit the planning of programs for the student which will meet the needs of the community. I fully recognize that these skills I have discussed require an intense evaluation of the educational and service processes. I am, however, confident that the goal of both nursing education and nursing service is the most skilled practitioner possible and that if we join forces we can and will accomplish this goal.

35 CURRICULUM IMPLICATIONS OF THE CHANGING ROLE OF THE PROFESSIONAL NURSE

Gertrude J. Torres, EdD, RN

The 1917 Standard Curriculum for Schools of Nursing, in speaking of the status of nursing education, declared, "The main difficulty is the lack of a clear understanding of what the function of a modern nurse is or what the purpose and scope of her training should be."[1] This statement demonstrates the concern of nursing educators over 50 years ago for the appropriate identification of the role of the nurse. The document continues by voicing concern that the value of the services given the nurse is being recognized in new fields of work and the character of the service she renders is rapidly changing.[2]

Both these statements seem appropriate for today, as we are also searching for a more vitalized place for nursing within the health care system, and they vividly remind us that nursing has historically been concerned with the identification of its specific role and functions. It seems we are destined inevitably to continue the search for our specific place in the health care system. We spiral or recycle concepts such as dependence-independence, a health-illness focus, or a generalist-specialist emphasis; we move back and forth with these concepts; but we make few real changes.

---

[1] National League of Nursing Education, Committee on Education, *Standard Curriculum for Schools of Nursing* (Baltimore: Waverly Press, 1917), p. 5.

[2] *Ibid.*, pp. 5-6.

Leaders in nursing education, through their influence on the nursing curriculum, have been most instrumental in affecting the course of nursing history. They have long struggled to find ways of improving the quality of the nursing service offered to the consumer by improving nursing education. However, their efforts have not always had a significant impact on the practice of nursing, especially in relation to reevaluating the role of the professional nurse. Stewart, in 1943, told nurse educators to keep their minds flexible and rid themselves of fixed patterns of thinking, narrow viewpoints, and even traditional loyalties.[3] It seems we still need to keep her suggestions in mind.

If we are to change the course of history in nursing as related to our roles, we must engage in effective and continual curriculum revision, both with a sense of real vigor and purpose. We must also recognize that curriculum revision requires us to be able to predict changes, so that we can prepare the professional nurse for the future—even if that future is viewed as only ten years hence. We can no longer emphasize merely the preparation of the professional nurse for today.

There are two concepts to keep in mind in discussing curriculum implications for the changing role of the professional nurse. These are the essence of *what* we teach and the identification of *where* the student will practice. Although both these concepts—the *what* and *where*—are essential aspects of any nursing program, the major thrust and emphasis needs to be on the *what*. We in nursing education have long oriented our courses and content around the medical model and the *where*; for instance, psychiatric nursing modelled from psychiatry and practiced in psychiatric settings. Today, recognizing that there will most likely continue to be changes in relation to the roles and functions of the professional nurse, as well as in the types of settings in which she will practice, we need to reorient ourselves to the *what* of nursing, so that the essence of nursing can be practiced in any setting or system and so that we are truly preparing a practitioner for today and tomorrow.

In focusing on the *what* of nursing education, which includes the concepts and theories we teach our students throughout the curriculum, let us review Model I which integrates the changing role into the curriculum process.

Philosophy

The philosophy or the statement of beliefs of the nursing program must be congruent with the philosophy of the parent institution. This is particularly significant in liberal arts colleges, which generally emphasize man in totality, a humanized world, and the development of

---

[3] Isabel M. Stewart, *The Education of Nurses* (New York: Macmillan Co., 1944), p. 380.

students in terms of their intellectual, cultural, and often spiritual potentials. Within this type of institution the beliefs about man and learning may differ significantly from those of a public institution of higher learning.

The philosophy is the base or foundation of the entire curriculum. If it is well developed, clear and complete, includes a glossary of terms, and truly reflects the beliefs of the entire faculty, it can be instrumental in guiding the faculty through the entire curriculum process. On the other hand, if it is vague, contradictory, confusing, or even too sophisticated for most people to comprehend, it will be almost useless, and the entire curriculum will demonstrate weaknesses.

One of the most significant parts of a philosophy relates to the unique present and future role of the professional nurse. This must be spoken to with great clarity and precision if it is to be useful to the public, the students, and the faculty. Frequently the philosophy describes or defines nursing in such general terms that one could superimpose names of other health care practitioners, such as social worker, in place of the word *nurse* and the description would still be appropriate.

In describing the changing and future role of the professional nurse, faculty need to be specific in relation to their beliefs as to the *what* of nursing and the *where* or settings in which nursing will be practiced; in addition, these beliefs must be realistic, so that they can be implemented. For example, faculty may believe that the emerging role of the professional nurse will involve her ability to function in extraterrestrial space and that man should be viewed more in terms of the universe rather than the limited environment of the earth. Such beliefs about the future may or may not be appropriate, depending on your frame of reference. But the question remains: Can they be implemented within the curriculum? Will the faculty require sophisticated courses in mathematics and physics to implement such beliefs? Will faculty be able to provide learning experiences appropriate to such beliefs?

In the statement of philosophy, the faculty need to describe the present and future health care system and identify the types of settings in which the professional nurse will practice. Thus, one should not merely identify health care settings that are presently available, but seriously and imaginatively look ahead to different types of settings in which the nurse may practice in the future, even though such settings are not yet available for practice within a given community. For instance, you may envision the professional nurse as functioning independently but collaboratively with other health care practitioners within ambulatory health care centers even though this is not currently the situation in your community.

Not only is it significant to look at changing health care settings, but it is also necessary to consider how the professional nurse functions

Model I
Components of Curriculum Process, Illustrating
Emphasis on the Changing Role of the Professional Nurse

Philosophy

Statement of beliefs incorporating man, society, health, nursing, and learning (inclusion of a glossary of terms is helpful):

Characteristics of man
  and society
Projection of present and
  future health care needs

Trends identified within the
  health care system
Present and emerging
  unique role and functions
  of the professional nurse

Characteristics of the Graduate

Broad behavioral objectives, which taken together describe the graduate:

Nursing Process
Research
Leadership for today
  and tomorrow
Professionalism in nursing

Utilization of scientific
  and nursing knowledge
  and theories
Changing society, health
  care system, and role of
  the professional

Conceptual Framework

Identifies scientific and nursing theories which support the changing role and functions of the professional nurse:

Role Theory
Change Theory
Decision-making Theory

Political Theory
Communication

Model I (Continued)

Horizontal and Vertical Strands

Identify knowledge, understanding, and skills progressively throughout the curriculum:

Nursing Process*	Dependent-independent- interdependent functions**
Health-illness care within the health care system**	Past-present-future role**

*Identified here as a horizontal strand.
**Identified here as a vertical strand.

Behavioral Level Objectives

Developed from Characteristics of the Graduate into various levels utilizing vertical and horizontal strands:

Characteristics of Graduate: Can utilize the nursing process in a variety of settings.
Understands the impact on the health care system of the changing role of the professional nurse.

Junior Level Objectives

Can utilize the nursing process in case of relatively "healthy" clients within the community in a dependent-independent manner.
Can identify the past and present role of the professional nurse in relation to the present health care system.

Senior Level Objectives

Can utilize the nursing process in the care of patients in a crisis setting interdependently with other health care professionals.
Can hypothesize about the future role of the professional nurse as related to the total health care system.

within the present, and will function in future, types of settings. Realistically, even if the health care system were to change dramatically, we would still have to use our present settings for some time. Different approaches to organizing nursing care, some of which have been identified by the other leaders within these settings, are being identified. Educators also need to state their beliefs about leadership, the change process, and interdisciplinary activities in terms of the changing and future role of the professional nurse rather than simply in terms of the past or the present. A glossary of terms is often helpful in clarifying the meaning of terms used in the philosophy. Examples might include such terms as "leadership" and "nursing process."

Let me suggest that every educator might profit from looking objectively at her nursing program's philosophy and reviewing it in terms of the changing role of the professional nurse.

Characteristics of the Graduate

Broad behavioral terminal objectives must support the developed philosophy and are instrumental in the development of level and course objectives. They need to be written with the concept of the changing role of the professional nurse clearly in mind. In the revised Statement of Charactistics of Baccalaureate Education in Nursing, devised by the NLN Council of Baccalaureate and Higher Degree Programs, the emphasis is on decision making, responsibility and accountability, hypothesizing and extending nursing science, interdisciplinary activities, improving the delivery of health care, and understanding the emerging role of the professional nurse.[4] All these characteristics strongly relate to the changing role of the professional nurse and need to be clearly stated within the developed terminal objectives. Since these objectives must be written broadly, they generally do not speak specifically to any particular setting (the *where* of nursing) but emphasize the *what* (although the content necessarily has implications for the choice of settings).

Conceptual Framework

The approach a particular faculty utilize to develop a conceptual framework is not as significant as the concepts or theories they identify within it. The philosophy of a nursing program speaks to the concepts of man, society, health, and nursing. It is essential that the conceptual framework encompass the specific theories under each of these concepts

---

[4] Council of Baccalaureate and Higher Degree Programs, *Characteristics of Baccalaureate Education in Nursing* (New York: National League for Nursing, 1974).

that speak to the essence and totality of nursing. Thus, within the conceptual framework one should be able to identify the relationships or connections between such concepts.

In terms of the changing role of the professional nurse within a dynamic health care system theories related to roles, change, decision making, and so forth, need to be made an intrinsic component of the curriculum; that is, they need to be identified within the conceptual framework. Here again, the *what* of professional nursing, rather than the *where,* is emphasized.

In identifying appropriate concepts or theories, as related to the changing role, it is sometimes helpful to work as a faculty group in a kind of brainstorming session. After many concepts and theories are identified, they can frequently be combined or synthesized and priorities can then be established in relation to the statements within the philosophy. This developed combination of concepts and theories within the conceptual framework gives us strong clues for the identification of course content.

Horizontal and Vertical Strands

In order to insure the integration of the philosophy, objectives, and conceptual framework into the level and course behavioral objectives, it is essential that pertinent knowledge, understanding, and skills be progressively identified. This can most easily be done through the utilization of horizontal and vertical strands. These strands, although expressed differently by various programs, usually relate to the major concepts identified within the philosophy. For example, the concepts of *man* and *society* are identified with the strand "individual-family-community," the concept *health* with the strand "health-illness continuum," the concept *nursing* with the vertical strands "dependent-independent-interdependent functions," "collaboration-coordination," and "leadership skills," as well as with the horizontal strand "nursing process."[5] Whether a strand is horizontal or vertical depends on the faculty's frame of reference. The strand "nursing process" in Model I has been identified as horizontal, since it is taught at each level within the nursing curriculum. The strands "health-illness care," "dependent-independent-interdependent functions," and "past-present-future role" are vertical strands. Following this model, the student would, in her initial clinical nursing experience, care for relatively healthy persons, utilizing the nursing process, and would function interdependently with other health care professionals.

---

[5] Gertrude Torres, "Curriculum Process and the Integrated Curriculum," *Faculty-Curriculum Development. Part IV: Unifying the Curriculum—The Integrated Approach* (New York: National League for Nursing, 1975), p. 27.

In identifying the changing role of the professional nurse, faculty need to insure that the appropriate strands are identified to guarantee their inclusion within the curriculum. Some of these strands might relate to the "simple is complex" phenomenon, to research, to implementation of the change process, to involvement in political and legislative systems within and outside institutions, or to interdisciplinary activities.

The diagramming of these strands can be a valuable tool in orienting students, faculty, and nursing service personnel to the approaches to content and learning experiences within the curriculum.

Curriculum Design

General education, as well as supporting course requirements, are based on the philosophy of the institution and the nursing program. For example, a Catholic, liberal arts college usually requires philosophy and religion courses, whereas a state college might require more history or government courses.

The identification in the philosophy of the emerging role of the professional nurse will give strong clues as to the general education or supporting courses that students may need. Faculty should look carefully through the entire school catalog for offerings that may be helpful in increasing students' awareness of concepts related to roles, change, and decision making. Some examples might include: interdisciplinary health courses on the changing health care system; women's role in the history of health care; experiences in communication systems; public opinion; consumer psychology; social change; and industrial sociology.

It is also important to identify the sequence of these course requirements: should they be parallel or prerequisite to particular clinical nursing courses? Generally, it is more appropriate to build on general education as supporting courses so that they can be totally incorporated into nursing theory and practice. Non-nursing courses in the upper division should be those more closely related to the student as a total personality with unique interests and needs.

Nursing course descriptions and content are developed from the course objectives, which stem, in turn, from the behavioral level objectives. Course descriptions that relate to course objectives should give strong clues to the content and should relate to changing roles. After all, it is through the course objectives and content that we ultimately meet our terminal objectives. If we as nurse educators believe that professional nurses will be leaders within and outside health care agencies, we need to incorporate this concept early, in each nursing course, and not wait until the very end of the student's learning experience. To offer an example: the student might, at an early stage in her learning experiences, lead in promoting health care of families and small groups of clients; at a subsequent point she might lead nonprofessional nurses and other students through the effective planning and evaluation of care; and at a later level she might lead an interdisciplinary team. (In this context "leadership" is meant to indicate utilizing the nursing process as a mechanism to improve health and nursing care.)

If faculty see the changing role of the professional nurse as related to more independent types of functions, it is essential that they take a careful look at the nursing courses, their content, and the methods utilized in teaching. A dependent, nonaggressive learner who is spoken to in the 50-minute lecture, who is given handouts for most of what is presented that is not in the textbook, and who infrequently has the opportunity to initiate an idea, can hardly be expected to function later as a professional nurse with great independence in a changing health care system. Also, a student who truly never evaluates her own nursing care or that of others can hardly be expected to function independently or with any degree of expertise. A student who never has an opportunity to do truly independent study projects or to search out data without direct guidance can hardly function as a leader later when such activities are essential.

I would like to reiterate three major points in relation to the *what* of the nursing curriculum. First, nursing educators have long been encouraged to incorporate into the curriculum the ever-changing role and functions of the professional nurse. Second, faculty need to identify specifically within each segment of the curriculum process the ways in which the changing role of the professional nurse is being incorporated in the curriculum. And last, new approaches to teaching need to be sought for a better integration of the concepts of changing roles into the nursing curriculum.

36 OFFERING LEARNING EXPERIENCES THAT REFLECT THE CHANGING ROLE OF THE PROFESSIONAL NURSE

Gertrude J. Torres, EdD, RN

One of the last and possibly most significant aspects of the curriculum development process is the identification of learning experiences as they relate to the formulated objectives. Learning experiences include those activities that support the meeting of the behavioral objectives and can occur within or outside the classroom. The emphasis in this presentation will be on the concept of clinical and nonclinical learning experiences outside the classroom and how they relate to the changing role of the professional nurse. In addition, an attempt will be made at some new approaches to these experiences.

We need to keep in mind that our beliefs about learning have a strong impact on the type and frequency of learning experiences we provide for the student. Let us look at a few learning theories and how they might influence the student's clinical learning experience.

Stimulus-response connections. This theory tells us that by providing the student with certain learning experiences and furnishing sufficient rewards for appropriate actions, specific behaviors will be elicited. Here reinforcement by the instructor is instrumental in the occurrence of learning.

Concept of imitation. Here the student is encouraged either overtly or covertly to utilize specific learning experiences to adopt or imitate a certain language, mannerism, or problem-solving strategy. In the clinical setting faculty would emphasize the use of role models. These role models are frequently identified as the faculty themselves, yet faculty are educators and not practitioners, which can cause confusion in the minds of the students.

Concept of repetition. The faculty's beliefs about repetition in relation to motor and cognitive skills have a significant impact on the frequency of experiences. Repetition needs to be identified more in terms of reinforcement for retention than in relation to progressive learning.

The stated philosophy of the nursing program should be a most valuable guide in understanding the faculty's beliefs about learning and should be carefully reviewed prior to the selection of clinical experiences. Beliefs about such concepts as motivation, individual differences, the development of attitudes, the transfer of learning, and the role of the learner—whether stated or not—will have a strong impact on the selection of learning experiences.

In the identification of learning experiences within a baccalaureate nursing program, especially as related to the changing role of the professional nurse and as an activity to assist the student in meeting objectives, we need to focus strongly on intellectual skills. These should be distinguished from the learning of verbal information and knowledge and should include observing, classifying, predicting, hypothesizing, and interpreting data. Such intellectual skills require a broad body of relevant knowledge and are essential if the motor skills are to be performed effectively. At present, the philosophies and conceptual frameworks of many programs emphasize the nursing process and require such intellectual skills as assessing, planning, diagnosing, and evaluating. Moreover, the Council of Baccalaureate and Higher Degree Programs has revised its characteristics of the baccalaureate graduate to stress such intellectual skills as decision making, hypothesizing, and data gathering. The assumption can therefore be made that these skills do in fact require a theoretical and empirical base of knowledge and are essential if nursing intervention is to be effective.

This emphasis on intellectual skills, however, results in much confusion in the minds of those who identify nursing as primarily involving interventive or performance skills focused on the art of nursing. In this view, performance skills seem to be in competition with intellectual skills, rather than both being perceived as essential components of the practice of nursing.

Part of the problem often seems to relate to the unidentified differences that necessarily exist between the evaluation of nursing care and the evaluation of a student's progress. Evaluation of care, which is meant to assist the student in learning, is different from evaluation for a grade.

Furthermore, it is often easier and more objective to evaluate physical care and performance skills than cognitive and intellectual skills, since we are not so sophisticated in the latter.

Tyler discusses five principles that should be remembered in selecting effective learning experiences:[1]

- They should give the student an opportunity to practice the kind of behavior implied by the objective.
- They should be satisfying to the student.
- They should be appropriate to the student's ability and level.
- They should differ from student to student while still attaining the same educational objective and thus giving the teacher a wide range of possibilities.
- They will usually bring about several outcomes related to more than one objective.

Nursing education has supported these principles to some extent. For example, we recognize that students can meet the same objective through a variety of clinical experiences within certain settings, such as acute-care settings where students deal with differing patients with distinct problems or needs. What we need to recognize more often is that the same objective can also be met in different types of settings. Skills relating to leadership, the nursing process, and collaboration, for instance, can all be practiced outside the acute-care system as well as within it.

We also consider clinical experiences as satisfying to students, especially if they are able to relate them to specific objectives and can view them as a means of progressing toward such objectives. It is only when students find an experience redundant to their previous experiences, or when objectives are not clearly spelled out, that frustrations arise. This is particularly true of registered-nurse students.

One of the objectives we frequently verbalize relates to developing skills in thinking. How many times have we said that we produce thinkers? If this is true, then we must offer clinical experiences in which students have the opportunity to think. Generally, *thinking* invovles more than simply remembering and repeating ideas; it entails inductive, deductive, logical processes.[2] We need to provide learning experiences that encourage relating ideas or concepts rather than merely memorizing them. We must not encourage ideas to be utilized and repeated without some type of analysis. Practice in problem-solving methodologies is essential in creating thinkers, and we must recognize

---

[1] Ralph W. Tyler, *Basic Principles of Curriculum and Instruction* (Chicago: University of Chicago Press, 1969), pp. 65-68.

[2] *Ibid.,* pp. 68-69.

that some settings more than others allow students the opportunity for such practice.

If the concepts relating to the changing role of the professional nurse are to be an integral part of the entire curriculum and are to affect learning experiences, it is essential that we review carefully not only the types of settings in which we place our students but also the characteristics of these settings that encourage or discourage thinking.

Let us now turn to the identification of some learning experiences for baccalaureate nursing students that support the changing or emerging role and functions of the professional nurse. Model II is an attempt to illustrate the relation of some typical concepts found in terminal objectives of nursing programs[3] to possible types of learning experiences which can be found outside the classroom. The model does not include areas related to research, professional responsibilities, or personal development, nor does it speak to the readiness or level of the student necessary for such experiences, which would have to be identified through the use of developed strands within the curriculum. The model represents only a sampling of ideas, and since the areas are broad in nature, the learning experiences frequently do not point out any specific specialty setting.

The first concept treated in the model relates to the professional nurse within the social system and suggests that the student be allowed exposure as a participant-observer in a variety of experiences relating to politics and organizations. If this is a major thrust within a curriculum, it might be well to encourage the student to take courses in politics or organizational theories. Inherent here also is the necessity for faculty members to be actively involved themselves in a variety of health care organizations. If the graduate of a baccalaureate nursing program is to do more than just accept the faculty's beliefs about the changing role, if she is required to develop her own concept, then she must be able to understand social systems. One of the most convenient institutions in which to understand social systems is the college or university itself. This whole area can be taken one step further by developing an interdisciplinary course with faculty from the political and social sciences in which students are offered relevant learning experiences.

One cannot educate for the changing role of the professional nurse without including concepts relating to role theory and the change process. Learning experiences should be offered in which the student can initially observe change and then become part of a changing process. Actually, almost any setting could be utilized to identify the presence or absence of change. The utilization of a mobile unit to offer health care to members of differing communities could afford an excellent opportunity for the student to observe the reactions of the consumers of

---

[3] For a more detailed treatment of this subject, see Gertrude Torres, "Composite of Program and/or Terminal Behavior Objectives of Baccalaureate Nursing Programs," *Faculty-Curriculum Development. Part I: The Process of Curriculum Development* (New York: National League for Nursing, 1974), pp. 14-16.

MODEL II
Learning Experiences Outside the Classroom and Terminal Objectives Related to the Changing Role and Function of the Professional Nurse

Concepts Related to Terminal Objectives	Possible Learning Experiences Outside the Classroom
The Professional Nurse within the Social System	• Observation of local or state legislatures in action, especially when health care issues are discussed. • Participating in official and nonofficial organizations involved in the improvement of health care. • Attendance at nursing organization meetings. • Participation in activities within the educational institution, especially those related to the health care of students.
Professional Nursing and the Change Process	• Observaton of current nursing practices within a variety of settings. • Participation in effecting change in relation to the present and emerging role of the professional nurse. • Participation in newly developed and differing health care settings within the community. • Utilization of a mobile unit, especially within communities that have inadequate health care facilities.
The Nursing Process	• Responsibility for comprehensive family care in the home on a continual long-term basis. • Twenty-four-hour client/patient caseload within acute or long-term settings. • Participate in health care organizations' mobile units stressing assessment and follow-up. • Assess the health care status of "well" individuals through college Health Days. • Evaluate nursing care given by peers and nursing care personnel within a variety of settings.
Leadership	• Participate in interdisciplinary activities within a variety of settings. • Provide consultation services to other members of the nursing team.

health care to the professional nurse offering such a service, while at the same time providing an opportunity for gaining an understanding of change.

Learning experiences generally relate to the area of the nursing process. It is only our lack of creativity that inhibits us from identifying innumerable other experiences, especially outside acute-care settings. If the nursing process is the structure of our discipline, the way the nurse thinks about nursing, every learning experience should assist the student in understanding the nursing process. Admittedly, we do focus on different aspects of the process at different times, relating to clients/patients with unique needs or problems. Also, we sometimes seek different settings based on the level of the student or the particular strands to be emphasized. Providing the student with a learning experience in which she follows a family for some two years would offer an opportunity to utilize the total nursing process, although certain aspects of it would be emphasized at different times. Thus, the student might spend months initially doing a total family assessment prior to the development of a specific plan of care. She might therefore not be able to evaluate long-term goals until later in her program.

Another example would be students who admit patients requiring surgery to acute-care settings; in this case, students could do what we frequently call "follow-through" care on a 24-hour basis until the patient returns home and could then visit the home later. Evaluation in relation to quality nursing care should be an integral part of this experience. This approach can be particularly effective in long-term settings, such as nursing homes.

We could also offer the student experiences working with a tuberculosis mobile unit or a Red Cross blood unit. Two helpful ways of identifying other such experiences are to consult the classified (yellow) pages of the telephone directory or to canvass local health care organizations.

Involving students in coordinating and collaborating activities, especially with other health care workers, is no easy matter. Yet these types of learning experiences are essential if we are to create true leaders. Having students interact on a one-to-one basis with physicians, social workers, or dietitians is an effective beginning, but more needs to be done. The student should observe interdisciplinary group activities early in her experiences so she can clearly identify the present role of the professional nurse; later, she will need to be a participant in such activities. This is a vivid reminder that experiences relating to the changing role of the professional nurse—however that is interpreted by a particular faculty—are not easy to offer and may first require changing other health care workers' attitudes about the nursing role.

If we are to engage in such experiences that relate to the changing role of the professional nurse, we need to be much more flexible in our approach to clinical laboratory experience in terms of time and the presence of the instructor. In relation to the latter, the instructor should always be available but not necessarily visible. We need to separate laying-on-of-hands time, where safety requires our presence, from those other times when we can and should encourage the student to function independently. For example, during assessment, planning, and evaluation (which relate to many cognitive-intellectual skills) the instructor need not always be visible. Actually, these are the most time-consuming aspects of the nursing process. On the other hand, during intervention, it may be *essential* that the instructor be present.

As an illustration, let us hypothesize a group of students who are doing a "24-hour caseload" with a client in a nursing home, with three hours of clinical laboratory time for the activity. If purposeful intervention is planned, the instructor's presence in the nursing home might be required for only one hour a week. The other two hours could be selected by the student at the appropriate times during the week, possibly when the client has visitors or needs special attention, and a diary of activities could be kept by the student to substantiate her activities. This may sound too loose and difficult to plan and control; yet, if we are to produce thinkers involved in an autonomous profession, we must reexamine our rigid approach to clinical hours. Apparently, we still think of the student as a worker who needs an eight-hour day to learn. I would like to ask, "After the first two or three hours in a particular setting, can you learn effectively?"

In essence, this presentation has attempted to encourage thinking of new ways of offering learning experiences within present clinical settings and also in the newly developing ones. We cannot continue to see the clinical laboratory experience as an eight-to-eleven-a.m., two-times-a-week experience, giving the same type of care (usually relating to comfort and hygiene) over and over again. I have tried to point out that some objectives in our programs can be met in many different ways and possibly in different settings that we have not yet even identified. To encourage creativity, we may need to forget how we ourselves were taught.

APPENDIX: WORKSHOP PANEL DISCUSSION

Dr. Stanton: If anyone from the audience wishes to participate in the panel discussion, just walk up, and when there's a gap in the conversation, just say, "I'd like to make a point here." We're going to discuss things, not in any order of importance and not necessarily because we know the answers, but we're going to try to answer some of the questions in some of the letters.

The first question was, "How can clinical nursing skills be maintained by full-time nursing faculty?" I'll start off by answering that. One of the things that can be encouraged is having faculty get involved in part-time clinical practice in their off-duty hours or during the summer, depending on the university's restrictions regarding moonlighting. There are some universities that provide joint appointments for their faculty/staff.

Dr. Torres: One of the things I think that administrators in nursing education need to truly believe in is continuing education for faculty. Frequently you will find deans or administrators supporting the mandating of continuing education in the state, but having little or no funds or time available for faculty to engage in such activities. The other thing is the question of role-model. As the faculty member is working with students in the clinical area, it would seem to me that she would be learning and updating herself. She is not blind to what the other nurses are doing and she has the opportunity to observe clinical specialists' functions. If she's awake, she can keep herself at least reasonably up-to-date.

307

People talk about updating skills. I wonder what they're really talking about. It reminds me of physical assessment skills. Some peole got really interested in this, as though we never used a stethoscope before, as though we never did these things on a night shift or in the emergency room. And you have continuing education for physical skills as though the psychomotor, intellectual, or interactive skills or psychological assessment or development assessment or economic assessment were things we didn't need updating on. In other words, people seem to overemphasize the physical assessment without the other components of assessment. I think if a faculty member wants to keep herself up-to-date, it is not that difficult. Now, being up-to-date does not, in my experience, mean being a skilled technician. I was brought up in a diploma program; I was a skilled technician. I don't need to maintain that level any longer.

Dr. Stanton: Related to that question was, "How does the demand for clinical nursing skills relate to the integrated teaching role?"

Dr. Torres: When faculties move from the medical model to the integrated curriculum, they frequently worry about "How do you teach?" Especially the physical skills. The first integrated course was nursing arts; that was some fifty or sixty years ago. They felt there was a body of knowledge that was truly nursing, and that it was nursing arts. I was a nursing arts instructor for years and I think you know what kind of nursing arts I'm talking about. Now, as we evolved into an integrated program, no longer was there nursing arts first, followed by Med-Surg and Psych, etc. Some schools decided that the first course should not be nursing arts, but fundamentals of nursing. They started out with understanding the nursing process for two weeks, followed by fourteen weeks of nursing arts. Then they felt the students had a base on which to function for the next group of courses. Some programs integrated to a much greater degree. When they talked about the process of oxygenation, that's when the "oxygen therapy" skill came up. When they talked about the concept of "adaptation and comfort," that's when the bath and bed came up. This naturally filled in the whole two or three years of nursing.

Now, there has been another thrust with the integration into the audiovisual, self-tutorial approach to skills. There was a point where I thought faculty had washed their hands of teaching any skillls. "You go into the library," or "You go into the learning lab and do your thing," and "Well, you know, you can do this audiovisual business, and then you can come into the clinical area and practice." So, we have gone from an overemphasis on skills fifty years ago to ignoring them today—to thinking students can do it themselves. Although I think some of us are holding back more toward the middle ground. Nevertheless, there are many programs that now teach the "skills of the nursing arts" prior to the student having the total composite of supporting science. For instance, before the students have had microbiology, they're being taught about personal hygiene, temperature, etc. Frequently the faculty is teaching. "There are bad germs, there are good germs, and when you take a temperature there are those bad ones you have to worry about." This gives the student only a smattering of the science, because they haven't had a strong science base. What I'm saying is, before you teach a skill, the student must have a scientific base.

Ms. Carlson: I'd like to comment on that. As a nursing inservice educator, I have taken nurse-assistant trainees, some with not even a high school education. (One of the requirements is that you may have to be able to read and write—period! Simple reading and writing skills.) Within four weeks they are capable of going onto units and doing a list of activities and functioning on the unit. Yet, we still insist on teaching these same skills in a university setting to people who are able to get into a collegiate program. We continue to perpetuate the same kind of programming for nursing. I find that very deplorable in terms of the intellectual skills that we ask our students to have. I emphasize again that the professional going into the clinical laboratory is not going in to learn to be a nursing assistant, which we have perpetuated over the years in terms of laboratory skills, but I suggest that their beginning activities should be assessment and the first part of the nursing process. This would apply to all activities throughout their entire education, in every area, whether it was neurological, obstetrical, surgical, etc. When you ask a student to do intervention or nursing therapy, you should remember that there is no profession which asks the student to develop therapy. The medical student does not give therapy to a patient; only someone with a license can give therapy. And yet we are constantly hearing comfort and caring called "intellectual nursing functions" on a university basis. We really have to think about what we're doing when we're teaching.

Dr. Stanton: Isn't it interesting that the nursing-service people here remind us about the intellectual part of nursing? We have an integrated program at our college and occasionally we get senior faculty members who feel that the student who begins her senior year knows everything. We have to remind ourselves that we have an integrated program, which means that at the senior level there may be some skills that students still have to learn.

309

Dr. Torres: I think we need to mention the push from students for these skills—and early—because their TV concept of nursing is the doing, the laying-on-of-hands, the performance of these skills. I have the feeling that if you could take a freshman class on the first day of college, put little white things on them, give them those Red Cross hats, and then let them go and wash and comfort people just for a week, out of context—just do the thing for a week and get it over with—then I think the next four years would be very profitable. I think sometimes you just have to meet the students' immediate needs and then carry on.

Dr. Stanton: That's an interesting point you make. I'm noticing a difference, however, in the students entering now. They are beginning to have a different concept of nursing. We have students who began their nursing experiences several years ago, who didn't think their patients were sick enough. They really expected that on the very first day they were going to see the oxygen tents around, since they had heard about all the calling for "Emergency!" and "Cardiac arrest!" They were very upset when they found that patients had ulcers and diabetes, and they needed a lot of teaching because their concept of nursing was from television. Actually, it was not nursing that they were looking at, but a medical model of a physician's assistant. But we're seeing a change, I think, in the student's conception.

Dr. Torres: Sometimes I think that faculty, when they get this reaction from students, would be more successful if they would just treat it and forget it, rather than trying to change the whole curriculum in relation to it. You'll get students who think that giving an injection is the ultimate in nursing. If it doesn't flow easily with the particular content and time, I would suggest that you just take them down to the allergy clinic and let them do this for the experience of the day.

Ms. Carlson: I think if we look at the medical model (it seems to be one of the things we're always looking at), we'll realize that the intern for the most part comes out with four years or even eight years of theory. It seems to me, it's the experienced nurse who ends up teaching him the skills. Am I correct? Apparently, we are doing that kind of programming for them. They learn certain skills, and the nurses kind of help them through.

Ms. O'Leary: The one thing I keep hearing is: "Where do you throw in the idea of the Nurse? And the role of the nurse?" When you think in terms of television and what the public is exposed to, you see that we not only have a student anticipating that her role is task oriented, but we also have the patient anticipating that the role is task oriented. As

310

educators we have to do something to combat such ideas. We need leadership in nursing that will get across to the public what they can expect the practitioner to do. Often, in home interviews with patients, when we try to determine how they interpreted the nurse's role in their health care, people have said, "She didn't do anyting but talk to me."

Dr. Stanton: Thank you, Helen. Another question here is, "With the current economic crunch and the cry for higher student-faculty ratio, how can nursing faculty monitor the clinical competence of students?"

Ms. Carlson: I suggest again that education and service have a joint venture. If you go back to your area and are able to work together, education with service and service with education, you will find that the problem isn't quite as bad as it might be. This assumes that you have service personnel who are qualified and you can utilize them. As Gertrude said, we must come back to the middle. No, not the old diploma school days and no, not the university days when there was a complete dichotomy. But there is a middle, and that is where the head nurse still has responsibility for students along with the instructor. The head nurse herself, as well as the staff nurses, would love—everyone likes to be a teacher—to work with student nurses. This is the philosophy of the service area. You would not need the ratio which is insisted upon by service people. You can't possibly have 10 to 1. We expect 6 to 1, or 8 to 1 at the most. But I don't think it's a question of numbers. If the student has had the theory and the practice back in the lab and the university, when they come onto the unit they should be able to function well enough so that they are safe, so that, for what they don't know, they know whom to go to. They should be able to go to any of the staff nurses and should be the eyes and ears for the safety of the patient.

The service people are responsible for the patient, not the educators. Medical students go around without the attending staff or their teachers on top of them. They go in to a patient, they do interviews, they look around, they get a lot of education, like doing independent work within the hospital. Your student nurse, if she moves off of the unit without an instructor, all hell breaks loose from service administration. "What are they doing without an instructor watching them?" We want nurses to be independent, yet they can't move without the instructor on top of them. I don't know what the liabilities are; that has to be looked into. I think we are very insurance conscious; how come the medical people aren't? This is a medical model you might want to look at for education.

Dr. Torres: We get a lot of letters at NLN asking what the teacher-student ratio should be. The criteria for accreditation speak to no ratio. People seem to feel that if the League were to say 1 to 6, then everybody out there would accept it. Now the League is a membership organization, and the membership has not come up with anything like this because it would be too constraining. When you talk about ratio, you're talking about several contexts. First, the budget. How many faculty do we need for how many students? In English or history, it might be 1 to 15 or 20. But in nursing it might be calculated at 1 to 8 or 1 to 10. Secondly, you have to separate budget concerns from the clinical area and what your objective and setting are. For instance, if the objective is nutritional assessment, one instructor could have 50 students all over town; she could be available, although not visible, and handle it quite effectively with preimposed, conference-type activities. Yet, it is also possible—in the premature nursery, for example—that only two students can enter a unit with an instructor; here the ratio would need to be 2 to 1. The idea of dictating 8 to 1 or 10 to 1 for every experience, for every instructor, is to fail to look at what you're trying to accomplish. I think this is essential if we're going to make our objectives effective for the student. Then you have to look at ratios in terms of safety. Where safety is a factor, ratio may have to be reduced.

Dr. Stanton: Another constraint on ratio is what the agency will allow. Although you might feel you could manage with 1 to 10, or 1 to 12, the agency has a right to set certain limits. Now, they're not telling you all they'll allow. And I think that agencies have a right to do this.

Ms. Carlson: I think the agency is really saying—and it has to look at this—that they're still really work oriented. Even though we say, "You're in for an educational experience," it's a dichotomy now and we know it. In reality, when you have ten students with one instructor from 8 to 12 a.m., the agency expects that by noon the patient that's been assigned to the student will have had the bath, the bed, and the 10 o'clock medication. This is not really the objective of education for those four hours, but it's the objective of the service agency. And that's why they say they want 10 to 1, 8 to 1, or 6 to 1, depending on the difficulty of the type of patient you're selecting and the safety required. You've got to change the thinking of the agency; they know that they're for education, but they still expect to take service from you. We have to say that we're going to come in and we're only going to do a history; we're going to have 10 students interview 10 patients; and there will not be any laying-on-of-hands. In this case, you could have 20 students or 1, and if you don't have any laying-on-of-hands, you don't need an instructor. Our concern is the physical. "Will they fall out of bed—are the side rails up?" "Can they ambulate without slipping?" We're so insurance- and malpractice-oriented that we don't allow freedom anywhere along the line.

312

Participant: I have to disagree with you. I'm a service person and I truly feel that the school has the right and the responsibility to the students to make the [ratio] assignment, to tell us what they're going to do. The only reason we limit 10 to 15 on an area is for physical reasons: you just can't have 50 students in one physical area. You would just be overwhelmed.

Ms. Carlson: Let's say that you have one instructor with a number of students scattered over several different units. You may have 5 students on the unit, and [administration] wants the instructor there. The instructor walks off for an hour and goes to another unit. Are they concerned that the instructor isn't physically present?

Participant: Yes. This has never been my philosophy. I feel that you should know your student. If you don't feel that she needs you to be physically present, then I should trust your judgment. If you feel that a student is presently all right in an area, then that's fine with me.

Ms. Carlson: That's beautiful. I wish everybody would feel the same way. Would you identify yourself?

Participant: I'm Maria Aperton, from the USPHS Hospital on Staten Island. We have had two agencies come in, and I must say we have excellent relationships. We speak to one another, we do preplanning, and I think it's been of mutual benefit. I don't expect beds to be made. We've had them come in and say, "We're going to do nothing this morning. We're just going to take a look around." And that's fine. I have no right to expect students to do the work we're being paid for.

Dr. Torres: I think that one thing the educator must keep in mind is that if you want students to assess, why pick the morning hours when all that activity's going on? Why not late in the afternoon or sometime when the students can really assess without getting in the way of service? You know what's going on, you know people must wash at 8 a.m.— there's just no other time!

Participant: Because of our physical set-up, we're not always in one building. We're out in the community, and we have 10 district offices. There are maybe 8 or 10 nurses assigned to each office, so we have to limit the number of students. When we have a student assigned to us for a beginning experience, we have a nurse assigned to that student. Now, it takes a while before the student is able to go out into the community on her own. When you're talking about clinical experiences, you have to

313

remember where you're getting that clinical experience. Also, as far as the hours are concerned, the agency does have hours, but our students don't always have the same hours. If it's more convenient for them, because of their educational requirements, to come in the afternoon, we welcome them to do this.

Participant: How do you close the reality gap between the NLN image of the nurse practitioner and actual practice?

Dr. Torres: If the NLN is to speak to it, you must have all the participants speak, because NLN is a membership organization. As a matter of fact, I'd have no vote at all, because I'm not an agency member. Aside from that, when membership try to describe the graduate, they tend to describe what the graduate *should* be. It's a kind of goal-oriented formula: A graduate should be this way, and this is what we should be educating for. If change occurs, it occurs slowly. If everybody thought that these characteristics were exciting and started to put them into their programs today, it would take four years to have the first graduates with those particular characteristics. We are educating for at least four years ahead, so there will be at least a four-year gap between education and service. In some areas of the country you get the feeling there's a fifty-year gap. The educational and service people, then, need to accept the fact that there is a gap and not feel guilty about it. Now, between the two gaps, whether it be four years or fifty years, there's a lag. The more education and service get together and the more they help each other, the more this lag is reduced. Do you support that, Sylvia?

Ms. Carlson: We try to close that as much as possible. Whenever an instructor or student identifies a gap, we have a conference with them. At one point we had something happen on a maternity area that the students felt was just terrible. They felt they just had to speak to this particular gap and their education in our particular service. We invited the physician who they felt was the culprit, the director of nurses, the instructor, and the group to meet and talk about it. It turned out that there was a reality situation that the students had to know about, as well as our hearing what they felt we were doing that was not according to Hoyle. At least we began to understand each other a little better, even though we couldn't close the gap completely. This is, I think, the gap we are talking about. But you must let the students know you're aware of it and not hiding what they see as deficiencies, for students pick these up very quickly. Students are usually very idealistic, and part of their understanding of the bureaucratic system has to be that there are certain restraints—as much as we'd like to eliminate them. At least they go

314

away feeling satisfied that we have tried and have listened to them, and they don't have the frustration of feeling that the agency is working at another level that they haven't been taught about.

Dr. Torres: It depends, though, on the sophistication of the personnel in the agency. If they're really clinical specialists and up-to-date in their own specialty field, the agency may be ahead of the educational institution. If the educational institution has young instructors just out of the graduate programs, who are very up-to-date in their specialty, then the agency may be behind. Here again is the interaction of trying to bring both up-to-date in terms of knowledge and practice.

Dr. Stanton: Thank you. Another question is, "What is a nurse and what should she be doing and how much should she get paid to do it in the ambulatory end of the program?" Now, the questioner is talking about articulating positions for nurses working in an ambulatory care setting in the community. Do you want to speak to that, Helen?

Ms. O'Leary: I think that recently we have allowed the question of money to really get in the way of what we are trying to do. If we think that working in certain settings implies more money, I'm beginning to worry a little bit. If you're talking about a specialist who has had graduate preparation in a certain area, then perhaps money becomes important. If you're talking about a practitioner working in a different setting, I don't know why she should be paid more in an ambulatory care center then in a hospital center.

Dr. Stanton: I'd take that question a little bit differently. First of all, I would say (and this is my personal opinion, although I think it has some basis in fact and in terms of the literature) that ambulatory care settings are the primary responsibility of nurses. Physicians, social workers, and others come in when they are needed. I think a nurse has to have at least a baccalaureate degree to work in this kind of setting. In fact, it seems to me that this is the one area where institutions could make changes. If you want baccalaureate nurses to practice to their full potential, give them the ambulatory care setting. In terms of what they should be doing, they should be doing, they should be doing everything they've been taught to do, using all their knowledge and skills with these patients. In terms of how much they should get paid, I think any nurse should get paid what she's worth. Now, that tends to be a problem. I think that in some areas of our country, professional nurses are being shortchanged. On the other hand, I think that, in a society that's supposed to be concerned about the people who live in it, it is unrealistic for any health professional to be making money off his services to people. However, I do think that every health professional should be paid in terms of his education and his contribution to the community. Because each community may be different, the community should determine the salary scales to some degree.

Dr. Torres: I think there is something we have to be careful about. Let's imagine ten years from now, with baccalaureate graduates in large numbers having their own little shingles out and being independent practitioners or family health practitioners. If they end up as the physicians did—the independent people charging what they please—and moving to such charges as physicians have, the theory is that they'll end up like the physician and the National Health Insurance is going to take care of that. So one of the things we have to be careful about is that, as Marge says, we don't make money because we become independent or autonomous and can charge as we please. That we are reasonable and that we give effective care and make a decent living is acceptable. But don't overdo it, which is what has happened to the physician. People are tired of having him make over $100,000 a year.

Dr. Stanton: That's a big gap between one professional and another—$10,000 and $100,000! I think we also have to be careful because, in every depression, somebody always comes out making money out of something. The health field is going to be one of the fields where somebody is going to try this, because it happens to be a very lucrative field. Everybody right now is trying to use the health field for upward mobility programs and things of that sort. I think we must be careful that nurses are not the ones to take advantage. But I think with National Health Insurance there will be more stability and less chance of someone going way up on the scale.

Dr. Torres: I remember back a few years ago they wanted the nurse to become a physician's assistant, and one of the attractive factors was that the nurse could make a bundle if she'd just relabel herself and work under the doctor's license. I'm glad to see nursing didn't buy it and give up its autonomy.

Dr. Stanton: The last question from the letters is, "What is the role of the nurse in diagnosis of human responses and intervention, and in the area of teacher-consultant and patient-family advocate?" Helen, do you want to speak to that?

Ms. O'Leary: My first reaction to that, when it was read to me, was, "What's the question that's being asked?" Because that's what nursing is all about. We anticipate that nursing does diagnosis of human responses with intervention, and I wasn't sure why the question was being asked. As far as teacher-consultant goes, in my own particular specialty, which is community health, we anticipate that all our nurses are teachers, and we anticipate that at certain given times they also are consultants. As for patient-family advocate, I think that is the goal of the nurse; I think that the nurse has to become stronger in this area, whether she's dealing with the community, the physician, a social agency, or even a hospital. This diagnosis of human responses and intervention is what it's all about. Sylvia, do you have a comment?

Ms. Carlson: No, but when Gertrude was talking about the physican and the nurse, it brought something to mind that I'd like to mention. Marge, I got a call recently from one of the instructors in the senior program that you set up with us at LIJ, where the seniors come onto the the unit independently with the instructor following them and just going around and saying "Hello." Our head nurses and our primary nurses are acting as preceptors in this program. This instructor said she had a student who was doing independent study with a physician. Now, this is a breakthrough, and I'd like to share that with you. The doctor is acting as preceptor, and the student is working with him and three other colleagues in the office. She will be following patients into our hospital as well as to other hospitals where they're working. She will be doing a senior experience in which she will actually follow patients in the hospital; she will do charts, psychosocial intervention, come back to the office, and follow patients into the home, working with the physician and his patients specifically. We have talked about independent nurse practitioners and we've also talked about doctors as colleagues—not the P.A. physicians, but the doctor working with the nurse as an independent practitioner in his office. In this relationship she shares the profits on a percentage basis because she can go out and see patients on the psychosocial follow-ups as well as physical follow-ups. I thought this was an interesting innovation. We're very pleased, and we can see a clinical specialist doing this, for example, with the obstetrician or the pediatrician in his office. We can see this in all areas, and we are very happy that one of your students is taking this role.

Dr. Stanton: We have two other students who are working with obstetricians and doing prenatal counseling. They will go into the hospital with the patient and will be on call during labor and delivery. We also have one student who has asked a physician about doing preoperative counseling, preparing patients for surgery and then doing follow-up care in the home. We feel that part of the role of the university is to help change the health care delivery system, to help physicians appreciate the role of the professional nurse. We are beginning to see

317

physicians thinking about the possibility of having a group practice with nurses in the community, because they see the value of having nurses invovled in this.

Participant: I'd like to speak to this, too, because I've just had three students who have completed this kind of situation in a physician's office. At the end of the experience, the physicians wrote letters to us saying they were satisfied with the experience. The students were highly satisfied and were able to do a great deal of assessment and to be of assistance to professionals.

Dr. Torres: If education and service were really united, we then could approach the interdisciplinary group and hopefully make some changes in their attitudes. I think—and this may be my bias—that service people tend to understand the position a little more closely, and if educators could get close to the service people and service people close to the physician, the whole circle could really support certain types of duty experiences that we're not able to get otherwise.

Participant: There are certain dangers in what is being discussed right now. We're still hanging onto the coattails of the physicians.

Ms. Carlson: I don't agree!

Participant: I don't question that. By the nurse and the student here [in a group practice], how many more patients could the physicain see? How much more money could we make a year?

Ms. Carlson: A lot! And for the nurses who get a percentage, you write a contract. There could be the MD, RN, social worker, and nutritionist in a group practice. The shingle would include all of them. It's a business contract, not an employee-employer relationship where the nurse is paid a certain amount of money per annum. On that basis, then, it's professional. The other way, you're absolutely right.

Participant: Another thing you should look at is: how much more effective is the care?

Ms. Carlson: It is very effective. I'm sure many of you are familiar with Dr. Barbara Bates in Rochester. She has reported on assessment by the physician and by the nurse working with the physician, and on the kind of things they come up with—what the differences are and how this integrates with the total care of the patient. She has written a great deal on this, and, as an M.D., hers should be an objective evaluation.
Another example happened when Malloy and Adelphi were coming

to LIJ as part of the "physical assessment push" for instructors a few years ago. One of instructors was in our OPD working with a pediatrician in neurology learning the assessment of the child. The pediatrician had seen a certain child a number of times and, neurologically, the child was still having some problems. But they were not identified from the physical point of view. The pediatrician told the mother to come back in three months, since he couldn't find anything definitive. The mother said, "If I live that long." And the doctor replied, "See you in three months!" The nurse, who did the same physical assessment in her practice session, asked the doctor if she might leave the room a few moments, went out, and, in speaking to the mother, identified the fact that she was suicidal. Just that one clue that the doctor never picked up! The mother has been suicidal three months before. This is nursing. While doing the same physical assessment as a physician, she picked up clues and heard things and was able to intervene. The child's condition was obviously not neurological; it was emotional with neurological manifestations. The nurse got the mother over to social service, and they were to help that particular family. In a clinic the difference between medicine and nursing is in terms of integration. They both did a physical assessment, but the story proves the point.

Dr. Torres: There's one thing we have to be careful about, and that is that we don't just keep track of what the doctor is doing and make up for his deficiencies. We must do what *we* are responsible for.

Participant: I'm very much concerned that what we're talking about is nurses making perfect the medical care of the already over-treated middle classes in this country. We're not talking about the terrible statistics of the poor and the disadvantaged.

Dr. Stanton: May I just say that all of us are right. However, we can't bend too far the other way; we can't just stay away from physicians altogether. When our students get involved with patients of physicians, they're involved in nursing, not medicine. I do not feel the physician should be involved with nursng. That's out of their realm. In terms of taking care of the disadvantaged, another experience that we offer students is in our nursing center, which is in a housing project in a disadvantaged area. This gives students a variety of experiences. And out in our area it is not unheard-of for people who are on Medicaid—which means that you are disadvantaged economically—to have to their own private physicians, so that you could be getting involved with patients who have private physicians, but who are at the same time disadvantaged. Other sections of the country probably have the same kinds of economic situations.

319

6 CURRICULUM REVISION IN BACCALAUREATE NURSING EDUCATION

37 CURRICULUM REVISION THE *WHAT, WHEN, WHY,* AND *WHO*

Gertrude J. Torres, EdD, RN

The title of this paper specifically relates to curriculum *revision*, not curriculum *change*, in order to emphasize a point. Nursing educators frequently, when speaking of curriculum, use the words *change* and *revision* interchangeably. Yet it is interesting to note that when we speak of change, we are more frequently confronted with a greater amount of subjectivity and resistance than when we use the word *revision*. Thus is seems appropriate, for this presentation at least, that we have a common frame of reference as to what concepts are being communicated by these words.

Instead of using them synonymously, we might recognize that, in truth, the two words have some rather different shades of meaning. To change means to make different, to transform, to replace, or to substitute one thing for another. Thus, to change a curriculum would mean to replace or make it different from what it was. To revise, on the other hand, means to look at something over again in order to correct or improve it or to create an updated version. It seems to me that in essence we do not *change* our curriculums, but *revise* them.

Our beliefs about nursing, health, and education have remained, for the most part, unchanged for over 50 years. The Curriculum Guides prepared by the National League of Nursing Education in 1917, 1927, and 1937 verify this fact. This is especially true if we accept the notion that while our terminology may differ from decade to decade, we are

323

frequently talking about the same things. Let me quote some revealing passages from the Curriculum Guides of 1917, 1927, and 1937:

> The steady expansion into new and exacting fields of effort is continually revealing to us both the strength and the weakness of our methods of training.[1] [Here the word *education* might be more appropriate than *training,* in relation to today's terminology.]

> The newer subjects dealing with the social and preventive aspects of disease are not introduced with the ideas of giving specialized training...but as a much-needed background for all branches of nursing.[2]

> Health nursing is just as fundamental as sick nursing and the prevention of disease is at least as important a function of the nurse in the care and treatment of the sick.[3]

> The subordination of the "human" element in our work to the physical and technical is one of the severest criticisms we have to meet in nursing today...We are dealing primarily with sick nursing and health nursing.[4]

> Our position is that "health" nursing is just as fundamental as "sick" nursing and the prevention of disease at least as important a function of the nurse.[5]

From these statements it is evident that we in nursing education have not changed our concept of stressing illness within the curriculum while also recognizing the need to encourage a more health-oriented approach to nursing. It seems we are still trying to improve the curriculum in terms of needs identified in the past.

Revising our curriculums should be viewed as an evolutionary process in which we update and improve them, even though we sometimes think we are totally changing the curriculum in a revolutionary manner. In speaking of the *what* of curriculum revision, we are referring to the improvement of the way we, as educators, organize our body of knowledge into learning activities and experiences. This involves updating our efforts to bring about improved, desired outcomes.

Recent improvements that can be identified relate to a change in emphasis from groups to individuals, from memory to inquiry, from telling to guiding, and from content to process values.[6] Other improvements more directly related to nursing are a greater interest in the emerging role

---

[1] National League of Nursing Education, Committee on Education, *Standard Curriculum for Schools of Nursing* (Baltimore: Waverly Press, 1917), p. 6.

[2] *Ibid.,* p. 7.

[3] National League of Nursing Education, Committee on Education, *A Curriculum Guide for Schools of Nursing* (New York: The League, 1925), p. 11.

[4] *Ibid.,* p. 11.

[5] National League of Nursing Education, Committee on Curriculum, *A Curriculum Guide for Schools of Nursing* (New York: The League, 1937), p. 21.

[6] Alice Miel, "Reassessment of the Curriculum—Why?" in Dwayne Huebner, ed., *A Reassessment of the Curriculum* (New York: Teachers College, Columbia University, 1964), pp. 12-13.

of the professional nurse, a greater acceptance of our responsibility in interdisciplinary activities, and an acceptance of the professional nurse as a participant in change within the social, health, and nursing care systems. These are not truly new interests, but renewed affirmation of previously held concepts.

In speaking about the *when* of curriculum revision, we must relate it to the *why*, for it is only the identification of the need to update or improve the curriculum that will cause it to take place. Let us identify some of the reasons that can encourage or even possibly discourage revision:

- A substantial number of nursing programs have recently expanded, resulting in greater increases in the number of nursing students and faculty. This yearly influx of new faculty, who come with differing beliefs, goals, and expectations, can strongly influence whether the curriculum will be revised. The same impact can also be felt in programs which have a high yearly attrition rate of faculty.
- Faculty are becoming more and more sophisticated in terms of curriculum and can more easily identify "weaknesses" within their present curriculums.
- Today, educational revision is viewed in terms of the total curriculum development process rather than the revision of a single course. Thus, there develops the recognition for a greater involvement on the part of the total faculty.
- Faculty's awareness of changing educational and social trends and their desire to implement these in the curriculum is increasing.
- Nursing educators are more actively engaged in a clearer delineation of the characteristics of their graduates, resulting in the recognition of a need to revise their present approaches to educating.
- More than ever, faculty are identifying themselves as being responsible for curriculum decisions.
- Social changes, especially economic ones, have demanded a greater amount of accountability on the part of nursing educators. These changes involve society's economic priorities, especially in relation to education and health care.

Generally, the time at which the faculty will identify the need for curriculum revision will vary from program to program and will more than likely be sporadic in nature. Viewing curriculum revision as evolutionary means that through formative and summative evaluation the curriculum can be constantly developing or, dramatically stated, "unfolding." Imagine the implications if we could convince our "change resistors" that the curriculum is never quite completed but is constantly unfolding before us!

The question of *who* is responsible for curriculum revision initially appears to have a rather simple answer. After all, the faculty who are responsible for the education of the nursing majors must *obviously* be responsible for the curriculum since they implement it. Yet, if things are that simple, why are there problems?

Although the professional educator is responsible for updating the curriculum, she cannot do it in isolation. She is influenced by the consumer of education and nursing care, by politicians, by other nursing and health care professionals, and by fellow educators within the university or college. These persons can often be identified as the "silent *who*" in curriculum revision. Yet often they are a powerful force, and the kinds of pressures they exert—either supportive or obstructive—can have a strong impact on a curriculum.

Some people believe that the educational administrator in nursing is the curriculum leader and the significant person in curriculum revision. Yet, one study has shown that faculty see *themselves,* not the administrators, as the curriculum leaders.[7] If this is correct, educational administrators in nursing are not presently part of the *who* in curriculum development, and leadership on curriculum matters is coming from within the faculty.

Nevertheless, the administrator can be a key person in supporting the faculty in their efforts. She should be regarded as an excellent resource person in terms of keeping the faculty up-to-date on outside issues and trends. As a leader, she can have a tremendous impact on the direction of the curriculum if she views this as one of her signficant functions. Theoretically, if she is the faculty "leader" and the faculty are responsible for the curriculum, it stands to reason that she should be the curriculum leader. Search committees interviewing for administrative as well as faculty positions should keep in mind their program's needs in relation to curriculum expertise.

Any given faculty needs some structure that will encourage and support the updating of the curriculum. The size of the faculty may strongly influence this structure. Faculties that function constantly as a committee of the whole are rare. In such situations, care needs to be taken in differentiating between the handling of present concerns and problems and the more evolutionary process of curriculum updating.

In larger institutions, where there are curriculum committees, the members of the faculty should be well represented within the committee. All curriculum committee recommendations should be brought to the faculty as a whole for decisions. Members of the committee should also represent both older and newer faculty members and include both identified resistors to change and those persons considered to be forces

---

[7] Audrey J. Conley, "Faculty Selection of Curriculum Leaders," (unpublished Ed.D. dissertation; New York: Teachers College, Columbia University, 1971).

326

for change. We need to keep in mind that both these characteristics—resistance to and desire for change—are present within most of us and are necessary for making sound decisions. A curriculum committee should develop effective mechanisms that will allow them to remain in touch with all faculty members; whatever the structure utilized for curriculum updating, it is essential that the total faculty be involved in the process at each step.

Whether we tend to view curriculum in terms of change or of revision, there are bound to be problems. These frequently stem from the faculty's difficulty in identifying curriculum revision as an essential responsibility on their part as nurse educators. Nursing faculty tend to have a high proportion of contact hours with their students; this, and their constant involvement in other related activities, makes it difficult for them to identify time to devote to curriculum revision. They are also frequently admonished to keep their clinical expertise updated, to publish, and to engage in research. Yet many of their frustrations would be reduced if they did spend time in redeveloping their curriculum, for a sound, well-developed, evolutionary curriculum that supports the faculty's beliefs is really the only way that a faculty group can be truly satisfied. This satisfaction will then allow faculty to engage in other activities more effectively.

Let me recapitulate the major points of this presentation. Curriculum revision is the evolutionary updating by the total faculty of the discipline's body of knowledge, organized into learning activities, and is generally influenced by changes in health, social, and educational patterns.

We, as nurse educators, have had a long, hard, but successful struggle in finding our way from training in acute-care settings to educating in institutions of higher learning. Now it is time to put our heads together in order to create truly dynamic curriculums which will better meet the needs of students as individuals and the needs of society as consumers of health care. This can only be done if we are strongly motivated to the continual updating of our curriculums.

38 THE PHILOSOPHY AS PART OF THE TOTAL CURRICULUM PROCESS

Jean Kelley, EdD, RN

Philosophy is a term with many different meanings. Traditionally it is viewed as an attitude or method of inquiry, or as a search for a unified picture which results from interrelating events. Some prefer to explain philosophy in terms of the type of problem under investigation. There are four major problems subjected to inquiry. First, there is inquiry into the nature of reality or being, otherwise known as metaphysics. Or there is an exploration into theories of knowledge which raises questions such as how man acquires knowledge, how far knowledge extends, and how knowledge can be tested. This approach to philosophy is known as epistemology. Next, there is concern for problems of values, known as axiology, which delves into what one values and how values are selected or excluded. Last, there is the problem of logic, or critical analysis, which uses a variety of modes of inquiry, ranging from experimental to quasi-theoretical, in its search for truth. This approach is sensitive to both language and logic. It is a method of inquiry that involves two distinct activities. First, there is the activity of clarifying the language used, and secondly, there is the activity of using logic to achieve order or to structure concepts which have been clarified.

Philosophy as part of the total curriculum process must consider all four major problems (i.e., reality, knowledge, values, and logic). analysis will be adopted in order to demonstrate the relationship of a philosophy to the process of revising a baccalaureate curriculum in nursing. To achieve this, an inquiry will be made into two issues:

- What is curriculum? This will question its meaning or syntactical expression.
- How does philosophy, or the beliefs and values of the faculty—which may be based on knowledge or on faith—reflect a unified picture of the total curriculum?

What is Curriculum?

Today, students of curriculum are faced with a verbal jungle containing much undergrowth due to variations in curriculum definitions, procedures, and designs. Once the undergrowth in this verbal jungle is cleared, students of curriculum will be able to travel an open road to curriculum revision. One approach suggested for the removal of this verbal jungle in curriculum is what may be named the Four-D attack. This campaign has four major phases, each of which is identified by a key word beginning with the letter "D":

- *Definition.* Defining curriculum or describing the nature of curriculum;
- *Determinants and their direction.* Identifying the basic determinants or elements of the curriculum (e.g., man, society, learning, knowledge) that serve as a basis for curriculum decisions and to assist in the achievement of curriculum goals;
- *Dimensions.* Using the components of the curriculum process (e.g., philosophy, objectives, learning experiences, evaluation) to revise the curriculum;
- *Design.* Developing a revised curriculum based upon definition and determinants of curriculum and the utilization of dimensions in the curriculum process.

The word curriculum, like the term philosophy, is subject to a wide range of intepretations. To a student of nursing, curriculum may mean instruction and clinical experiences; to the teacher of nursing, curriculum may mean courses and behavioral objectives; while to the educational administrator, curriculum may mean the total efforts of the school or provision of an environment conducive to learning.

A review of the literature on curriculum, however, revealed that at least three different major concepts of curriculum are prevalent.[1] They are outlined in the following paragraphs.

---

[1] George Beauchamp, *Curriculum Theory,* 2nd ed. (Wilmette, IL: Kagg Press, 1968), p. 80. Also see, by the same author, *Basic Dimensions of Elementary Method,* 2nd ed. (Boston: Allyn and Bacon, 1965), pp. 54-55.

1. *The Experience or Activity Concept* views curriculum as a sequence of potential experiences selected by the school for the purpose of preparing learners to think and to act in generally accepted ways. Examples of curriculum writers who might be placed under this classification, based on their definition of curriculum, are: Caswell and Campbell, Goodlad, Neagley and Evans, Saylor and Alexander, and Smith, Stanley, and Shores.

2. *The Psychological Concept* of curriculum sees it as a psychological process concerned with interaction of the learner and his environment in order to produce the outcome of maximum development of individual potentialities. Typical curriculum writers supporting this approach are: Douglas and Hobson, Downey, King and Brownell, and Tyler.

3. *The Social Concept* maintains that curriculum is a contrived environment directing an influence upon individual learners, with the prime goal of teaching them to function in groups and to solve problems of society. MacDonald, and to a certain extent Taba and Beauchamp, support this concept of curriculum.

If three such varied concepts of curriculum are prominent in the literature, what is the best way for faculty to revise a baccalaureate curriculum in nursing? Should the curriculum be revised around one of these concepts, around two of them, or should all three concepts be considered and given equal treatment? Inlow[2] maintains that the social concepts should be the major focus in revising a curriculum. More specifically, Inlow proposed that society's values cause a curriculum to emerge. This approach is based on the belief that society's values determine the educational goals, content, instructional methods and evaluation of the nursing program. Taba, on the other hand, took a more comprehensive stand by viewing curriculum as a *plan for learning*.[3] That plan has four determinants, or elements. They are one's beliefs about: man; society with its cultural demands; the learning process; and knowledge or content of a discipline. Faculty statements of beliefs about these four determinants constitute a philosophy from which curriculum objectives are derived; from which learning experiences are planned, selected, and implemented; and upon which evaluation of the plan for learning is built. Taba's interpretation of curriculum takes into account all three concepts of curriculum prevalent in the literature. She considers the social, the psychological, and the experience concepts of curriculum. The problem facing faculty in the process of revising a curriculum is to determine what

---

[2] Gail Inlow, the *Emergent in Curriculum* (New York: Wiley, 1966).

[3] Hilda Taba, *Curriculum Development: Theory and Practice* (New York: Harcourt Brace & World, Inc., 1962), pp. 293-294.

concept or concepts of curriculum has or have the highest priority in their development of a master plan for facilitating students' learning to practice the discipline of nursing.

George Beauchamp summarizes the literature on curriculum with a definition which embodies the three major concepts.[4] His definition states: a curriculum is a design of a *social group* for the educational *experiences* of its *learners* in a school and that design is a realistic document having four specific structures: (1) a written statement of intent or philosophy; (2) written goals or objectives; (3) a written guide for instructional activities; and (4) a written evaluation scheme. The curriculum is analogous to the *U.S. Constitution* in that the latter is a written guide to the political structure of this country, while the former is a written guide to the educational structure in a school of nursing.

In revising a curriculum, the first giant step to be taken by a faculty is to agree upon a definition of curriculum and its accompanying determinants. If the four major determinants of man, society, learning, and knowledge are accepted, then the faculty will need to explore what each element means and the direction it should take. For the determinant *man*, the faculty needs to have certain information about "man-the-learner" in order to make sound curriculum decisions, such as where the student population comes from; the characteristics, personalities, abilities, talents, and potentialities of the learners; the learners' needs, behaviors, and achievements. With this information in hand, the faculty is in an excellent position to revise the plan for learning so that it is directed toward helping man-the-learner to develop as an individual to his maximum potential.

For the determinant *society*, the faculty may need to explore society's values in terms of education for a profession and its values concerning health. Society's concept of the function of education influences the kind of schools it supports. Therefore, it is important to know whether society believes that professional schools of nursing exist to transmit the current culture, to cure all of society's health ills, or to socialize professionals into a role that is constantly changing. How does society view health and health care—as a right or privilege? What does society think about the health care system—as a fragmented, inefficient monster that serves only the needs of the deliverers of health care or a comprehensive, economical, consumer-sensitive system? With answers to these and other similar questions, the faculty should be able to redesign a plan for learning directed toward helping learners achieve social awareness.

For the determinant *learning,* the faculty needs to reach consensus on its theoretical focus for learning the profession of nursing because each theory of learning provides a different frame of reference. Once

---

[4] Beauchamp, *Curriculum Theory,* p. 79. Also see, by the same author, *The Curriculum of the Elementary School* (Boston: Allyn and Bacon, 1956), pp. 41-42.

332

agreement is reached on what learning is and how it is best achieved, the faculty can translate it into action. In learning nursing, three crucial questions must be examined. *What is the role of the nurse that must be learned?* Is it preparation for a single role, such as in primary care, or for a multiple role in primary and secondary care? *What are the outstanding factors that most influence learning nursing*—individual differences, motivation, content, or sequence? *How do you prepare nurses to solve problems that have not as yet been identified?* Is it through providing learners with basic principles, concepts, and the ability to discriminate knowledge or is there a more effective process?

In relation to the determinant *knowledge,* the faculty must realize that nursing as a practice-oriented profession has two notable characteristics: (1) it has a unique body of knowledge that is expanding and increasing in complexity, and (2) it has a method of inquiry, often referred to as the nursing process, which needs to be transmitted into action.

Two further issues regarding knowledge are in need of exploration. Is it possible to translate relevant nursing knowledge through present instructional methods, or are new instructional media and materials needed? Is our transmission of nursing knowledge providing a base upon which the professional nurse can continue to grow and develop, or is it providing competency for a graduate's first job, which may be training for obsolesence?

With reliable information and answers to the questions raised in relation to the learning process and knowledge as determinants of the nursing curriculum, the faculty should be able to revise the curriculum in the direction of preparing learners to continue to learn for a lifetime in the profession.

Figure 1 presents a summary of the four major determinants of the curriculum and the direction for striving toward achieving them.

Philosophy as a Part of the Curriculum Process

Determinant	Direction or Goal
Man-the-Learner	Self Development
Society	Social Development
Learning } Knowledge	Continuous Development

Figure 1. Determinants and goals of the curriculum.

A philosophy for a school of nursing presents a point of view, an expression of beliefs, or speculation about the nature and value of the curriculum and its major determinants. It is a putting together of perceptions about the determinants or related phenomena. It is the foundation and materials from which the total curriculum structure is devised. It is the picture window for the conceptual framework. It is a commitment by the school of nursing to prepare professional nurses for a practice-oriented discipline based on its own unique setting, faculty, and students. If the philsophy for a curriculum is clear, detailed, and written, it becomes a chart or blueprint for curriculum decisions on program objectives, content, learning experiences, and evaluation.

Excerpts from the philosophy of a mature, traditional baccalaureate program (the School of Nursing of the University of Alabama, Birmingham) and its recently revised, soon-to-be-implemented curriculum are presented to illustrate how the philosophy describes the major elements and serves as a picture window for the total curriculum structure:

Philosophic Statements about Man

Old: The faculty believes in the dignity and worth of each individual; the curriculum is designed to serve students who are intellectually capable and curious and who are seeking opportunities for maximum development of their individual potentialities.

New: Man is a biophysical, psychological, spiritual and linguistic being who posseses adaptive mechanisms through which he strives toward self-actualization. Man is unique, unified, valuing and constantly interacting with his environment.

Philosophic Statements about Society

Old: Nursing is an important social force and makes an essential contribution to the total health program of society.

New: Society possesses structure, values, belief and morals which influence individual behavior. Society changes as it adapts to changing knowledge, technology and human resources...Quality health care is a basic human right and is provided in harmony with the individual's lifestyle to the extent desired by him and allowed by his health state.

Philosophic Statements about Learning

Old: Learning is an ongoing and lifelong process which best occurs when all persons involved share in the objectives of the program.

New: Learning is a continuous lifelong process through which the individual changes his behavior. It occurs in individuals through active participation in the learning process and results from integration of cognitive, affective and psychomotor experiences.

Philosophic Statements about Knowledge

Old: In a period of rapid and progressive change in response to new

334

knowledge and demands for health services, the faculty believes that the student must be able to analyze, synthesize and transfer knowledge from one situation to another. . . Nursing is an intellectual discipline and requires vigorous study of its components as well as practice of its skills.

New: Nursing is a discipline which exists as a social force acting in man's behalf when individuals or groups are vulnerable to stress. It operationalizes its functions by employing a scientifically based, goal-directed, interpersonal process.

Philosophic Statements about Professional Nursing Education

Old: By combining general education with nursing education in an academic setting, students will be better prepared to make continuing contributions toward improvement of the nursing profession and of communities they serve.

New: Preparation for professional nursing includes experiences in primary and secondary health care settings with clients of various age groups and socio-economic strata. Interdisciplinary collaboration essential to health care is promoted through shared learning experiences among students in the health professions. Nursing education strategies are required which foster commitment, accountability, decision-making, self-awareness and continued self-enrichment.

In summary, the philosophy as a part of the total curriculum process is a set of mind or habitual approach to curriculum implementation and improvement. A philosophy for a school of nursing is the faculty's belief and values on which the curriculum is based; it is the faculty's current statement of intent. In revising a baccalaureate curriculum in nursing, one needs to avoid two philosophic sins: identifying faculty beliefs but not putting them into action (i.e., thought without action); and taking action, such as revising the curriculum, without first identifying the faculty beliefs (i.e., action without thought).[5] To revise a curriculum, faculty need to be bold and courageous in working with new beliefs and values; to have confidence in handling mistakes, frustration, and embarrassment; to be tolerant of ambiguity yet able to develop specific statements of beliefs; to have a healthy respect for old beliefs and values, for much can be learned from the past; and to have patience and vision to seek a unified picture of the revised curriculum.

BIBLIOGRAPHY

Beauchamp, George. *Curriculum Theory*. 2nd ed. Wilmette, IL: Kagg Press, 1968.

---

[5] James Dickoff and Patricia James, "Beliefs and Values: Bases for Curriculum Design," *Nursing Research* 19: 415-426, September-October, 1970.

_____. *Basic Dimensions of Elementary Method,* 2nd ed. Boston: Allyn and Bacon, Inc., 1965.

_____. *The Curriculum of the Elementary School.* Boston:Allyn and Bacon, Inc., 1964.

_____. *Planning the Elemenary School Curriculum.* Boston: Allyn and Bacon, Inc., 1956.

Caswell, Hollis, and Campbell, Doak S. *Curriculum Development.* New York: American Book Company, 1935.

Dickoff, James, and James, Patricia. "Beliefs and Values: Bases for Curriculum Design." *Nursing Research* 19:415-526, September-October 1970.

Douglass, Harl R., and Hobson, Clay S. "The Function and Nature of the Curriculum." *The High School Curriculum,* 3rd ed. New York: The Ronald Press, 1964.

Downey, Lawrence. *The Secondary Phase of Education.* New York: Blaisdell Publishing Company, 1965.

Firth, Gerald. "Youth Education: A Curriculum Perspective." *Youth Education: Problems, Perspective, Promises.* Washington, DC: ASCD, 1968.

Goodlad, John I. *The Changing School of Curriculum.* New York: Fund for the Advancement of Education, 1966.

_____. "Curriculum: The State of the Field." *Review of Educational Research* 30:85, June 1960.

Inlow, Gail M. *The Emergent in Curriculum.* New York: John Wiley & Sons, 1966.

King, Arthur R., and Brownell, John A. *The Curriculum and the Disciplines of Knowledge.* New York: John Wiley & Sons, 1966.

MacDonald, James B. "The Person in the Curriculum." *Precedents and Promise in the Curriculum Field.* Helen F. Robison, ed. New York: Teachers College Press, 1966.

Mayhew, Lewis B., and Ford, Patrick J. *Reform in Graduate and Professional Education.* San Francisco: Jossey-Bass Publishers, 1974.

Neagley, Ross L., and Evans, N. Dean. *Handbook for Effective Curriculum Development.* Englewood Cliffs, NJ: Prentice-Hall, Inc., 1967.

Saylor, J. Galen, and Alexander, William M. *Curriculum Planning.* New York: Holt, Rinehart and Winston, 1966.

Smith, B. Othanel; Stanley, William O.; and Shores, J. Harlan. *Fundamentals of Curriculum Development.* New York: Harcourt, Brace & World, 1957.

Soltis, Jonas. *An Introduction to the Analysis of Educational Concepts.* Reading, MA: Addison-Wesley Publishing Company, 1968.

Taba, Hilda. *Curriculum Development: Theory and Practice.* New York: Harcourt, Brace & World, 1962.

Tyler, Ralph W. *Basic Principles of Curriculum and Instruction.* Chicago: University of Chicago Press, 1950.

39 THE CONCEPTUAL FRAMEWORK IN NURSING EDUCATION

Jean Kelley, EdD, RN

The 1972 version of the NLN *Criteria for the Appraisal of Baccalaureate and Higher Degree Programs in Nursing* included a new criterion stating, "The curriculum plan is based on a conceptual framework(s) consistent with the stated philosophy, purposes, and objectives of the program(s)."[1] Since that time nurse educators throughout the nation have been involved in a search to identify their program's unique frame of reference. For many this search has been a difficult one because considerable confusion exists over what is meant by "a conceptual framework." The verbal vegetation surrounding the term "conceptual framework" is as dense as the underbrush encircling the words "philosophy" and "curriculum." Often the term conceptual framework is used interchangeably with theoretical framework, curriculum theory, theory of education, or nursing theory.[2] Before a conceptual framework can be located and identified successfully, it is necessary to stipulate a definition of this elusive object in order that it function to provide direction for the curriculum-building process.

A conceptual framework is the *rationale* for the curriculum. It is an expression of the faculty's ideas on what nursing is and what education is, as concerns the practice of professional nursing. It is the way the faculty *looks at data and groups facts into a rationale* that makes explicit what is implicit in a school of nursing's statement of philosophy.[3] A con-

---

[1] National League for Nursing, Department of Baccalaureate and Higher Degree Programs, *Criteria for the Appraisal of Baccalaureate and Higher Degree Programs in Nursing* (New York: The League, 1972), p. 8.

[2] Em Bevis, *Curriculum Building in Nursing: A Process* (St. Louis: C.V. Mosby Company, 1973), p. 18.

[3] Faye Abdellah and Eugene Levine, *Better Patient Care through Nursing Research* (New York: Macmillan Company, 1965), p. 69.

ceptual framework, through its major ideas or concepts, mirrors the philosophy, objectives, and terminal outcomes of the curriculum. It is also a predictive tool in that it tells what will happen to a student of nursing as a result of exposure to and experiences in a specific educational program. A conceptual framework may be viewed as evidence that faculty can use to justify why certain content and learning experiences are selected for and others excluded from their program. Meanwhile, a baccalaureate program next door may use another framework with a different set of learning experiences.

Ideally, the conceptual framework is a clear and concise narrative or diagram depicting the basic concepts or ideas of the faculty that give shape and form to the curriculum in nursing. A conceptual framework differs from a theoretical one in that the latter is an approach to problems which are scientifically based and involve hypotheses.[4] This approach (theoretical) may be on one of several different levels (i.e., descriptive, explanatory, predictive, or prescriptive).[5]

A conceptual framework, on the other hand, reflects the faculty's major concepts of the curriculum. These concepts, identified by the faculty as being intrinsic to the practice of professional nursing, give rise to subconcepts, which in turn suggest certain theories containing hypotheses about the concepts. Thus, through a conceptual framework the faculty clarifies the fundamental concepts of the baccalaureate curriculum in nursing, as well as relevant subconcepts and theories.[6]

The conceptual framework for each professional school of nursing is similar, yet different. A recent analysis of the conceptual framework from fifty baccalaureate programs in nursing revealed a common core of concepts underlying the curriculum.[7] The core consisted of four major concepts: Man, Society, Health, and Nursing. Conceptual frameworks for baccalaureate curriculums in nursing are similar to each other in that they tend to contain one or more of these concepts. However, conceptual frameworks differ in how a faculty develops, emphasizes, or gives priority to the concepts selected for a specific curriculum and in the way they are articulated with subconcepts and theories. For example, if faculty identify Man as a major concept, an accompanying subconcept might be man as a biophysical, psychological, spiritual, and linguistic being, while the theories to be articulated might include: adaptation, interaction, human development, communication. Should the conceptual framework for a school of nursing speak to the concept of Society, a subconcept might be man in the midst of an everchanging society, while theories in need of articulation with that concept might be: group,

---

[4] *Ibid.*

[5] James Dickoff and Patricia James, "A Theory of Theories: A Position Paper," *Nursing Research* 17: 196-227, May-June, 1968.

[6] Bevis, *loc. cit.*

[7] Gertrude Torres and Helen Yura, *Today's Conceptual Framework: Its Relationship for the Curriculum Process* (New York: National League for Nursing, 1974) pp. 2-5.

change, communication, and organizational theories. When Health is recognized as a principal concept in a conceptual framework, an attendant subconcept is that health may be viewed as levels or cycles ranging from wellness to illness, and the theories in need of articulation may be: adaptation, health care systems. When Nursing is acknowledged as a concept, a concomitant subconcept might be that there is a unique body of nursing knowledge and a specific method of inquiry known as the nursing process. Theories in need of articulation with this concept are: role, change, communication, decision making, leadership, group and organizational theories.

An illustration of a conceptual framework for one baccalaureate program in nursing appears in Figure 1. The narrative accompanying the diagram stresses the primary curriculum outcome as being a generalist professional nurse who has had an opportunity for psychosocial develop-

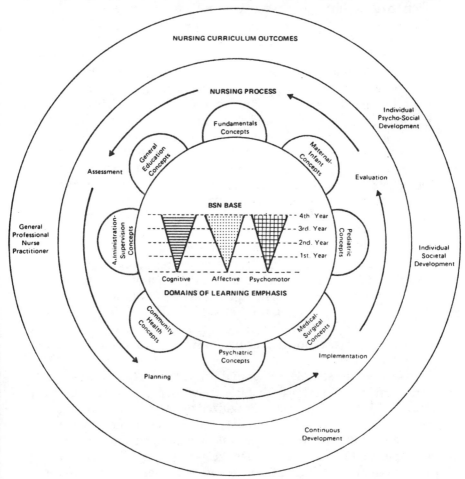

Figure 1. Conceptual framework for the bachelor of science in nursing curriculum, University of Alabama in Birmingham School of Nursing, 1974.

ment, societal development, and preparation to continue to learn for a lifetime during the practice of professional nursing. To attain the curriculum outcomes, nursing is viewed as a dynamic process of interaction with individuals and their families in order to assist them in achieving a maximum level of wellness. This process is most effectively used when cognitive, affective, and psychomotor learnings from general education and from nursing education are selected, organized, and used by learners while assessing, planning, implementing, and evaluating health care. From the beginning of the undergraduate program in nursing, emphasis is placed on increasing the student's acquisition of learnings from the three domains of cognitive, affective, and psychomotor. This emphasis, along with appropriate learning experiences, continues to increase throughout the four years of the educational program, so that upon graduation the nurse possesses a wide learning foundation, or baccalaureate base, from which to draw during the practice of nursing as a generalist and upon which graduate education or continuing education can be built. The diagram appearing in Figure 2 shows the conceptual framework for a master of science in nursing curriculum. It begins with baccalaureate preparation in nursing as its base. Its aim is to increase the breadth and depth of learning from the cognitive, affective, and psychomotor domains, but in one major area of nursing. By focusing on increasing the knowledge, understanding, and skills in one nursing major, learners become more competent in utilizing the nursing process with the individuals and families they encounter. In addition to acquiring expertise or specialization as a nurse in one clinical field, students also receive theoretical preparation for roles as teachers of clinical nursing, as administrators of nursing theories, or as consultants on nursing. To facilitate this expansion of knowledge, understanding, skills, and preparation for a multifaceted role, supportive courses from general education are used throughout the length of the one-year educational program.

The diagram in Figure 2 illustrates that the master of science in nursing curriculum is based upon baccalaureate preparation; it has mastery of nursing knowledge, understanding, and skills as its major focus; and its overall concept is preparation for a professional field, with the outcome being a clinical specialist who has been prepared to render services to the nursing profession and society, as well as to teach and conduct research in nursing.

Analysis of the sample conceptual framework from a baccalaureate curriculum in nursing reveals that it acknowledges the four common concepts: (1) Man-the-Learner is recognized through the three domains of learning, psychosocial development, and continuous development; (2) Society is realized through societal development and psychosocial development; (3) Health is noted in the narrative in relation to the levels or cycles of health ranging from wellness to illness; and (4) Nursing is described as a dynamic process of interaction with individuals and

340

families which is used to assist others in achieving a level of health and which is a process that has assessment, planning, implementation, and evaluation phases. Theories articulated with these concepts include: interaction, adaptation, group or family, change, systems, role, and learning. In addition to clarifying the philosophy for the baccalaureate program in nursing, this conceptual framework also depicts the major goals and terminal behaviors of the curriculum (i.e., a general professional nurse practitioner who has had an opportunity for three types of development: psychosocial, societal, and continuous).

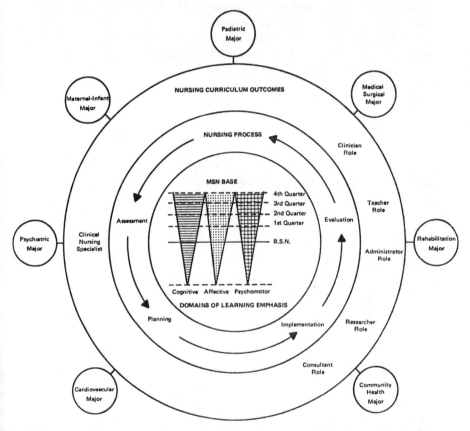

Figure 2. Conceptual framework for the master of science in nursing curriculum. University of Alabama in Birmingham School of Nursing, 1974

Conceptual Framework as Part of
The Total Curriculum Process

How does the conceptual framework fit into the total curriculum process? You will recall that the conceptual framework is the rationale for the curriculum. That rationale flows from the philosophy or beliefs and values of the faculty which specify the major determinants or concepts that will be systematically followed throughout the curriculum. The conceptual framework goes further than just naming concepts, notions, and ideas. It clarifies those concepts through the identification of specific subconcepts and pertinent theories that need to be articulated throughout the curriculum. As a result of this clarification and identification of concepts, subconcepts, and theories, the conceptual framework gives direction to the development of courses and to the selection of pertinent content and learning experiences in the nursing and general education components. The end-product or terminal outcomes of the curriculum may be communicated more effectively to students, employers, and new instructors through the use of a clear, logical, and detailed framework. In addition, such as framework provides a guideline to faculty in their evaluation of the curriculum. A conceptual framework, therefore, pervades all dimensions of the curriculum process (i.e., the philosophy, objectives, design, approach to courses, content, and learning experiences), as well as the evaluation process.

A major deterrent to undergraduate education in the profession of nursing is the lack of distinct conceptual frameworks for curriculums. The building of discernible conceptual frameworks for revised baccalaureate curriculums in nursing will directly influence the degree to which the nursing profession progresses in the preparation of its members for a practice-oriented discipline dedicated to making a contribution to the health care needs of mankind.

40 THE DEVELOPMENT OF BEHAVIORAL OBJECTIVES THROUGH CURRICULUM STRANDS

Gertrude J. Torres, EdD, RN

Curriculum strands represent the elements that are interwoven throughout the organized body of knowledge presented in an educational program. Those strands should support the philosophy and conceptual framework of the program and can be identified within the characteristics of the graduate. The purpose of this presentation is twofold: first, to discuss the utilization and development of objectives; and second, to demonstrate how the identification of curriculum strands can be helpful in the development of level and course objectives.

Words, unless defined from a common frame of reference, can impede understanding. Thus, we first need to look at the words that will be utilized for this presentation before preceeding. Mager believes that "an objective is an *intent* communicated by a statement describing a proposed change in a learner."[1] It should be noted that the words *objective, goal* and *aim* are frequently used synonymously. Nursing programs often speak of their goals or aims in relation to meeting the community's need for professional nurses or having the student take the licensure examinations. They refer to objectives when they speak of student characteristics or behaviors. It might be helpful to view

---

[1] Ralph F. Mager, *Preparing Instructional Objectives* (Palo Alto, CA: Fearson Publishers, 1962), p. 3.

343

objectives as a means to achieve programs, aims or goals. They also should be viewed as a means for building skills and knowledge progressively to higher levels of achievement. As a result, the characteristics of the graduate, stated in terms of behaviors, can be seen involving a lifelong process of learning and improving one's expertise.

A behavior objective can be thought of as a manner of conducting oneself in order to reach a goal; this usually involves some modification or change in behavior on the part of the learner, which often relates to the basic aim of education and the criteria for measuring learning. In terms of the components of objectives, Tyler feels that clearly formulated objectives have a behavioral and content aspect. These components really speak to behavior in relation to cognitive and psychomotor skills and to content in terms of the essence and structure of the discipline of nursing, such as the nursing process. He encourages the development of a two-dimensional chart which speaks to both these aspects.[2] The development of such a chart would identify the knowledge related to nursing science or theory and the behaviors that would result from the use of this knowledge. Whether one develops a chart or not is less significant than realizing the need to ensure that these two dimensions are components of all objectives.

In discussing the development of objectives, it would be rather short-sighted not to include the works of Benjamin S. Bloom and his associates. Their taxonomies of educational objectives related to the cognitive and affective domains can be very helpful to the nurse educator.[3][4] We in baccalaureate nursing education frequently utilize some of the concepts noted in these taxonomies in the development of our characteristics of the graduate. For example, in relation to knowledge, we stress its use in summarizing, predicting, judging and determining directions rather than merely in knowing specific facts. In the area of comprehension, we mean more than understanding demonstrated through communication; we stress interpretation, relationships, and the identification of trends. We also stress synthesis and evaluation through comparison.[5]

The revised Characteristics of the Baccalaureate Graduate, as set forth by the Council of Baccalaureate and Higher Degree Programs, demonstrate the use of these taxonomies. For example, in relation to the affective domain, Bloom stresses the acceptance of responsibility under a willingness to respond and a commitment to a position or cause,[6] while the Characteristics similarly speak to accountability and

[2] Ralph W. Tyler, *Basic Principles of Curriculum and Instruction* (Chicago: University of Chicago Press, 1969), pp. 47-48.

[3] Benjamin S. Bloom, ed., *Taxonomy of Educational Objectives. Handbook I—Cognitive Domain* (New York: David McKay Co., 1967).

[4] Benjamin S. Bloom, ed., *Taxonomy of Educational Objectives. Handbook II—Affective Domain* (New York: David McKay Co., 1967).

[5] Bloom, *Cognitive Domain*, pp. 204-207.

[6] Bloom, *Affective Domain*, pp. 179-181.

the sharing of responsibility. In relation to the cognitive domain, Bloom speaks to application in relation to the ability to predict,[7] as do the Characteristics. It is evident that the taxonomies can be helpful tools for a faculty as it develops objectives.

In the development of all behavioral objectives within a program it is essential that we view them as one part of the entire curriculum process. Objectives *cannot* be developed within courses in isolation and without any interrelatedness to the philosophy or conceptual framework. The lack of interrelatedness of objectives is probably one of the greatest curriculum weaknesses that can be identified in nursing programs.

Model I attempts to demonstrate this relationship between objectives and the other major components of the curriculum process. As noted, the philosophy of the program gives direction to the characteristics of the graduate, which will lead to the development of a conceptual framework and curriculum strands and will be followed by the development of level and course objectives. What is also significant to note is that the characteristics lead to level objectives which lead to course objectives. For purposes of simplifying this presentation, Model I uses a total of only four nursing courses, two under Level III and two under Level IV, which really represent the junior and senior years. (It is recognized that this would not be suitable for all institutions, especially those using the trimester approach.) If the curriculum process is followed as indicated in Model I, what should follow is a curriculum that is totally connected in relationship to its parts. Thus, if one were to place all the objectives within a given program on a large table and set them up as demonstrated in the Model, one should be able to identify progressive learning from course to course and level to level. This approach can be most helpful as a way of avoiding redundancy as well as ensuring the teaching of certain knowledge.

In developing level and course objectives from terminal objectives, the question sometimes arises as to the necessary degree of specificity. Objectives that represent graduate behaviors are of necessity broad in nature. The deeper you go into the curriculum process, the greater the specificity required. Some faculty develop not only course objectives but specific behavioral outcomes for each unit of content or for each week of clinical learning experience. No matter what position a faculty takes in relation to the need for more or less specificity, what is essential is that all objectives interrelate and demonstrate progression within the program.

Let us now look at Model II, which represents but one sample of possible approaches to utilizing the Characteristics in developing curriculum strands. It is assumed that if this presentation related to a specific program, a stated philosophy and conceptual framework

[7] Bloom, *Cognitive Domain,* p. 205.

would be developed which would support the identified characteristics and strands. (Words and phrases in the Characteristics of particular pertinence to the strands in the model have been italicized for emphasis.)

The curriculum strands are identified as either vertical or horizontal within the last two years of the program, when clinical nursing courses are generally taught. Generally, since vertical strands speak best to the concept of progression, it is essential to have a substantial number of them in order to achieve progressive learnig. Horizontal strands are those concepts which the student needs to utilize during most of her learning experiences and include assessing, planning, implementing, and evaluating nursing care. Recognized as the nursing process, this particular strand truly has its concepts incorporated into all the characteristics that are identified for a graduate. It would be difficult to teach the nursing process vertically, which would mean that the student would initially only assess health status or health potential without intervention and would later evaluate nursing care during the senior year. The only other horizontal strand identified is the acceptance of personal responsibility and accountability (Characteristic 5 in Model II), concepts that need to be incorporated continuously in all aspects of the nursing curriculum. Let me repeat at this point that this is a sample approach and that groups of faculty may differ strongly on which strands might be vertical or horizontal, depending on their beliefs about nursing and learning.

In Model II the first two levels relate to the general education and supporting courses in which the theoretical and empirical knowledge relating to the humanities and sciences are learned. Seven vertical strands are shown in Levels III and IV; in parentheses next to these strands are the numbers of the Characteristics supported by these strands.

Model III is an example of how a broadly stated behavioral characteristic can be utilized to develop level and course objectives in light of the strands identified. In a sense, this is utilizing a broad objective to develop more specific, workable objectives at the course level. This approach can be helpful in the development of program objectives.

Note that the level objectives follow the horizontal strand of the nursing process and vertical strands concerning the individual, family, community, and the health continuum. Following this line of reasoning, using strands to develop objectives, identify for yourself in Model III which level is represented in each of these objectives:

1. Understands the present role of the professional nurse in utilizing the nursing process.

MODEL I
FLOW OF BEHAVIORAL OBJECTIVES
AS PART OF THE TOTAL CURRICULUM PROCESS

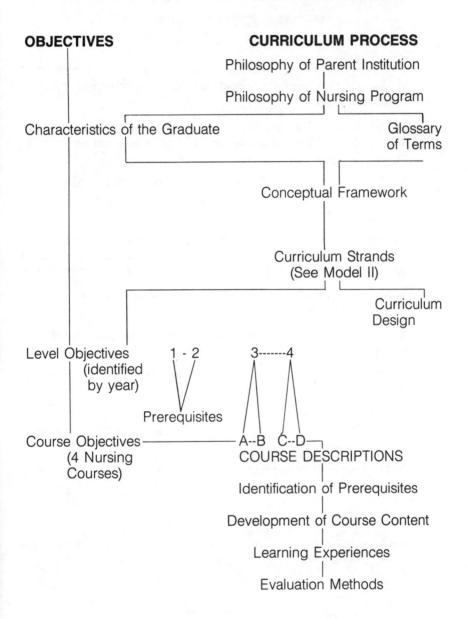

OBJECTIVES

CURRICULUM PROCESS

Philosophy of Parent Institution

Philosophy of Nursing Program

Characteristics of the Graduate

Glossary
of Terms

Conceptual Framework

Curriculum Strands
(See Model II)

Curriculum
Design

Level Objectives
(identified
by year)

1 - 2   3-------4

Prerequisites

Course Objectives ———————— A--B C--D
(4 Nursing   COURSE DESCRIPTIONS
Courses)

Identification of Prerequisites

Development of Course Content

Learning Experiences

Evaluation Methods

MODEL II
UTILIZING THE CHARACTERISTICS OF THE GRADUATE TO IDENTIFY CURRICULUM STRANDS

CHARACTERISTICS OF BACCALAUREATE GRADUATE*

1. *Assess health* status and health potential; *plan, implement,* and *evaluate* nursing care in concert with clients—*individuals, families,* and *communities.*

2. *Utilize theoretical* and *empirical knowledge* from the physical and behavioral sciences and the humanities as a source for making nursing practice decisions.

3. Utilize *decision-making theories* in determining care plans, designs, or interventions for achieving comprehensive nursing goals.

4. Utilize nursing interventions as *hypotheses* to be tested; anticipate a variety of consequences and make *predictions;* and select and *evaluate* the effectiveness of alternative approaches.

5. Accept individual *responsibility* and *accountability* for nursing interventions and their results.

6. Use nursing practice as a means of *gathering data* for refining and extending nursing science.

7. Share in the responsibility for the health and welfare of all people with citizens and colleagues on the *interdisciplinary health team* by *collaborating, coordinating,* and *consulting* with them.

8. Assist in implementing *change* to improve delivery of health care.

9. Understand *present* and *emerging roles* of the professional nurse.

---

* National League for Nursing, Department of Baccalaureate and Higher Degree Programs, *Characteristics of Baccalaureate Education in Nursing* (New York: The League, 1974).

MODEL II (Continued)

CURRICULUM STRANDS

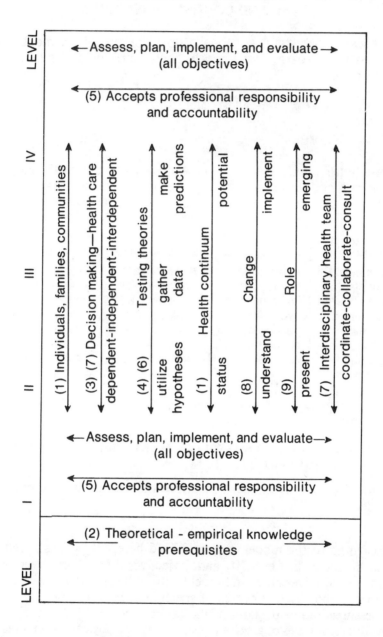

(The number noted next to the strand identifies the specific characteristic(s) to which it speaks)

MODEL III
THE UTILIZATION OF A CHARACTERISTIC IN KEEPING WITH THE CURRICULUM STRANDS TO DEVELOP LEVEL AND COURSE OBJECTIVES

"Assess health status and health potential; plan, implement, and evaluate nursing care in concert with clients—individuals, families, and communities."

THE NURSING PROCESS

LEVEL III	LEVEL IV
Assess health status: plan, implement, and evaluate nursing care in concert with clients and families.	Assess health potential; plan, implement nursing care in concert with families and communities.

Course A	Course B	Course C	Course D
Assess health status; plan, implement and evaluate nursing care in concert with individuals	Assess health status; plan, implement and evaluate nursing care in concert with families	Assess health potential; plan, implement and evaluate nursing care in concert with individuals and families	Assess health potential; plan, implement and evaluate nursing care in concert with families and the community

2. Assesses community needs in relation to potential health hazards.

3. Implements planned change through consultation with other nursing personnel.

4. Understands the need to utilize theories in making nursing decisions.

According to the model conceptualized here, Objectives 1 and 4 would be found in Level III, and Objectives 2 and 3 in Level IV.

Course objectives noted in Model III are still somewhat generalized and in need of a higher degree of specificity. For example, the area of assessment of health status might lead to specific objectives relating to the different types of assessment such as psychological, developmental, physical, and economic. Greater specificity is needed in order to guide both faculty and students more effectively through each learn-

350

ing experience. Later, greater specificity of objectives is crucial in helping to develop evaluation tools.

The development of objectives within any program is time-consuming and at times frustrating. One of the major reasons is that objectives—especially course objectives—are often developed in isolation by the individual faculty members or by groups of faculty teaching certain courses and are frequently slanted toward specific course content rather than toward those behaviors relating to nursing science. The more time spent by the total faculty in the development of the objectives, the better; the efforts will be paid back a hundredfold, since well-organized and well-stated objectives make the identification of course content, learning experiences, and evaluation methods much easier.

Let me summarize by reminding the reader of several major points to be kept in mind in dealing with the curriculum:

- Objectives should contain a behavioral and content aspect and should reflect changes in a learner.
- The development of objectives must always be viewed in relationship to the entire curriculum process and show progression from the general to the specific.
- Curriculum strands that can be identified within the philosophy and conceptual framework, and later in the characteristics of the graduate, are helpful in the development of more specific objectives for each level and course.
- Well-developed behaviorial objectives are essential if the program is to implement its philosophy and conceptual framework.

41 CURRICULUM DESIGN AND APPROACHES TO NURSING COURSES AND CONTENT

Jean Kelley, EdD, RN

Faculty involved with the revision of a baccalaureate curriculum in nursing must make many crucial decisions. One such major decision is to reach agreement on a philosophy and a conceptual framework for the new curriculum, as well as on compatible behavioral objectives. Another milestone is for faculty to move from a philosophy, framework, and objectives into a concrete curriculum design that dictates an appropriate approach to nursing courses and content.

For faculty to transfer their beliefs and wishes into a house of action, it will be necessary for them to review the four major determinants of the curriculum and to decide which one or ones take priority in designing a new curriculum. These four major determinants are generally accepted to be: Man-the-learner; Society and its health care needs; Learning to function as a professional nurse; and Knowledge of professional nursing. One faculty group might decide that who the learner is and where he aims to go in professional nursing should be of prime importance, while another faculty group might determine as paramount what product of a nursing education program would contribute most to the health care needs of society as a whole or best serve the varying needs of our many societies. Other faculty groups might decide that certain factors which influence learning the role of the professional nurse should be the main focus of the curriculum design. Still others might choose as the principal thrust of the curriculum how the body of nursing knowledge is organized and how its method of inquiry is transmitted.

Importance of Determinant Priority

In order to clarify the importance of such choices, examples will be presented from selected school of nursing faculty groups that have made a decision on the priority of one of the four determinants in designing a baccalaureate curriculum in nursing.

"Man-the-Learner" as a Priority in Curriculum Design

When Man-the-learner is adopted as a primary focus in the design of a nursing curriculum, the faculty is expressing concern for who the learner is and where he intends to go during a career in professional nursing practice. One faculty group (the Department of Nursing, State College of Arkansas, Conway) designed a Career Options in Nursing Education curriculum which had as its philosophic source the economic needs of the learner. There were other bases such as man and his motivating needs, the nursing process, the health-illness continuum, and specific nursing content, but the economic needs of man-the-learner took precedence. With this belief in mind, the faculty designed a curriculum so that a learner could acquire fundamental nursing knowledge, skills, and understanding during one year of study and then drop out to work as a practical nurse, or could continue during a second year of study to acquire necessary nursing knowledge, skills, and understanding, receive an A.D.N. degree, and drop out to work as a registered nurse. The option existed for these learners to return at a later date to complete requirements for a baccalaureate degree in nursing. Nursing courses and content for this curriculum design were selected and organized based on the assumption that all nurse practitioners have a need for similar basic concepts, knowledge, skills, and understanding. Therefore, certain nursing content and concepts were reintroduced year after year. For example, man and his motivating needs were introduced in the first year and reintroduced in the second year. This curriculum design and approach to nursing courses and content present two potential problems. The first is the repetition of some of the same concepts year after year. Secondly, this approach presupposes a determination by faculty of the extent to which the economic and learning needs of students are being met when completion of a four-year baccalaureate program spans a period of time greater than five years and the knowledge imparted risks becoming outdated.

"Society" as a Priority in Curriculum Design

When Society is accepted as a primary determinant in designing a collegiate curriculum in nursing, the faculty is recognizing that a registered nurse needs to be prepared through baccalaureate education to function in a changing health care system in order to meet the health needs of society as a whole or the varying health needs of the many societies that comprise our nation. One faculty group (the School of Nursing of the University of Wisconsin-Madison) designed a curriculum based on the belief that the product of a baccalaureate program should be able to function differently from graduates of other types of nursing programs. Specifically, they declared the end-product should be prepared to function independently in performing nursing activities, but interdependently or collaboratively with other disciplines in the delivery of health care. Subsequently, a curriculum was designed with the assumption that the professional nurse of the future needs a college education which provides opportunities to acquire the following:

1. General as well as higher level of knowledge and skills essential to nursing practice;

2. Expertise in primary or secondary health care, as opposed to learning to care for clients at all levels of health and illness and in all types of settings;

3. Knowledge about health care systems and the roles of health professionals functioning in such social systems; and

4. A personal autonomy and identity in addition to meeting societal expectations of the nursing profession.

The resulting curriculum was organized around four components: general education, nursing practice, health services, and electives. All four components, including nursing practice, were introduced in the freshman year and continued throughout the remainder of the four-year program. The structure of the nursing component is of particular interest to faculty considering a curriculum revision. During the first two years of the curriculum, students were provided with a preconcentration nursing practice core, which emphasized content and learning experiences needed by all levels of practitioners in nursing. Use of the nursing process in helping man adapt to his environment was stressed during this core.

The last two years of the nursing component, on the other hand, accentuated professional nursing practice by providing: (1) a concentration core dealing with health and illness, health issues, nursing research, and group dynamics; and (2) an area of concentration in primary or secondary health care.[1] This type of nursing component prepared graduates to change nursing practice and the health care system as well as to participate in research on nursing practice. One advantage of this curriculum design and approach to nursing courses and content is that the learner receives experiences in nursing situations throughout the entire four-year curriculum, rather than the two- or three-year exposure that is typical of many baccalaureate programs. However, there are at least two problems inherent in this curriculum design: (1) faculty must determine the nature of that common core of nursing knowledge, understanding, and skills needed by all levels of nurse practitioners; and (2) they must determine the extent to which graduates of the program have changed or might change nursing practice and the health care system.

Learning as a Priority in Curriculum Design

When Learning is viewed as a major determinant in designing a baccalaureate curriculum, the faculty is acknowledging that certain factors—such as motivation, readiness, or transfer—influence learning the role of a professional nurse, or that the best way to prepare a registered nurse is through teaching a specific process or processes. One faculty group (the College of Nursing, Arizona State University) designed a Continuous Progress Curriculum based on the concept of mastery. In this curriculum design, sequential learning in nursing practice, along with appropriate materials and facilities, was provided so that students had the freedom and time, within limits, to proceed to learn at their own rate, as well as to assume responsibility for their own learning. This faculty group believes that progress with learning stimulates a student's motivation. Although motivation for learning occurs within a student, faculty can facilitate it by giving positive reinforcement to the student whenever learning tasks are achieved or completed. Mastery in nursing was defined by the faculty as "achievement of all stated goals for which criteria are defined behaviorally and which goals are determined by the faculty to be essential to the practice of nursing."[2] With this type of curriculum design, it is crucial for faculty to identify the essential content for the practice of nursing and to provide time for the student to master the content. This curriculum based on the concept of mastery was organized around four levels:

Level One. Expanding and contracting families; patients with a communication problem; community resources; basic nursing care.

---

[1] Rose Marie Chioni and Eugenia Schoen, "Preparing Tomorrow's Nurse Practitioner,"*Nursing Outlook* 18:50-53, October 1970.

[2] Dorothy F. Corona, "Continuous-Progress Curriculum: A Format for Change," in Joyce Crane, ed., *Theoretical Approaches and Innovative Practices in Curriculum Development* (Durham, NC: Duke University School of Nursing, 1971), p. 143.

Level Two. Hospital care of children with genetic conditions; adults with change in body image or self-concept; patients with a psychiatric disorder.

Level Three. Complex nursing care problems with hospitalized patients who require use of community resources.

Level Four. Student-centered experiences in leadership and research.

Objectives for nursing competence at each level were developed. These were further broken down into specific objectives for two nursing courses that were offered at each level. One course was concerned with core concepts, while the other contained clinical-specialty content and learning experiences. Within each course, more specific objectives were identified for each learning unit. Mastery of one learning unit served as the entry into the next. The usual time frame for mastery of all learning units on a level was one semester; if more time was needed by a particular student, another semester was allowed. Learners who mastered the material in less than one semester progressed to the next level.[3]

Another faculty group (the School of Nursing, University of California, San Francisco), which viewed learning as a priority in designing a baccalaureate curriculum, selected a process-oriented approach. In this design, the problem-solving process was seen as the core of professional nurse behavior.[4] As a result the curriculum was geared to teaching the process of problem-solving activities. To implement this type of curriculum design, the faculty defined the steps in the problem-solving process and planned for students to be exposed to selected, genuine nursing problems while learning the problem-solving cycle of inquiry. In addition, nursing practice was described by the faculty as a decision-making process in that most nursing problems require a student to make a decision and to test actions. The aim of this type of curriculum design was to teach students of nursing how to solve problems in a decision-making frame of reference and to become aware of the hypothetical character of nursing interventions, which in turn might serve to stimulate students further to learn the problem-solving cycle.

This problem-solving model offered a common mode for organizing knowledge in the curriculum. It provided a tool that evoked the nursing process and directed students to learn the decision-making process. The sequence in this problem-solving model was from patient problem to nursing problem to nursing intervention. Content emerged from analysis of each typical clinical situation. The essential

---

[3] Corona, *op. cit.,* pp. 141-161.

[4] Marlene Kramer, "Operationalizing Curriculum Theory: Process as Content—Implementation of a Process Oriented Curriculum," in Joyce Crane, ed. *Theoretical Approaches and Innovative Practices in Curriculum Development* (Durham, NC: Duke University School of Nursing, 1971), p. 118.

content in the curriculum was a set of nursing problems which represented a wide range and diversity of situations that crossed clinical lines, age groups, and health care settings. Thus the problems presented the core concepts of nursing or basic principles of nursing and illustrated nursing interventions in a variety of situations; relevant knowledge and technical skills were introduced when appropriate during the analysis of a nursing problem.

The curriculum was organized so that three nursing courses were offered over a period of three years; each course was three quarters in length. The titles of the courses were: Introduction to Nursing Problems; Nursing Process in Major Health Interruptions; and Introduction to the World of Work.

In each course the Problem-Solving and Decision-Making Process was taught to a class of 80 students by a faculty team of from nine to twelve, with one serving as the course coordinator. Due to this unique curriculum design, there were no traditional clinical departments or blocks of time to study clinical specialties, such as medical-surgical or psychiatric nursing.

One outstanding feature of this curriculum design is that nursing knowledge, understanding, and skills are taught in relation to specific problems in need of solution. Thus, essential content is taught when learners need to know it, and not in isolation of nursing situations. Problems innate to this curriculum design are:

1. The identification of problems that will bring forth essential nursing content and skills;

2. Faculty loss of identity with a clinical specialty; and

3. The need to change the role of the teacher from lecturer to facilitator of learning.[5]

Knowledge as a Priority in Curriculum Design

When Knowledge is perceived as the main focus in the design of a curriculum, the faculty is declaring that nursing has a unique body of knowledge and a method of inquiry that can be taught so that graduates are prepared to continue to learn for the lifetime of their career in the profession. In this approach to curriculum revision, faculty must reach accord on the major concepts from the expanding body of nursing knowledge that a student of nursing needs to learn. Typical concepts that are often selected are *body image, stress, self-concept,* and *adaptation.* Once agreement on the concepts is reached, relevant content and learning experiences need to be selected and integrated into

---

[5] Kramer, *op. cit.,* pp. 115-139.

the curriculum, which will bring about interaction between the learner and his environment and produce positive behavioral changes. Decisions will need to be made on what concepts, content, and clinical experiences are to be stressed at what level or year. Generally, nursing content and learning experiences are selected based on the concepts faculty assign to a specific level. In an integrated curriculum design, most nursing courses are taught by faculty teams that cut across clinical areas, since major nursing concepts are readily taught in many settings. For example, the concept of body image may be learned by a student rendering care to a pregnant client or to one who has undergone radical head and neck surgery. One outstanding problem with a curriculum design in which nursing knowledge is integrated is: When do you teach what to whom?

Summary

When faculty adopt one of the four classical determinants as a priority in designing a baccalaureate curriculum in nursing, several implications for curriculum development ensue. First, faculty beliefs about the determinant must be translated into a curriculum model, such as the Career Options in Nursing Education model, the Continuous Progress model, the Problem-Solving and Decision-Making Process model, the Health Care Systems Product model, or the Integrated model. Next, decisions must be made on how to organize the curriculum so that relevant content and learning experiences can be selected, arranged, implemented, and evaluated. Lastly, the faculty as teachers may need to change their roles and instructional strategies and perhaps the entire faculty organizational structure. There is no one universally effective curriculum design and approach to nursing courses and content for baccalaureate education. Instead, there are a number of curriculum designs and approaches from which a faculty group may choose in revising a baccalaureate curriculum that will prepare registered nurses with some competence for an initial job as well as provide them with a broad base for professional practice upon which a challenging and rewarding career may be built.

42 LEARNING EXPERIENCES WITHIN AND OUTSIDE THE CLASSROOM

Gertrude Torres, EdD, RN

We in nursing education have a strong commitment to learning experiences that are planned to meet specific objectives. This commitment is often seen by other educators as unnecessary and too rigid an approach to learning. The chemist, biologist, or historian has few overt problems teaching without stated or written objectives, and such disciplines often approach learning experiences rather loosely. When their objectives are stated they tend to be broad in nature and may therefore be of little assistance in daily teaching activities.

The rationale for the development of appropriate and significant objectives and learning experiences in nursing education is that we are strongly committed to educating the student for self-development and for a professional role which serves society. We recognize that we are accountable for producing professionals who can meet the health and nursing needs of society. Through the development and identification of learning experiences to meet objectives, we are able to accomplish this charge; we cannot support a hit-or-miss approach to teaching and learning and still be accountable for our product.

Implied in the identification of learning experiences that support the meeting of objectives is that they offer an opportunity for the student to learn. Learning involves discovery of new knowledge, understanding, and skills. A learning experience, in its broadest sense, involves all those activities inside and outside the classroom that assist the student to meet specifically identified objectives.

After the development of course objectives and the identification of content within the nursing courses, faculty need to identify the appropriate teaching methods to be utilized. Clinical laboratory experiences are an obvious example of a teaching method and will be discussed later. However, several principles need to be kept in mind in identifying methods to approach the teaching of content.

Approach to Teaching Methods

No one teaching method is appropriate for assisting the student to meet the broad range of stated behavioral objectives. Also, no one teaching method is an effective way of approaching all content. Thus, a variety of teaching methods is usually more effective than a single approach.

Teaching methods need to bear a relation to the student's past experiences. Dramatic and sudden changes in teaching methods require orientation and a period of time for the student to adapt. Also, the student's ability and level of sophistication needs to be taken into consideration.

Groups, too, have "personalities" and differ significantly. Thus, what may have been an effective teaching strategy in relation to certain objectives for one class may not be effective for another.

Teaching methods need to be identified in terms of available supporting resources. Some resources that need be reviewed prior to the selection of teaching methods include: classroom facilities, seating arrangements, size and availability of learning centers, and teacher availability.

Teaching methods should support educators' strengths rather than weaknesses. In the team-teaching approach, faculty expertise needs to be carefully assessed in terms of individual abilities to utilize certain teaching methods.

Teaching methods need to be realistic in terms of the amount of time available to educate. Since time is limited, it is essential to identify the appropriate teaching methods; the more appropriate the teaching method is to program objectives and course content, the less time will be needed for the student to learn.

The teaching methods chosen should reflect the faculty's beliefs about learning as stated in the program's philosophy.

We are all aware of the many teaching methods available—panel presentations, role playing, case presentation, autotutorial and other independent study approaches, small and large group discussions, and many others. Yet it seems that our approach too often reflects the way we ourselves have been educated. The lecture or "formal handing out" of knowledge or skills in some cases continues to be the sole teaching approach to all content. There seems to be some unwritten agreement that we must teach via the lecture method unless there is some special reason for a change. If you don't believe this, may I suggest that, the next time you walk into a classroom, you take a careful, objective look at your students and see what teaching method they expect will be utilized. Creativity and flexibility—not commitment to tradition—are essential components in identifying effective teaching methods.

Clinical Laboratory Experiences

Clinical laboratory experiences also need to be chosen with the same regard for the specific behavioral objectives. This statement may seem simple enough on the surface, but let us examine two problems which often interfere. First of all, experiences are *not* identified or planned until all the other components of the curriculum process are well developed. Although early during curriculum revision different health care settings may be identified in relation to the changing role and function of the professional nurse as identified in the philosophy, the specific activities which will be carried out by the students during frequent use of these settings cannot be identified until much later in the revision.

The second problem arises from the fact that certain clinical settings should not be utilized unless they offer the student an opportunity to practice the kind of behavior implied in the behavioral objective. For example, if certain settings are rigid and bureaucratic in nature and do not allow for the meeting of specific objectives that speak to independence of performance or thought, other settings must be utilized.

The greatest amount of educationally oriented time is spent by faculty and students engaged in activities related to clinical laboratory experiences. The activities before and after the experience frequently involve a greater amount of time than the experience itself. This being the case, it is essential that these activities be carefully identified to ensure success. Few would argue with this line of reasoning, yet we frequently approach this responsibility with rigidity, almost like a habit, and with little or no imagination. Admittedly, we have progressed since the Curriculum Guides were published; in 1937, the most difficult problem in relationship to curriculum administration was the correlation of theory with practice.[1] For the most part, with the evolution of the integrated curriculum and more broadly stated objectives relating to

---

[1] National League of Nursing Education, Committee on Curriculum, *A Curriculum Guide for Schools of Nursing* (New York: The League, 1937), p. 127.

a variety of settings, it is easier now to correlate theory and practice. We need to go further at this point, however, and become more sophisticated in selecting clinical activities.

Utilizing two objectives that might be found in a nursing program, let us identify some of the appropriate clinical laboratory settings.

Objective (appropriate at Level III in Model II). *Can assess the developmental status of a healthy individual.* Content or knowledge to be imparted (not to be viewed as complete) might include: assessment as part of the nursing process; understanding of the concept of health; theories—psychological, developmental, interactive.

Laboratory settings in which the student would have an opportunity to practice the behavior meeting this objective might include:

- Schools at all levels.
- Industry.
- Diagnostic clinics.
- Meetings of groups such as Golden Age Clubs.
- Nursing homes.
- Community environments, such as hotel lobbies, bus depots.
- Assigned families within the home.
- Community clinics such as immunization centers and newborn clinics.
- Screening units such as T.B. mobile units.

(Note: Since the objective does not speak to any particular age group, all age levels are included.)

Objective (appropriate at Level IV in Model II). *Can evaluate health restoration services to an individual in conjunction with other health care practitioners.* Assumed content or knowledge (not to be viewed as complete) might include: theories or concepts—role, group, decision, leadership, interpersonal, interactive; understanding of community resources related to health care; understanding present and emerging role of health practitioners; pathophysiology.

Laboratory settings in which the student would have an opportunity to practice the behavior (sampling only) might include:

- Interdisciplinary team conferences in hospitals, long-term settings, clinics, health and medical centers.
- Interaction of individually planned meetings with dieticians, physiotherapists, social workers, physicians, etc.
- Home visits in which other health care practitioners are actively involved.

What is significant to note in the discussion of these objectives and experiences is that there is a variety of settings in which a specific objective can be met. Thus, unless the objective relates to a particular setting, students can be placed in very different environments to meet the same objective. Also, it is essential that we identify the content or knowledge needed to carry out the behavior identified within the objective in order to know where such content or knowledge can be provided.

One's initial reaction to this particular approach may be to cite the difficulty of finding settings where these behaviors can be practiced. There is no easy way out of this dilemma. Experiences are available relating to both the objectives cited, even if they may be to some extent limited. For example, it might be quite challenging to identify a setting in which a large number of nursing majors can function in an interdisciplinary manner to evaluate health care, although health and medical care institutions might need leadership from faculty to engage in such activities and it might take months or even years to get such activities organized.

Yet it is possible to find these experiences, if perhaps on a more limited scale. For example, encouraging students to call physicians, to go to dieticians to discuss health restoration, and to speak with social workers about available resources are some behaviors appropriate to the second objective.

Within any given course related to a specific group of objectives, it is helpful to identify what may be called *critical* and *less critical* experiences. Clinical experiences may be identified as those specific learning experiences in which all students should be involved, for example, observation and follow-through care of a patient in labor and delivery or a patient experiencing surgery. Less critical experiences would include other experiences in which the same objective can be met.

Objectives related to a client's ability to adapt to new environments could be met in almost any clinical environment. Thus, all students would not be required to meet objectives in the same setting. Generally, we need to recognize that most experiences need not be critical in nature since objectives are not usually that specific. This will allow us greater flexibility in our approaches to clinical types of learning experiences.

In planning clinical experiences we should also identify those experiences in which students need to function independently and those in which direct guidance is necessary. We can think of this as laying-on-of-hands time which is within the interventive aspect of the nursing process. Students who are to be practitioners in an autonomous profession need learning experiences similar to those experienced by the medical intern—the freedom to assess, diagnose, plan and evaluate care, and also guidance in intervening. In terms of safety and care, this is most significant during the laying-on-of-hands time. Both faculty and students must use professional judgment in decisions relating to the need for faculty presence, as has always been done. Faculty must always be available but need not always be visible in any approach to learning experiences.

We also need to revise the way we schedule clinical learning experiences in terms of time commitments. If we are in fact producing independent and interdependent practitioners, then students need to be more accountable for their own use of clinical time. If a particular nursing course requires six hours of laboratory experiences per week, maybe two hours could be utilized by the student in terms of her own responsibilities as related to a particular objective. For example, in order to provide opportunities for the student to utilize the nursing process on a long-term basis with a nursing home client, the student could visit the client whenever it is most appropriate for meeting objectives—possibly in the evening to meet the client's family. A diary could be kept by the student so that the faculty can be kept informed of these activities. This approach could also be used with a student who is responsible for the care of a family in terms of health promotion, and so forth, for a two-year period. Too often we are committed to the concept of total comprehensive care involving continuity, but do little to allow for such experiences.

Let me close by saying that we need to take an about-face in the planning of learning experiences and let our historical background fade into the wind. We need to change our thinking in relation to such concepts as: the student is a learner, not a worker; the student needs guidance in the clinical area, not supervision; the time spent in the clinical laboratory does not directly relate to the concepts learned; the ratio of faculty to students depends on objectives, not on predetermined rigid habits; the student cannot give total care the first day of her experience; clinical experiences produce a generalist, not a specialist.

43 SOME COMPONENTS OF CURRICULUM EVALUATION

Gertrude Torres, EdD, RN

It seems safe to assume that prior to any curriculum revision, some form of curriculum evaluation has taken place. Therefore, curriculum evaluation would seem to be the force that really leads the curriculum process, rather than being its least component. Since some type of evaluation, whether formative or summative, must have occurred in order to identify the need for revision, the direction of the revision needs to be based on data concerning the strengths and weaknesses of the previous curriculum approach.

Let us view the curriculum process in a cyclic manner, going from evaluation to the development of the philosophy to learning experiences and then back to evaluation and the philosophy. This approach supports the notion that, in the curriculum process as in the nursing process, we are in a constant state of revision, attempting through evaluation to keep our activities up-to-date and relevant.

Let me state that, from my experience, faculty generally do not revise their curriculums based on any in-depth study of their previous curriculums, but instead base their revisions on new theories and concepts of learning and nursing, which tends to encourage the "band-wagon" approach.

Evaluation, in terms of curriculum development and revision, needs to be viewed in the context of program objectives and the expected characteristics of the graduate. Ongoing evaluation of students and faculty is an essential component of any program, but is indirectly rather than directly related to evaluation for purposes of curriculum development. We evaluate students for both learning and grading, and faculty for teaching effectiveness. We evaluate the curriculum for the improvement of the program of studies. This type of evaluation is essential if we are to be accountable to the community at large; consumers of professional nursing care, taxpayers, donors, and boards of trustees expect us to commit ourselves to the achievement of our program goals and to be accountable in relationship to the characteristics we maintain our graduates will demonstrate. Thus, the term *evaluation* involves a process in which we gather data or evidence in relation to the attainment of specific objectives for which we are accountable. We therefore cannot take this responsibility lightly or approach evaluation in a haphazard manner.

One of our greatest weaknesses in curriculum evaluation is that we usually lack a systematic, total, and comprehensive approach. We also lack sophistication in the utilization of appropriate tools with which to measure our successes or failures. Our resistance to this approach to evaluation is often based on our lack of understanding, our insecurity, or possibly our fear of its results.

Another force which may encourage our resistance is a lack of commitment to our program objectives and the characteristics of our graduates. We often state them well but fail to utilize them properly in the development of course objectives. For the past decade or so, characteristics of baccalaureate graduates have included areas related to research and preparation for graduate education. Yet today few nurses even read the reports of nursing research, and we still have a tremendous shortage of nurses with graduate preparation. Another problem is that some objectives have been written so vaguely or are so ill-defined that one would find them almost impossible to use in measuring results for success or failure.

The process of curriculum evaluation needs to include at least the following three components if it is to be in any way complete:[1]

- Identification of critical and minimum levels of achievement.
- Validation of previous knowledge, skills, and beliefs.
- Validation of levels of achievement, both present and future.

Involved in the identification of critical and minimum levels of achievement is the utilization of a criterion-referenced test which identifies an individual's ability in relation to an established standard of performance. This differs from norm-referenced approaches, which

---

[1] For a fuller discussion, see Gertrude Torres, "Curriculum Evaluation for Today and Tomorrow," in *Faculty-Curriculum Development, Part II—Curriculum Evaluation* (New York: National League for Nursing, 1974), pp. 17-19.

measure success in relation to the performance of others on the same measure. Only with criterion-referenced measures can we guarantee the critical and minimum level of achievement essential to the practice of professional nursing and the realization of the characteristics of the graduate. We should not assume that the norm of a group in which success may be achieved is adequate.

Let us relate this to the tools, written and clinical, which a faculty have developed to measure success at the junior level for the purpose of curriculum evaluation and not for grading of students. In both these tools the faculty, through consensus, have identified essential critical knowledge and behaviors that must be demonstrated clinically. Students' success would be measured against these specific criteria, and curriculum content and learning experiences would be revised, based on the data received. With this approach it is essential to keep in mind that knowledge and skills relate directly to the level objectives, which in turn support the meeting of the behavioral characteristics of the graduate.

The data resulting from the use of such tools could have useful purposes other than the revision of curriculum. Results might validate the need for additional resources relating to funds, faculty, or resources. Also, decisions relating to admission criteria, course requirements, or number of students might be influenced by such data.

If we believe that education involves a change in behavior, it seems essential that we be able to validate that a change has in fact occurred. Change involves some type of modification from the entry of the student into the program to the exit of the student from the program. Therefore, we need to measure, through some type of validation, the knowledge, skills, and beliefs possessed by the student when she enters the program. These can be thought of as significant diagnostic tools in terms of both curriculum evaluation and student achievement. The major focus would be the mean achievement of the group in relation to curriculum decisions, although the achievements of an individual student could be utilized to assist or guide her during the program.

We must keep in mind that we are measuring entering students' abilities in relation to the stated characteristics. Measurement could take place when students enter the college or when they enter the first clinical nursing course, depending on the faculty's frame of reference. If faculty view the total curriculum design as supporting the meeting of the characteristics, they would validate appropriate knowledge, skills, and beliefs at the beginning of the program. The data on students would then support changes in nonnursing requirements as well as in nursing courses. If the faculty are more interested in data related to the professional content of the program, validation would be done at the beginning of the nursing curriculum. Since the characteristics relate to cognitive, psychomotor, and affective domains, validation tools might be needed to reflect all these areas.

Instruments for such evaluation could include both teacher-made and standardized tests in the form of objective and essay tests, tests utilizing audiovisual aids, and performance evaluation methods.

Admittedly, these tools take time and effort to develop. But they should be well worth the effort, supplying us with quantitative data for identifying priorities and areas we need to emphasize within the curriculum. These decisions are often based on professional or qualitative judgments, unsupported by measurement data; such judgments are, of course, an essential component of any evaluation. However, they need to be balanced with quantitative judgments, based on measurement data when possible.

The last component—the validation of levels of achievement—reflects the need for measurement that truly reflects the graduate's achievement of the characteristics and verifies that change has in fact occurred from previously established levels of knowledge and skills. By such means, faculty can truly be accountable and can offer data in proof that education has occurred. Comprehensive examinations, as suggested previously for the junior level, need to be given prior to graduation. Also, longitudinal studies of the graduates should be carried out. Such studies should include a variety of approaches, all relating specifically to the characteristics; some possible methods include questionnaires to and interviews with graduates, their employers, and possibly even with faculty of the graduate programs in which they enroll. Again, collection of this sort of information is no easy matter and is quite time consuming. Yet without such data, how do we prove our accountability and on what basis do we revise our curriculums? Since many programs have similar types of characteristics, they might develop consortia for the purpose of sharing tools and approaches to such types of evaluation.

In the process of curriculum evaluation, other areas need to be considered. Responsibility for such evaluation must be identified and belongs to the faculty who develop the characteristics and who are the experts in the discipline. Faculty who are committed to evaluation need administrative support, and that involves more than simply the recognition that it is a good idea. Resources such as funds, computer time, and supporting as well as consulting services are vital.

It is also important to understand who is involved in evaluation, both within and outside the system of higher education.[2] Faculty in nursing and other disciplines, as well as students, are within the system, while consumers of care and employers are outside the system. All need to be involved in the process if it is to be comprehensive.

In order to assure an ongoing program of curriculum evaluation,

---

[2] For a more detailed discussion of this subject, see Helen Yura, "The 'Who' in Curriculum Evaluation," in *Faculty-Curriculum Development, Part II—Curriculum Evaluation* (New York: National League for Nursing, 1974), pp. 35-41.

a committee of the faculty may need to be part of the structure of the school or department. A curriculum committee should relate to curriculum; a committee that deals primarily with student or faculty affairs is not sufficient. While evaluation may be considered a part of the regular curriculum committee's responsibilities, measures need to be taken to ensure that the curriculum process is carried out. With ongoing curriculum development and resulting problems, it is easy to see how evaluation might get little or no attention.

Summary

The curriculum process and its components may be viewed as a cyclic process and curriculum revision as a constant force necessary to keep education dynamic, vital, and up to date. Curriculum revision must be based on quantitative data as well as qualitative judgments. Evaluation of the *what* of curriculum revision relates to the ability of the educational program to cause a change in behavior on the part of the student in terms of the characteristics of the graduate. Student and teacher evaluation should be separated from curriculum evaluation, even though some of the evaluative tools may be similar.

It is through curriculum evaluation that we can demonstrate our accountability as educators. Faculty are responsible for curriculum evaluation and must include interested persons from both the internal and external environments of the college.